COMBINATION VACCINES

COMBINATION VACCINES

DEVELOPMENT, CLINICAL RESEARCH, AND APPROVAL

Edited by

RONALD W. ELLIS

BioChem Pharma, Inc., Northborough, MA

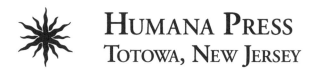

HUMANA PRESS
TOTOWA, NEW JERSEY

© 1999 Humana Press Inc.
999 Riverview Drive, Suite 208
Totowa, New Jersey 07512

This publication is printed on acid-free paper. ∞
ANSI Z39.48-1984 (American National Standards Institute)
Permanence of Paper for Printed Library Materials.

Cover design by Patricia F. Cleary.

For additional copies, pricing for bulk purchases, and/or information about other Humana titles, contact Humana at the above address or at any of the following numbers: Tel: 973-256-1699; Fax: 973-256-8341; E-mail: humana@humanapr.com or visit our website at http://humanapress.com

Printed in the United States of America.   10 9 8 7 6 5 4 3 2 1
Combination vaccines: development, clinical research, and approval / edited by Ronald W. Ellis.
        p. cm. --
    Includes index.
    ISBN 0-89603-717-7 (alk. paper)
    1. Combined vaccines. I. Ellis, Ronald W.
        [DNLM: 1. Vaccines, Combined. QW 805 C7308 1999]
    RM281.C65 1999
    615'.372–dc21
    DNLM/DLC
    for Library of Congress   98-55262
                                                                        CIP

To my wife, Danielle, and children, Jacob and Miriam,
for their love, patience, and support.

PREFACE

Breakthroughs in immunology, molecular biology, biochemistry, and other related fields coupled with a greater understanding of pathogenesis have resulted in the research and development (R&D) of many new vaccines as well as improvements in several existing ones. If such vaccines are widely used in at-risk populations, then it should be possible to prevent much morbidity and mortality. Combination vaccines (defined as two or more vaccines in a physically mixed preparation) provide a way in which to encourage increased use of a wide range of vaccines in a broad population. The combination vaccine usually is mixed at the time of manufacture, but also may be mixed immediately before being given to the subject.

The schedule for routine pediatric immunization used to be relatively simple, consisting of four doses of diphtheria-tetanus-pertussis (DTP) and one of measles-mumps-rubella (MMR) as injected vaccines as well as oral polio vaccine (OPV). This schedule had remained unchanged until about the last 10 years. During the 1990s, several new vaccines have been introduced into the routine immunization schedule for the first two years of life and are becoming more widely used. Conjugated polysaccharide vaccines for *Haemophilus influenzae* type *b* (Hib), given in three to four doses, were demonstrated effective for preventing disease in young infants. Immunization with recombinant hepatitis B (HB) vaccines (three doses) also became recommended during the first year of life, since immunization of high-risk adult populations had failed to reduce the rate of new HB infections. More recently inactivated polio vaccine (IPV), another injected vaccine, has been recommended in the US to replace the first two doses of OPV in order to reduce the incidence of already rare cases of vaccine-associated polio following the initial dose(s) of OPV. Finally, varicella (V) vaccine, now given as a single dose in the second year of life, was introduced to prevent chickenpox. As a consequence, what started as five injections in the first two years of life has become as high as 15, leading parents and health-care practitioners to become concerned that young children could become like pincushions! This plethora of vaccines creates increased needs for recordkeeping and storage that could discourage health-care providers from administering the full range of indicated vaccines. These issues have stimulated major efforts toward the development of *multidisease* combination vaccines that could reduce the number of injections in children.

The foregoing individual vaccines are monovalent, i.e., each one is directed against a viral or bacterial pathogen that has a single antigenic type, meaning that its major antigenic determinants are group-common. However, there are many significant pathogens that have multiple serotypes or serogroups. There are *multivalent* combination vaccines available for several such pathogens, including poliovirus (3 types), influenza virus (3 types), *Streptococcus pneumoniae* (pneumococcal; 23 types), and rotavirus (4 types). Ongoing R&D efforts are directed toward the development of additional multivalent combination vaccines against pathogens such as *Neiserria meningitidis* (meningococcal), *Streptococcus agalactiae* (Group B Streptococcus or GBS), and dengue virus. The development of such multivalent vaccines avoids the use of multiple injections for individual serotypes. Thus, multivalent combination vaccines typically are developed as such from the outset rather than developing and licensing each individual serotype vaccine on its own. Furthermore, multivalent vaccines themselves may become part of multidisease combination vaccines, as already has happened for IPV.

The concept of combination vaccines has been developed and exploited throughout most of the 20th century. DTP vaccines have been available as multidisease combinations for about half a century, while pneumococcal, influenza, and polio vaccines have been available as multivalent combinations for several decades. Combination vaccines can be both live (e.g., MMR, polio) or inactivated/nonlive/killed subunit (e.g., DTP, HB, Hib). The main thrust in the development of new combination vaccines has been DTP-based multidisease combinations for pediatric use, with the prospect of reducing (up to) 13 shots down to 4. There is also interest in a combined MMRV vaccine for use during the second year of life and eventually a booster dose in childhood. At the same time, new pediatric multivalent combination vaccines are being developed, the newest being rotavirus vaccine, which was approved in the US in 1998. There also is interest in developing new multidisease combination vaccines (such as hepatitis A–hepatitis B) for adolescents and adults, groups that ordinarily are less approachable for routine immunizations, such that combining vaccines may increase the immunization rates for these general age groups.

There are many challenges in the development of new combination vaccines, as are discussed in *Combination Vaccines: Development, Clinical Research, and Approval*. These include technical, clinical, regulatory, manufacturing, marketing, and clinical-use issues. The key to the successful development of combination vaccines lay in identifying all such issues for each proposed combination and developing a comprehensive integrated plan that addresses all these challenges toward the beginning of the program.

There are a large number of combination vaccines both in current use as well as in development (Chapter 1). For combination-inactivated vaccines based on DTP, the pertussis component has been the whole-cell vaccine until recently. However, with the recent licensures of acellular pertussis vaccines, this new component has become the basis of future DTP combinations. DTP vaccine is not used for the immunization of adults (due to reactogenicity of the P component). Nevertheless, there has been a wide range of other combination vaccines for adults and adolescents (Chapter 2). Some of these vaccines are used in infants and children, whereas others are used exclusively in the older age groups. Immunization schedules have been developed for both adults and adolescents.

A key challenge for combination vaccines is that vaccine antigens, which have been developed and licensed separately as vaccines, are brought together into physical mixtures that are not always stable and potent. Thus, pharmaceutical and technical developments of combinations must be performed in a way that an immunogenic and stable mixture in appropriate containers is developed according to accepted regulatory standards (Chapter 3). The available combination vaccines and the schedules for routine pediatric immunization are listed, which reinforce the complexity of the technical task involved in their development. Similarly, there are many clinical challenges in developing combinations (Chapter 4). More specifically, the immunogenicity of a particular component when given individually often is not the same as in a combination; when diminished in combination, this phenomenon is known as *interference*. There are key statistical considerations in determining the appropriate size of consistency trials for proving that the combination is as immunogenic as its components given individually. Since it is not usually possible or ethically acceptable to test the clinical efficacy of a combination vaccine in terms of some or all of its components, it is very useful to define a type of immune response associated with protection, i.e., *immunological correlate of efficacy* (Chapter 5). Such correlates may be used effectively in place of efficacy for the evaluation and licensure of combinations. The ideal correlate of efficacy is one for which there is an assay (*surrogate assay*) and a defined quantitative level of antibodies (*seroprotective level*) associated with protection.

There are three multivalent and one multidisease combination vaccines that serve as models for the development of future combinations. The trivalent influenza vaccine is unique in that its antigenic composition is changed every year according to the most prevalent strains expected to be in circulation around the world (Chapter 6). Having two major surface antigens that play a role in protection, antigenic competition between these antigens appears to be important in the efficacy of these vaccines. The pneumococcal polysaccharide vaccine for older adults, being 23-valent, has the most antigens of any combination vaccine (Chapter 7). Many of these same polysaccharides are being developed into multivalent pediatric vaccines following conjugation to carrier protein, as has been done for the Hib conjugate vaccine. The quadrivalent rotavirus vaccine is the newest combination vaccine as well as the first new multivalent live combination vaccine developed for routine use since the 1950s (Chapter 8). This vaccine was developed without the benefit of knowing a correlate of efficacy. There are intertypic interactions among the component viruses in multivalent rotavirus vaccines that have been studied. The MMR vaccine was the first multidisease live combination vaccine (Chapter 9). The mixing of three live viruses presented significant challenges in formulation and clinical interference during its development.

Regulatory guidelines have been developing for combination vaccines. A vaccine developer needs to anticipate multiple issues during development (Chapter 10). It is clear that consultation with regulatory agencies early in the development program can be very beneficial for assuring that the final formulation and its associated clinical data meet regulatory expectations. From the perspective of the regulatory agency itself, issues regarding the control of manufacturing and clinical safety and efficacy (immunogenicity) are paramount (Chapter 11). The mere saving of additional injections entailed by the combination vaccine may not be sufficient for licensure if safety or immunogenicity is compromised significantly.

Combination vaccines present many special challenges for the health-care practitioner (Chapter 12). These issues include how to deal with an increasing number of products from different manufacturers, interchangeability among combination products within a regimen, concomitant use with other vaccines, giving extra doses of a particular antigen in combination relative to separately, the tracking of immunization status, and safety followup.

I hope that *Combination Vaccines: Development, Clinical Research, and Approval* will serve as a comprehensive reference on significant aspects of combination vaccines. Since immunization remains the most practical and cost-effective way to prevent many infectious diseases, the development of additional multidisease combination vaccines may lead to increased rates of immunization and thereby population-wide control of such diseases. New diseases may be able to be prevented by new multivalent combination vaccines. As developers, clinicians, and health-care practitioners gain more experience with combinations, future development efforts may be expected to become more efficient and rapid in terms of time to market.

I thank my many colleagues in the field of combination vaccines. I am especially grateful to Jacques Armand, John Boslego, Kenneth Brown, George

Chryssomalis, Ian Gust, Carlton Mescievitz, Stanley Plotkin, Patrick Poirot, David Ryan, John Ryan, Robert Sitrin, Howard Six, and John Vose for their many stimulating discussions with me and insights into the field during the course of our collaborations in developing combination vaccines. The loving support and encouragement of my wife, Danielle, and children, Jacob and Miriam, have been very important to me throughout the course of the preparation of this book. Most importantly, I would like to thank all the authors for their excellent contributions that should make this volume the key reference in the field of combination vaccines.

Ronald W. Ellis

CONTENTS

CONTRIBUTORS

KENNETH R. BROWN, MD, *Merck Research Laboratories (retired), Philadelphia, PA*

H. FRED CLARK, PhD, *Associate Professor, Section of Infectious Diseases, University of Pennsylvania School of Medicine, Children's Hospital of Philadelphia, Philadelphia, PA*

MICHAEL D. DECKER, MD, *Associate Professor, Department of Preventive Medicine and Medicine, Division of Infectious Diseases, Vanderbilt University, Nashville, TN*

KATHRYN M. EDWARDS, MD, *Professor, Department of Pediatrics, Division of Infectious Diseases, Vanderbilt University, Nashville, TN*

RONALD W. ELLIS, PhD, *Vice-President, Vaccine Development; General Manager, BioChem Pharma, Inc., Northborough, MA*

LYDIA A. FALK, PhD, *Center for Biologics Evaluation and Research, Food and Drug Administration, Rockville, MD*

KAREN L. GOLDENTHAL, MD, *Center for Biologics Evaluation and Research, Food and Drug Administration, Rockville, MD*

PETER A. GROSS, MD, *Vice-Chair and Professor of Medicine, New Jersey Medical School; Chair, Department of Medicine, Hackensack University Medical Center, Hackensack, NJ*

MAURICE R. HILLEMAN, PhD, *Merck Institute for Therapeutic Research, Merck Research Laboratories, West Point, PA*

AGNES HOFFENBACH, MD, PhD, *Clinical Program Director, Pasteur Mérieux Connaught, Marnes-la-Coquette, France*

CHIA-LUNG HSIEH, PhD, *Wyeth-Lederle Vaccines & Pediatrics, Sanford, NC*

BERT E. JOHANSSON, MD, *Department of Pediatrics, Babies' and Children's Hospital, Columbia-Presbyterian Medical Center, New York, NY*

DENNIS M. KATKOCIN, PhD, *Wyeth-Lederle Vaccines & Pediatrics, Pearl River, NY*

ROBERT KOHBERGER, , PhD, *Wyeth-Lederle Vaccines & Pediatrics, Pearl River, NY*

LORIS D. MCVITTIE, MD, *Center for Biologics Evaluation and Research, Food and Drug Administration, Rockville, MD*

KAREN MIDTHUN, MD, *Center for Biologics Evaluation and Research, Food and Drug Administration, Rockville, MD*

PAUL A. OFFIT, MD, *Professor, Section of Infectious Diseases, University of Pennsylvania School of Medicine, Children's Hospital of Philadelphia, Philadelphia, PA*

PETER PARADISO, PhD, *Vice-President, Scientific Affairs and Research Strategy, Wyeth-Lederle Vaccines & Pediatrics, West Henrietta, NY*

STANLEY PLOTKIN, MD, *Pasteur Mérieux Connaught, Doylestown, PA*

FRANCIS M. RICCI, PhD, *Department of Regulatory Affairs, Merck Research Laboratories, West Point, PA*

EMMANUEL VIDOR, MD, PhD, *Clinical Program Director, Pasteur Mérieux Connaught, Marnes-la-Coquette, France*

JOHN R. VOSE, PhD, *Executive Director, Scientific and Regulatory Affairs, Pasteur Mérieux MSD, Lyon Cedex, France*

1

Pediatric Combination Vaccines

Emmanuel Vidor, Agnes Hoffenbach, and Stanley Plotkin

Introduction

The idea of combining more than one vaccine into a single product to be administered by injection or by other means is far from new, as the first attempts were made over 70 years ago. The obvious advantage of combining vaccines against diphtheria (D), tetanus (T), pertussis (P), *Haemophilus influenzae* type *b* (Hib), poliomyelitis and hepatitis B (HB) into a single product for use in children has promoted the further study in recent years of both pharmaceutical and immunological interactions between vaccines. On the pharmaceutical side, factors such as pH and ionic strength of the medium, the presence and type of adjuvant, and the type of preservative used influence the immunogenicity of the different components making up a combination vaccine. The rules of the game are only partly known: consider that while adsorption of D and T toxoids to aluminum compounds is needed in order to enhance their immunogenicity *(1)*, conversely adsorption of Hib polysaccharide (PRP) conjugates to aluminum salts decreases Hib immunogenicity *(2)*. Another example is the decreased immunogenicity of inactivated poliovirus vaccine (IPV) in the presence of thiomersal (also known as thimerosal), which is used as a preservative in diphtheria-tetanus-whole-cell-pertussis combination vaccines (DTwP) *(3)*.

Little is known about the immunological interactions among vaccine components. Animal studies have revealed phenomena such as epitopic competition and induction of suppressor T-cells *(4)*. From empirical clinical data, we know that interference between vaccine valences does occur *(5)*, often unpredictably *(6)*. One interaction that has been seen repeatedly, although it is presently unclear if it is a pharmaceutical or immunological problem, is the marked depression of responses to Hib conjugates in combinations also containing diphtheria-tetanus-acellular pertussis (DTaP) components *(7–9)*. Nevertheless, one particular

From: *Combination Vaccines: Development, Clinical Research, and Approval*
Edited by: R. W. Ellis © Humana Press Inc., Totowa, NJ

DTaP, discussed as follows, exerted no insidious effect on Hib immunogenicity in combination (10).

Thus, every novel combination must be tested in the clinic to be certain that all of its components remain immunogenic. As our vaccines have grown more sophisticated, two messages have emerged. First, each combination must be tested in comparison to its individual components, or at least to combinations that already have been shown to be equivalent to individual components. In practice, that means a quadrivalent product such as DTP-Hib must be compared to DTP + Hib given separately, and a pentavalent product such as DTP-Hib-IPV must be compared to DTP-Hib + IPV or to DTP-IPV + Hib or to DTP + Hib + IPV. Each group of vaccinated subjects must contain 200–500 children for statistical reasons, depending on the number of comparisons to be evaluated and the statistical endpoints to be used (11).

Second, consistency among vaccine lots must be demonstrated. At least three lots of each combination must be tested in groups of children, and the immune responses obtained should not differ statistically from lot to lot. This also requires approx 200–500 children per group to obtain meaningful results (11). In addition, large safety trials are necessary to show that the combination vaccine does not cause more reactions than its constituent components.

In brief, the clinical development of combination vaccines is arduous, time consuming, and expensive.

Types of Combinations

When two vaccines are given simultaneously to the same individual but through separate administrations at different injection sites, the vaccines are said to be *associated*. When the vaccines are mixed in the same syringe and administered as a single injection, they have been *combined*. Liquid vaccines, e.g., DTwP or DTaP, can be used to reconstitute a lyophilized vaccine, such as Hib capsular polysaccharide conjugated to tetanus toxoid (PRP-T). Reconstitution can be performed extemporaneously in the lyophilisate vial, then taken up into a syringe and injected. In some cases, this process has been simplified by the introduction of a "bypass" syringe. In this presentation, the lyophilized and liquid vaccines are housed in the same syringe but are separated by a rubber partition, with the liquid vaccine distal to the needle. When the syringe plunger is depressed, the liquid vaccine passes via a side channel into the lower chamber where mixing takes place instantaneously in real time as the vaccine is injected. Only when two liquid vaccines are stably contained in the same suspension, ready for injection or oral administration, can one speak of a true combined vaccine.

DT and DTP: The First Combinations

The father of combined vaccination was undoubtedly Gustav Ramon of the Pasteur Institute (Marnes la Coquette, France). In the early 1920s, Ramon developed chemical methods to convert D and T toxins into toxoids to produce the first vaccines against these deadly diseases *(12)*. In the 1930s, he began clinical studies combining the D and T antigens *(13)*, despite the prevailing notion that antigenic competition would prevent joint immunization *(14)*. By the late 1930s and during the time of World War II, inactivated *Bordetella pertussis* bacteria were added to D and T, giving birth to the diphtheria-tetanus-whole-cell pertussis combination, otherwise known as whole-cell DTP or DTwP. No attempt was made to determine whether the components interfered with one another, but rather antibody responses were taken as proof of efficacy, based on arbitrary levels. This acceptance was aided by the adjuvant effect of whole pertussis bacteria, which heightened the responses to D and T, convincing investigators that no field studies were necessary *(15)*.

Whole-Cell Pertussis Vaccine Combinations

In recent years, several other vaccines have been added to DTwP vaccine.

DTwP-Hib

Three Hib conjugate vaccines (PRP-D, HbOC, and PRP-T) have been used in combination with a number of DTwPs, either for primary immunization during the first year of life or for booster immunization. The PRP-D vaccine has been used in combination with several DTwPs *(16–18)*. However, because of its inherent poor immunogenicity in infants below the age of 1 yr, this vaccine has been used mainly for booster immunization. The DTwP-HbOC vaccine is produced by Wyeth-Lederle (WL) in the United States, whereas DTwP-PRP-T combination is produced by Pasteur Mérieux Connaught (PMC) in Mancy P' Etoile, France, Swiftwater, PA, and Willowdale, Ontario, Canada. The PRP-T vaccine also has been used in combination with DTwP vaccines of other origins. In the DTwP-PRP-T vaccines, the PRP-T component is lyophilized and must be reconstituted by a liquid DTwP vaccine just before injection. In contrast, the PRP-D and HbOC conjugate antigens are both liquid vaccines. Recently, a fully liquid formulation of PRP-T in combination with a DTwP vaccine was developed *(19)*.

Data from controlled studies on these combination vaccines reveal that their safety profiles are comparable to those of the component vaccines given at separate sites *(5,16,20–29)*, and no increase in the incidence of adverse events was observed. The same controlled studies also showed that the immune responses to D, T, and P antigens observed after the third vaccine injection given during the first year of life were generally similar between the associated and the combined vaccines. In a few instances, higher immune responses to the combined vaccine or inconsistent evidence of interference was shown (21–23,25,27,28), for which the clinical relevance has not been demonstrated (see Table 1 for details). The only potentially clinically relevant decrease in immune response was observed for antibodies to PRP (anti-PRP). In most of the controlled studies using PRP-T (5,20,23–25,29), the anti-PRP geometric mean titer (GMT) observed after the third dose was lower in infants given combined DTwP-PRP-T compared with those who received associated vaccines, except for two studies (21,28) in which the anti-PRP GMT actually was higher in the infants who received combined DTwP-PRP-T. In some studies, the group of infants who were given the combined vaccine had statistically significantly lower anti-PRP GMT values and lower percentages of subjects with antibody titers above the levels of 0.15 or 1.0 μg/mL.

The use of DTwP-Hib combinations as booster vaccines also has been evaluated on several occasions (17,29–31). All vaccines, without exception, showed a strong ability to boost antibody levels against all antigens. Controlled studies revealed no differences between the responses observed in children given the combination and those given the associated vaccines (17,30). One study demonstrated that DTwP-PRP-T could adequately boost anti-PRP levels even in children primed with the HbOC conjugate vaccine (31).

DTwP-Hib combination vaccines are administered to children in many countries following different immunization schedules, and as yet no epidemiological evidence has emerged to support the clinical relevance of the apparent interference with the anti-PRP responses.

DTwP-HB

One HB vaccine, developed by SmithKline Beecham Biologicals (SB; Rixensart, Belgium), containing 10 μg of recombinant HB surface antigen (HBsAg), has been combined with a DTwP vaccine. This combination has been used for primary immunization during the first year of life using a three-dose regimen according to either a 2–4–6-month or a 3–5–7-month schedule. Few published data on this vaccine are available (32–35). In one controlled study (34), where the safety profile of this combination vaccine was compared to the safety profile of the same vaccines given at separate sites, no increase in the incidence of adverse events in the combination group was shown. This controlled study also showed that after the third vaccine dose, the immune responses to all antigens were similar between the two groups when evaluated by the percentage of infants who had achieved protective levels of antibodies. The GMT values for the D, T, and P antigens were slightly lower in the combination group, but this between-group difference did not achieve statistical significance. The low statistical

Table 1. Effect of Combinations Based on Whole-Cell Pertussis Vaccine on the Immunogenicity of Individual Antigens[a]

Vaccine seroprotective criterion (ref.)	Diphtheria ≥0.01 IU/mL	Tetanus ≥0.01 IU/mL	Pertussis agglutinin titer	PRP ≥1.0 μg/mL	Polio DA ≥ 1:4	HBsAg ≥10 mIU/mL
DTwP-Hib (5, 20–25, 27–29)	± or +	± or +	– or ± or +	± or – or – – (+ in rare occasion)	NR	NR
DTwP-HB (34)	0 (– on GMT)	0 (– on GMT)	0 (– on GMT)	NR	NR	0
DTwP-eIPV (42,43)	0	0	0	NR	0 (– on GMT)	0
DTwP-HB-Hib (29,36,37)	NA	NA	NA	NA	NA	NA
DTwP-Hib-eIPV (46,48,50,51)	0	– or 0	– or 0	– – or – or 0 or + (+ in dual-chamber)	0 (+ on GMT)	NR

[a]As evaluated by geometric mean titer (GMT) values and percentage of subjects achieving seroprotective levels of antibodies. Review of data from controlled studies.

0, no difference in the immune response between the combination vaccine and the two vaccines administered separately.

±, increase or decrease in the immune response between the combination vaccine and the two vaccines administered separately: <10% variation.

+ or –, increase or decrease in the immune response between the combination vaccine and the two vaccines administered separately: ≤25% variation.

++ or – –, increase or decrease in the immune response between the combination vaccine and the two vaccines administered separately: ≤50% variation.

+++ or – – –, increase or decrease in the immune response between the combination vaccine and the two vaccines administered separately >50% to ≤80% variation.

NA, not available.

NR, not relevant.

power of this study, not designed as an equivalence study, prevents any definitive conclusions on this interference to be drawn, for which the clinical relevance again has not been demonstrated *(see Table 1)*. Immune responses to HBsAg largely exceeded the level considered as indicative of long-term clinical protection (94.9–100% of infants reached titers $\geq$ 10 mIU/mL, and the GMT values were 1175–2318 mIU/mL).

The DTwP-HB combination vaccines were designed for developing countries where the integration of HB into the Expanded Program on Immunization (EPI) has been recommended by the World Health Organization (WHO), and some of them (mainly in Southeast Asia and in South America) have started to use this combination.

DTwP-HB-Hib

A recombinant HB vaccine developed by Merck Research Laboratories (Merck; West Point, PA), containing 5 µg of HBsAg, has been developed in collaboration with Commonwealth Serum Laboratories (Parkville, Victoria, Australia) into a combination with DTwP and Hib for primary immunization during the first year of life using a three-dose regimen. The Hib component in this vaccine is the conjugate PRP-OMP, enabling a fully liquid combination to be prepared. This combination vaccine has been given as a primary immunization series at 2–4–6 months, followed by a booster at 18 months of age. Few data are available on this vaccine, designed for use in the Pacific region, but preliminary immunogenicity results seem promising, with no evidence of a decrease in immune response to any of the antigens *(29,36,37)*.

DTwP-eIPV

A vaccine combining DTwP with an enhanced-potency IPV (eIPV) was developed in the late 1970s in Canada *(38)*, France *(39)*, and The Netherlands and was historically the first pediatric combination to extend beyond DTwP. The main problem encountered during its development was the detrimental effect of thiomersal, the preservative classically used in the DTwP vaccine, on the potency and the long-term stability of the eIPV antigens. This led to the development of two types of DTwP-eIPV vaccines. To overcome formulation incompatibilities *(29,40)*, the first vaccine used the dual-chamber syringe technology, while the second used an alternative preservative (2-phenoxyethanol) for the DTwP vaccine, which permitted the development of a fully liquid combination vaccine containing all antigens *(39)*. The eIPV antigens derived from various cell cultures (primary monkey kidney cells, MRC-5, Vero cells) have been used in combination with several DTwPs, either for primary immunization during the first year of life or for subsequent boosters.

No well-designed, controlled studies have been performed to compare the safety and the immunogenicity of the DTwP-eIPV combination vaccine to the associated DTwP and eIPV vaccines given at separate sites. The descriptive data available reveal this combination vaccine has a similar safety profile to that anticipated for the individual DTwP and eIPV vaccines based on historical comparisons *(29,40–45)*. The descriptive studies also showed that the responses to D, T, and P antigens observed after the third injection given during the first year of life were similar to those seen in children given DTwP alone *(42,43) (Table 1)*. The percentages of infants reaching neutralizing antibody titers of 1:4 to poliovirus types 1, 2, and 3 also were similar to those seen when the eIPV vaccine was given alone *(39)*.

DTwP-eIPV combination vaccines have been used on a large scale for more than 10 years in several countries, where all infants have received primary immunization with these vaccines. More recently, this combination vaccine has been replaced in some countries by the DTwP-eIPV-Hib combination. Poliomyelitis has not been resurgent in countries where most children are immunized with DTwP-eIPV vaccines.

DTwP-eIPV-Hib

A pentavalent combination vaccine containing PRP-T and eIPV was developed and tested in Canada *(46)* and France *(29,47–51)*. In these combinations, the lyophilized PRP-T vaccine is reconstituted by a fully liquid DTwP-eIPV vaccine just prior to injection. The bypass dual-chamber syringe technology also was used to allow direct reconstitution of the lyophilized PRP-T vaccine concomitantly with the injection maneuver.

When the safety profile of this combination vaccine was compared in controlled studies to that of DTwP-eIPV and PRP-T vaccines given in association *(29,46,48,50,51)*, no increase in reactogenicity was noted for the combination. These initial trials were further supported by results from a large-scale observational two-year study done in >20,000 French infants *(49)*. The controlled studies on DTwP-eIPV-PRP-T also showed that the immune responses to D, T, and P antigens observed after the third injection given during the first year of life were generally similar to those obtained when the vaccines were given in association. Inconsistent interference in the immune responses to T and P antigens was shown in some cases *(46)*, for which the clinical relevance has not been demonstrated *(Table 1)*. As with the DTwP-Hib vaccine, a possibly clinically relevant reduction in the level of anti-PRP was observed. In all controlled studies *(46,48,50,51)*, the anti-PRP levels observed after the third dose were lower in the group of infants who received the combination vaccine compared to those who received the associated vaccines. Lower anti-PRP GMT values or lower percentages of infants reaching anti-PRP titers ≥ 0.15 or 1.0 µg/mL in the group given the combination vaccine reached statistical significance in some studies.

In two controlled trials, the dual-chamber vaccine performed better than the reconstituted vaccine in terms of immunogenicity *(48,50,51)*.

A version of this combination vaccine not including the P antigens (DT-eIPV used to reconstitute PRP-T) has been tested in Sweden using the northern European primary immunization schedule (3–5–12-months) *(52)*. The introduction of the eIPV antigens had no effect on the immune responses to the other antigens.

DTwP-eIPV-Hib combination vaccines have been introduced in several European countries and in Canada under several vaccination schedules (2–3–4, 3–4–5, or 2–4–6 months) and as yet there is no epidemiological evidence to suggest that the observed interference with the anti-PRP immune responses is medically important in terms of the observed incidence of invasive Hib diseases.

Acellular Pertussis Vaccine Combinations

Although wP vaccines generally have been remarkably successful, the use of certain of them have been associated with reports of high reactogenicity and variable efficacy *(53,54)*. The questionable safety profile of some of these vaccines led to discontinuation of their use in several countries *(55)*.

Over the years, research on the immunogenicity of the *B. pertussis* bacterium has identified at least five protective antigens: pertussis toxin (PT), filamentous hemagglutinin (FHA), pertactin (PRN), and agglutinogens (Fim 2 and 3). Different aP vaccines, containing one to five of these purified antigenic components, have been developed and combined with D and T antigens (DTaP). Fortunately, although wP acted as an adjuvant for the D and T toxoids, its substitution by the aP vaccine has not appeared to diminish the immunogenicity of these components *(56)*.

Different DTaP combinations have been tested in efficacy trials, and all appear better tolerated than their wP equivalents. However, although it had a considerable degree of efficacy, only one of the aP combinations was as good as the best wP vaccine *(57,58)*. Nevertheless, these data, accumulated from many large-scale studies, have convinced some authorities to recommend aP vaccines for routine immunization of infants. Specifically, Japan, United States, Canada, Sweden, Germany, and Italy all are using aP vaccines on a national basis.

No clear serological correlate of protection against disease for the aP vaccine has yet emerged from the large-scale efficacy studies and, in view of the many different P antigens in use, manufacturers have labored to define criteria to demonstrate equivalence of DTaP in combinations with DTaP when administered alone *(57)*. Although this problem has dogged the development of combination vaccines containing an aP component, immunogenic equivalence of the P antigens has been generally accepted by authorities as being indicative of efficacy *(59)*. Vaccine combinations based on aP vaccines are described as follows.

DTaP-Hib

Several vaccine manufacturers have prepared combinations of DTaP and Hib vaccines to be administered to infants in a primary immunization series during the first year of life. Four different DTaP vaccines of varying pertussis antigen compositions have been used to reconstitute the lyophilized PRP-T vaccine. Two vaccines contain two P components (PT and FHA), both developed by PMC (one produced by Biken (Osaka, Japan) for the United States, the other produced by PMC in France). A three-component vaccine (PT, FHA, and PRN) is produced by SB, and a five-component vaccine (PT, FHA, PRN, and Fim 2, 3) is produced by PMC in Canada.

Controlled studies were performed comparing the safety and immunogenicity of DTaP and PRP-T vaccines given to infants, either combined or given separately in two injection sites *(7–9,60–63)*. No study revealed any significant increase in the incidence rate of local and systemic reactions associated with the combined vaccine *(9,62)*. The immunogenicity of the D, T, and P components was not affected by their combination with PRP-T *(8,9,62,64)*. In contrast, anti-PRP responses were significantly reduced in infants given the reconstituted mixture of DTaP and PRP-T compared to those in children who had received the two associated vaccines *(7–9) (Table 2)*. The percentage reduction in anti-PRP GMT values following administration of DTaP-PRP-T compared to the associated vaccines ranged from 33 to 92%, depending on the combination under study *(7,61)*. However the percentage of infants with seroprotective titers of anti-PRP (≥0.15 µg/mL) was not affected, regardless of the vaccine used. This negative influence on the anti-PRP GMT values was observed only for the three combinations based on aP vaccines containing two to three components. No diminution in GMT values or percentages of seroprotected infants (≥0.15 or ≥1.0 µg/mL) was seen in vaccinees given a DTaP-PRP-T combination based on the five-component aP vaccine *(63)*. The explanation for this difference in the behavior of the five-component vaccine is unclear.

The lower anti-PRP levels induced following primary immunization with most combined DTaP-PRP-T vaccines persists up until the time of the booster. Nevertheless, the evidence indicates that infants are still protected against disease despite these lower titers. A booster dose of DTaP-PRP-T has been shown to elicit a strong anti-PRP responses, irrespective of whether infants had previously received the Hib conjugate alone or in combination, suggesting that the combined vaccine efficiently primed these infants *(8,65)*. Further support that immunological memory can be elicited by a primary immunization series with DTaP-PRP-T follows the observation that high anti-PRP levels were achieved in response to a booster dose of unconjugated PRP administered at 12-15 months of age to previously immunized children *(8)*.

Table 2. Effect of Combinations Based on Acellular Pertussis Vaccines on the Immunogenicity of Individual Antigens[a]

Vaccine seroprotective criterion (ref.)	Diphtheria ≥ 0.01 IU/mL	Tetanus ≥ 0.01 IU/mL	Pertussis (PT) fourfold increase	Pertussis (FHA) fourfold increase	Pertussis (PRN) fourfold increase	PRP ≥ 1.0 µg/mL	Polio DA ≥ 1:4	HBsAg ≥ 10 mIU/mL
DTaP-Hib (7–9,60–64)	0	0	0	0	0	± (−− or −−− on GMT)	NR	NR
DTaP-HB (73–78)	0 or + (0 or − on GMT)	0 or + (0 or − on GMT)	0 or +	0 or +	0 or +	NR	NR	0 or −
DTaP-eIPV (83–86)	0 or − (0 or − on GMT)	0 (0 or − on GMT)	0 (0 or − on GMT)	0 (0 or − on GMT)	0 (0 or − on GMT)	NR	0	NR
DTaP-eIPV-Hib (10,29,60, 83–86,96,97)	0 (0 or − on GMT)	0 (0 or − on GMT)	0 (0 or − on GMT)	0 (0 or − on GMT)	0 (0 or − on GMT)	0 or − or −− (0 in full liquid)	0	NR
DTaP-HB-Hib (98–101)	0 (+ on GMT)	0	0	0	0 (−− on GMT)	− or −− (−−−) on GMT	NR	0
DTaP-Hib-eIPV-HB (102)	0	0 (+ on GMT)	0 (− on GMT)	0 (− or + on GMT)	NR	− or ± (−− on GMT)	0 (+ on GMT)	0 or ± (−− or ++ on GMT)

[a]As Evaluated by Geometric Mean Titer (GMT) values and percentage of subjects achieving seroprotective levels of antibodies. Review of data from controlled studies.
0, no difference in the immune response between the combination vaccine and the two vaccines administered separately.
±, increase or decrease in the immune response between the combination vaccine and the two vaccines administered separately: <10% variation.
+ or −, increase or decrease in the immune response between the combination vaccine and the two vaccines administered separately: ≤25% variation.
++ or −−, increase or decrease in the immune response between the combination vaccine and the two vaccines administered separately: ≤50% variation.
+++ or −−−, increase or decrease in the immune response between the combination vaccine and the two vaccines administered separately >50% to ≤80% variation.
NR, not relevant.

The immunogenicity of another Hib conjugate vaccine (PRP-D) was shown not to be reduced when combined with the Biken DTaP *(66)*. When booster doses of PRP-D were given to toddlers who had been primed either with the same aP vaccine *(67)* or with a wP vaccine *(68)*, anamnestic responses were seen. These same studies showed that there was no increase of reactogenicity when the Hib conjugate and DTaP vaccines were combined as a single injection *(67)*. In some trials in Iceland, Germany, and the United States, where the GMT anti-PRP response to PRP-D or PRP-OMP was diminished when combined with a DTaP vaccine, protective efficacy against disease was obtained nevertheless *(69–72)*.

Thus, administration to children of combined DTaP-Hib vaccines tends to be associated with lower anti-PRP responses, although the clinical relevance of this observation is not clear, particularly when a booster dose is recommended during the second year of life.

DTaP-HB

A DTaP combination vaccine containing HB antigen was developed by SB and has been licensed in Europe since 1997 *(73)* for active primary immunization of infants from the age of 2 months. Most studies on this vaccine have assessed the 2–4–6-month schedule. The combination of DTaP and HB did not result in an increased incidence of reactions when compared with the same vaccines given separately *(74,75)*. The safety profile compared favorably to that observed after administration of other commercial DTaP vaccines.

In controlled comparative studies, DTaP-HB did not affect the immune responses to the D, T, and P antigens *(74,76)*. Antibody titers were at least as high in the group of infants given the combined vaccine as in the group given separate vaccines. One month after the third dose, all infants from both the separate and combined vaccine groups achieved seroprotective antibody titers to D and T, and similar vaccine response rates for the three pertussis antigens *(74,76)*. In another randomized study, DTaP-HB vaccine elicited higher antibody responses to all the vaccine antigens compared to when DTaP was given alone *(75) (Table 2)*.

In comparative studies, the anti-HBsAg response following primary immunization of infants given DTaP-HB at 2–4–6 months was comparable to that observed in those given the associated vaccines. The proportions of infants with seroprotective levels of antibody to HBsAg ($\geq$10 mIU/mL) were high (>98%) *(73,75)*, although the GMT anti-HBsAg responses were lower than those observed one month after the third dose of a HB vaccine (produced by the same manufacturer) but given alone to infants at 2–4–6 months of age *(77,78)*. Moreover, when the 2–4–6-month schedule was compared to the 0–1–6-month schedule that is widely used for HB immunization, significantly higher immune responses (greater than a threefold difference in antibody titers) was observed with the latter schedule *(79)*. The proportions of subjects who achieved seroprotective levels of anti-HBsAg were 98 and 100% for the 2–4–6-month and 0–1–6-month schedules, respectively *(75)*.

The good safety profile and the relatively maintained immunogenicity of each component in the DTaP-HB vaccine has led to its approval by the European Medical Evaluation Agency for infant immunization from the age of 2 months.

DTaP-eIPV

Combined vaccines have been developed in Denmark by North American Vaccines (Columbia, MD) *(29)* and by PMC in Canada *(80)* and France *(29,81–86)*. In order to avoid the known interaction of eIPV with thiomersal, DTaP antigens were preserved in 2-phenoxyethanol, enabling the development of fully liquid vaccines containing all vaccine components. Antigens of eIPV of two cell-culture origins (MRC-5 and Vero) were combined with DTaP vaccines containing one, two or five components for primary immunization during the first year of life and for subsequent boosters.

One well-designed, controlled study *(83)* compared the safety and the immunogenicity of the DTaP-eIPV combination to the associated vaccines and showed no increase in reactogenicity associated with the combination vaccine. Other studies also have shown safety profiles consistent with expected results from the two vaccines given alone *(29,84)*. In addition, the immune responses to D, T, and P antigens observed after the third dose of DTaP-eIPV given during the first year of life were similar to those obtained when the vaccines were given separately *(83–86) (Table 2)*. Furthermore, the percentages of infants reaching neutralizing antibody titers of 1:4 against polio virus types 1, 2, and 3 were similar to those obtained when the eIPV vaccine was given alone *(39)*.

The use of DTaP-eIPV combinations as booster vaccines given during the second year of life *(80,83,84)*, at 4–7 years of age *(82)*, or later in life *(81)*, also has been evaluated. All vaccines showed a strong ability to boost antibody levels for all antigens, with no difference between the combination group and the associated vaccine group, whether evaluated in controlled trials *(83)* or compared to historical values. This combination is expected to be introduced on a widespread basis in 1998.

DTaP-eIPV-Hib

This pentavalent vaccine has been developed by PMC in Canada *(10,87)* and France *(83–86,88–93)* and by SB *(60,87,94–96)*. As for the analogous wP combination vaccine, only PRP-T is used in these combinations. Either the lyophilized PRP-T component is reconstituted by a fully liquid DTaP-eIPV vaccine just prior to injection, or a liquid PRP-T vaccine is used to create a fully liquid combination vaccine *(10)*. Comparison of DTaP-eIPV-PRP-T developed by SB with DTwP-eIPV-PRP-T by PMC showed comparable responses to all components *(96)*.

When the safety profile of DTaP-eIPV-PRP-T was compared in controlled studies to that of associated DTaP-eIPV and PRP-T vaccines *(60,84,85,96,97)*, combination of the vaccines did not appear to increase overall reactogenicity. The same controlled studies also showed that the immune responses to D, T, and aP antigens observed after the third vaccine injection given during the first year of life were generally similar between the two groups, although small reductions in the immune responses to D, T, and aP antigens were shown in rare instances *(29,83)* *(Table 2)*. As with the DTaP-Hib vaccine, the only possibly clinically relevant difference concerned the anti-PRP response. In four controlled studies, the anti-PRP level observed after the third dose was lower in the groups of infants who received the combination vaccine than those who received the associated vaccines *(60,83,85,86)*. In some studies, the between-group differences in GMT values or the percentages of infants attaining anti-PRP levels of 0.15 or 1.0 µg/mL reached statistical significance. However, the pentavalent combination containing the five-component DTaP produced by PMC in Canada, which is a fully liquid vaccine, performed better than the two associated vaccines *(10)*.

The use of DTaP-eIPV-PRP-T combinations as booster vaccines also has been evaluated *(10,84,86,89–91,93–95)*. Without exception, they showed a strong ability to boost antibody levels for all antigens, even when very low levels of anti-PRP were present prior to the booster vaccination *(29)*. A DTaP-IPV-PRP-T combination vaccine is now licensed in Canada, and two others are in the final stages of approval for European countries.

DTaP-HB-Hib

The combined DTaP-HB vaccine manufactured by SB has been used to reconstitute a lyophilized Hib conjugate vaccine (PRP-T). This combination was tested for infant primary immunization at 2–4–6 months of age *(98,99)* or at 3–4–5 months of age *(100)*.

Controlled studies compared the combined DTaP-HB-PRP-T vaccine with DTaP-HB and PRP-T vaccines given at two separate sites *(100)* or with the DTaP, HB, and Hib vaccines given at three separate sites *(98,99)*. Although some differences were noted among the vaccine groups, antibody responses to most of the D, T, P and HB components were adequate and within the expected range compared to DTaP-HB vaccine given alone *(99)*. More than 94% of infants had seroprotective levels of anti-HBsAg ($\geq$10 mIU/mL), and over 98% were seroprotected against D and T ($\geq$0.1 IU/mL) *(98,100)*. Fourfold increases in antibody titers to aP components were observed in >92% of subjects from each vaccine group *(101)*.

However, all of the comparative studies revealed interference with the anti-PRP response *(98,99,101)*. GMTs in infants immunized with DTaP-HB-PRP-T were decreased by up to 80% compared to the control vaccines. GMT values were 1.2–1.5 µg/mL in the DTaP-HB-PRP-T vaccine group and 5.5–6.4 µg/mL in those who had received the DTaP, HB, and PRP-T vaccines as three separate injections. The proportion of children who reached anti-PRP levels of 0.15 or 1.0 µg/mL also was reduced when DTaP-HB was combined with PRP-T vaccine compared to responses in vaccinees who received DTaP, HBV, and PRP-T vaccines separately *(98,99)*. Furthermore, by the time of the booster in the second year of life, the proportion of subjects with persistent anti-PRP levels ≥0.15 µg/mL was lower in the group given combined DTaP-HB-PRP-T vaccine than in the group given separate injections *(100)*.

However, there is evidence to suggest that the lowered levels of anti-PRP obtained after immunization are not clinically important. The anti-PRP response to a booster injection of Hib conjugate vaccine was assessed in 10- to 15-month-old children who had been immunized previously with either DTaP-HB-Hib or the associated vaccines and who had achieved low (<1.0 µg/mL) or undetectable (<0.10 µg/mL) levels of anti-PRP at the end of primary immunization *(98,99)*. Nearly all children who had received the DTaP-HB-Hib vaccine showed a rise in the level of anti-PRP IgG following the Hib booster dose, reaching titers ≥1.0 µg/mL *(98)*. Children who had received the combined vaccine in their primary series responded to the booster dose of Hib as robustly as those who had received the DTaP-HB and Hib vaccines separately or the DTaP, HB, and Hib vaccines administered in different sites *(99)*. In addition, the existence of PRP-specific immunological memory at the time of a booster dose of unconjugated PRP vaccine was assessed in toddlers aged 15–22 months who had received either DTaP-HB-Hib vaccine or the associated injections as a primary series at 3-4–5 months of age *(101)*. Children were boosted with the DTaP-HB and unconjugated PRP, either mixed together or in separate injections. The booster dose of PRP elicited anti-PRP levels ≥0.15 µg/mL in >97.5% of subjects, and 86% of vaccinees had levels ≥1.0 µg/mL regardless of the type of booster given. However, a smaller increase in anti-PRP GMT values was observed in the group given the combined booster. Among infants who did not have detectable anti-PRP after the primary series, most attained anti-PRP titers ≥0.5 µg/mL after the PRP booster. The kinetics of the anti-PRP response were rapid, with all children achieving anti-PRP levels ≥0.5 µg/mL within 7–14 days of the booster with no further increase one month thereafter, indicative of an anamnestic response to vaccination. Furthermore, the booster dose induced predominantly anti-PRP IgG, which is also compatible with a response to a T-cell-dependent antigen. These observations suggest that primary immunization with DTaP-HB-Hib had induced immunological memory to Hib, despite the absence of detectable circulating anti-PRP after the third vaccine dose. Nevertheless, given the relatively little data available regarding the anti-PRP response to a DTaP-HB-Hib vaccine, further studies are required in order to support the widespread use of this vaccine.

DTaP-eIPV-HB-Hib

At present, fully liquid hexavalent DTaP-eIPV-HB-Hib combined vaccines are under clinical development (by PMC in partnership with Merck, and by SB). One of the two PMC-Merck fully liquid hexavalent vaccines was shown to have a good safety profile after primary immunization (102) and after a fourth dose administered as a booster (29). Reactogenicity rates were comparable to those noted after administration of the PMC DTaP-eIPV-PRP-T vaccine (29). Primary immunization at 2–3–4 months of age elicited acceptable antibody responses to all antigens (Table 3). Over 92% of infants achieved seroprotective titers to HBsAg ($\geq$10 mlU/mL) and to PRP ($\geq$0.15 µg/mL), and >99% of infants developed protective titers to D and T toxins ($\geq$0.01 IU/mL). All infants had detectable neutralizing antibodies to poliovirus types 1, 2, and 3. At least 87% of infants showed a fourfold increase in antibody titers to P antigens after completion of the primary series (102). The levels of antibody responses to all components, including PRP, were within the range of those observed following primary simultaneous immunization with the separate vaccines (29). A strong anamnestic response to all components of the hexavalent combination was induced by the fourth dose administered to 12- to 15-month-old toddlers, which attests to the effective priming provided by primary immunization with this vaccine (103).

Thus, the combination of DTaP-eIPV-HB-PRP-T given as a single injection in the same syringe seemed safe and immunogenic when used in primary immunization followed by a booster dose during the second year of life. Further data will be needed to establish a basis for the routine use of this hexavalent vaccine.

Combined Vaccines Not Including Pertussis Antigens

Although whole-cell or acellular DTP is the fulcrum of many pediatric combinations, the principle of combination can be applied to other vaccines that do not include P components.

Hib-HB

Merck has combined their recombinant HB vaccine with PRP-OMP for primary immunization (29,40,104,107). The combination is given in two doses during the first year of life, followed by a booster dose in the second year.

In a controlled study (104), the safety profile of this combination vaccine was compared to that of its associated component vaccines. No increase in reactogenicity was observed in the combination group. This study also showed

Table 3. Immunogenicity of Four Doses of a Hexavalent, Fully Liquid, Acellular Pertussis Combination Vaccine Given to Infants at 2, 3, 4, and 12–14 Months of Age[a]

Antigen	Criterion for positive response	Postdose three		Postdose four	
		Responder (%)	GMT	Responder (%)	GMT
Diphtheria	% ≥ 0.01 IU/mL	99.0	0.2 IU/mL	100.0	1.2 IU/mL
Tetanus	% ≥0.01 IU/mL	100.0	0.7 IU/mL	100.0	7.1 IU/mL
PT	% fourfold rise (EU/mL)[b]	88.3	53.3 EU/mL	69.0	87.7 EU/mL
FHA	% fourfold rise (EU/mL)[b]	87.7	97.7 EU/mL	69.0	149.0 EU/mL
Polio 1	% DA ≥ 5 (Neut.)	100.0	254.0 (i/dil)[c]	100.0	3113.0 (1/dil)
Polio 2	% DA ≥ 5 (Neut.)	100.0	115.0 (i/dil)	100.0	2496.0 (1/dil)
Polio 3	% DA ≥ 5 (Neut.)	100.0	290.0 (i/dil)	100.0	3938.0 (1/dil)
PRP-T	% ≥ 0.15 μg/mL	91.7	1.5 μg/mL	100.0	28.6 μg/mL
HBsAg	% ≥ 10 mIU/mL	91.6	142.0 mIU/mL	98.5	1458.0 mIU/mL

[a]Based on ref. 102.
[b]With fourfold rise between pre- and postprimary series titers of the pre- and post-fourth-dose titers.
[c]Inverse of dilution.

16

Table 4. Effect of the Combination of HB
with Two Other Vaccines on the Immunogenicity of Individual Antigens[a]

Vaccine seroprotective criterion (ref.)	HA % >20 mIU/mL	HBsAg % >10 mIU/mL	PRP % >1.0 μg/mL
HA-HB (108–112)	0[b]	0[b]	NR
Hib-HB (104)	NR	0[b] (– on GMT)	0

[a]Evaluated by the percentages of subjects achieving seroprotective levels of antibodies. Review of data from controlled studies.

[b]0: no difference in the immune response between the combination vaccine and the two vaccines administered separately.

that the anti-PRP responses observed after the second vaccine injection, and to HBsAg after the third vaccine injection, were similar in the two combined vs associated groups of vaccinees according to the percentages of infants achieving seroprotective antibody titers. The anti-HBsAg GMT level was slightly lower after immunization with the combination vaccine, and the between-group difference was statistically significant (Table 4). Nevertheless, anti-HBsAg response largely exceeded the level considered as indicative of a long-term clinical protection (98.4% of infants in the combination group obtained anti-HBsAg titers ≥10 mIU/mL; GMT = 4468 mIU/mL).

The development of Hib-HB vaccine, now licensed in the United States (106,107), has opened up new options for childhood vaccination by offering the possibility of association with DTwP or DTaP, thus avoiding the issue of possible deleterious effects on the immunogenicity of P-containing combinations.

HA-HB

A combination of hepatitis A (HA) and HB vaccines has been developed by SB and is licensed in many countries. Clinical studies comparing HA-HB to the associated vaccines (108–112) have shown that the combination of the vaccines does not adversely affect reactogenicity. Furthermore, the antibody responses obtained against the HA and HB antigens were quite satisfactory, with no evidence for interference (Table 4).

MMR and MMR-V

Measles, mumps, and rubella attenuated viruses have long been administered as a combined vaccine (MMR). In this case, specific studies were done to show that the combination was no less immunogenic than the individual vaccines (Table 5) (113). Equivalent safety also was demonstrated in studies leading up

Table 5. Antibody Responses
to MMR Vaccines Given Separately or as Combined MMR[a]

	% Seroconversion (GMT)[b]		
	Measles	*Mumps*	*Rubella*
Monovalent	100% (82)	92% (19)	100% (306)
Combined	99% (89)	90% (31)	100% (301)

[a]Based on ref. *113*.
[b]Measles and rubella titers determined by hemagglutination-inhibition, mumps titer by neutralization *(152)*.

to licensure, which involved approximately 10,000 children. This result was not obviously expected, because many people had argued that three live viruses would interfere with one another if given simultaneously. The excellent immunogenicity and effectiveness record of MMR testifies to the contrary *(114,115)*.

Bivalent measles-rubella and measles-mumps combinations also were developed to provide a flexible approach to child vaccination, and studies are in progress to develop a quadrivalent measles-mumps-rubella-varicella (V) vaccine (MMR-V) *(116)*. Interestingly, early data show that anti-V responses are diminished when combined with MMR, whereas V vaccination in association with MMR poses no problem *(117)*. Although the lability of varicella-zoster virus may account for this difficulty, other factors might be at work. Augmenting the dose of V vaccine in the combination may provide a practical solution.

Multivalent Combinations

At this point, it is worthwhile drawing attention to the distinction between combining vaccines and combining antigens from different strains of the same pathogen. Although a combined vaccine is a mixture of different vaccines in a single product that can protect against several diseases, multivalent combinations protect against just one disease by combining the different antigens relevant for protection. In some cases, multiple purified antigens from a pathogen may be required to provide immunity against disease. For example, the aP vaccines are often produced by purifying the different P antigens separately and then mixing them in various combinations to form the final vaccine. In other cases, immunity to more than one bacterial or viral strain may be necessary to protect against disease. This necessitates the combination of antigens from the different strains into a single vaccine, known as a multivalent vaccine.

Viral Vaccines

INFLUENZA

The oldest multivalent vaccine is the influenza vaccine, which contains three different viral strains *(118)*. Two of the strains are type A viruses, differing in their hemagglutinin (H) and neuraminadase (N) proteins, and the third is a type B virus. The strains are chosen based on those in current worldwide circulation; in recent years, both an H1N1 strain and an H3N2 strain of Type A have been included. Although few data are available, it does not appear that the combination of strains interferes with their individual immunogenic properties *(119)*. A multivalent intranasal influenza vaccine is undergoing phase III clinical trials in the United States. Although early data have shown interference between the live attenuated viruses used in this vaccine *(120)*, more recent results suggest that the problem has been overcome *(121)*.

POLIO

The polio vaccine developed by Salk is a trivalent vaccine, containing serotypes 1, 2 and 3. Likewise, the live attenuated oral polio vaccine (OPV) also contains these three serotypes. OPV originally was given as three sequential administrations of the individual serotypes because of interference among the viruses when they were given together at a dose of about 10^6 $TCID_{50}$ for each virus *(122)*. Moreover, it was found to be preferable to give the attenuated poliovirus types in the order 1-3-2 in order to avoid the stronger interference caused by type 2 *(123)*. Eventually, research showed that by adjusting the dosage of each serotype, interference was sufficiently reduced so that after two doses of a trivalent vaccine seroconversion to all three serotypes could be guaranteed *(124)*. In practice, three doses are given in the primary immunization series to provide high and long-lasting antibody responses. The OPV formula used in the United States now consists of about $10^{6.7}$ $TCID_{50}$ of type 1, $10^{5.8}$ $TCID_{50}$ of type 2, and $10^{6.5}$ $TCID_{50}$ of type 3 per dose. Nevertheless, even today, problems with OPV vaccination in tropical areas justifies experimentation with other dosage formulas *(125)*.

ROTAVIRUS

Another live attenuated multivalent viral vaccine given orally is the rotavirus vaccine. This vaccine, which was licensed recently in the United States, contains four different attenuated viruses, representing the G-protein serotypes 1–4 of Group A rotavirus, that are those most commonly found in human infections. Serotype 3 in the vaccine is a natural monkey virus, while serotypes 1, 2, and 4 are reassortants containing the gene for the G protein from those serotypes together with a background of 10 other genes contained in the genome of the serotype 3 monkey virus. Each virus in the mixture is given at a dose of

10^5 TCID$_{50}$, and three doses are given to ensure immunization against all sero-types *(126,127)*.

Bacterial Capsular Polysaccharide Vaccines

Capsular polysaccharides from organisms that cause frequent bacteremia have long been used as vaccines. Whereas Hib is by far the most important *H. influenzae* serotype *(128)*, the meningococci have many serogroups, of which at least five are clinically important *(129)*, and the pneumococci include many serotypes that cause disease *(130)*.

MENINGOCOCCAL

Meningococcal polysaccharide vaccine contains antigens for Groups A, C, W-135, and Y. As yet, no protective antigen is available for Group B. This mixture of polysaccharide antigens is highly immunogenic from the age of 18 months, and the multivalent combination does not diminish individual immunogenicity.

PNEUMOCOCCAL

Twenty-three serotypes of pneumococcus have been identified to be the most frequent causes of bacteremic or localized pneumococcal disease in adults. Early versions, produced before World War II, only contained a few serotypes, but more recent versions of the vaccine contained first 14 and then 23 serotypes. Although the 14- and 23-valent vaccines never were formally compared, the immunogenicity of each serotype in the more comprehensive combination seems to be unimpaired.

Dosing Schedule

Each combination vaccine component, and the combination itself, must provide optimal safety and immunogenicity profiles when integrated into the routine immunization schedules previously used with the single products. Indeed, given the possible interference on immune responses resulting from the combination of multiple antigens and because the routine schedule is not necessarily optimal for each component, the time-interval between doses and/or the number of doses must be assessed for each new vaccine combination.

Vaccination schedules for infant immunization are based on the epidemiology of the diseases against which the vaccines are developed. They also are designed in order to optimize compliance to vaccination, vaccine coverage, and protection. With current inactivated or subunit vaccines, a primary series of at least three doses generally is needed to elicit protective primary antibody responses in infants. A fourth dose of vaccine also may be required to ensure mid- or long-term protection by inducing a memory response in infants whose immune system is still maturing.

Immunization schedules have been shown to markedly influence the level of immune response. In particular, important issues are the age of the vaccinees and the immaturity of their immune systems at the initiation of vaccination, the presence of high levels of passively transferred maternal antibodies in younger infants *(131)*, and the time interval between the immune system stimulations by the vaccine components.

For most components of combination vaccines used for infant immunization, the so-called "extended schedule," with a two-month interval between doses (e.g., 2–4–6 months), is more immunogenic than the "accelerated schedule," in which the interval is only one month (e.g., 2–3–4 months). For aP combination vaccines containing Hib and eIPV components, the immunogenic advantage of the 2–4–6-month schedule as compared with the 2–3–4 month regimen has been clearly demonstrated *(86,132)*. However, although levels of antibodies were still higher in the 2–4–6-month primary schedule group before the booster, there was no apparent advantage after the booster dose. Immune responses were similarly strong after the booster dose in the children immunized by the 2–3–4-month schedule *(90)*, attesting to the induction of an efficient immune memory after the primary series, regardless of the immunization schedule. Similarly, a 3–5–9 month primary immunization regimen was shown to be more immunogenic for the D and T components of a DTwP vaccine compared to immunization at 2–3–4 months *(133,134)*. However, no differences in the levels of antibodies to D, T, and P were observed at the age when the preschool booster was given *(135)*. The lower antibody concentrations following a accelerated immunization course might have implications for long-term protection, especially if a booster in the second year of life is not given. However, three doses of DTaP-eIPV-Hib vaccine given on a 3–5–12-month schedule were shown to be as immunogenic as four doses given at 2–4–6–12 months of age *(93)*.

The impact of immunization schedule was extensively studied for the plasma- and yeast-derived HB vaccines. Various immunization regimens with HB vaccines have been assessed in adults and children *(136,137)*. Two schedules for HB vaccination are predominantly used in healthy individuals, regardless of age: either three doses at 0–1–6 months, or four doses at 0–1–2–12 months *(136,137)*. However, HB vaccination administered by these two schedules cannot be integrated into the routine pediatric schedules used in most countries for either DTwP- or DTaP-containing vaccines. HB vaccine administered to infants at 2–4–6 months of age thus was demonstrated *(77,78)* to induce seroprotective titers of anti-HBsAg (≥10 mIU/mL) in 99% of vaccinees, even if the GMT values were lower than those expected following the established schedules. Immunological memory to HBsAg has been demonstrated to persist for at least 5–12 years after primary immunization (although the level of anti-HBsAg does wane after vaccination), provided that a seroprotective titer of 10 mIU/mL was reached after primary immunization *(138–140)*. A booster dose of HB vaccine elicits a high and rapid anamnestic response, suggesting the presence of a persistent immunological memory afforded by the primary vaccination could mean long-lasting protection. However, although a booster with HB vaccine is not thought to be necessary to sustain immunity and because of the need to give boosters of other components, current combinations incorporating HB being developed will be administered at 2, 4, 6, and 12–15 months of age in order to optimize the rate of protection of the infant population against all diseases covered by the combination vaccine.

Thus, although more potent vaccines and changing epidemiology may permit a reduction in the number of doses administered during infancy, for the time being it appears that three immunizations before one year of age are still necessary.

Future Combinations

The future holds possibilities of combining vaccines that go beyond mere mechanical mixing. For example, genetic engineering enables genes from one organism to be inserted into the genome of another. Genes encoding proteins that induce protective immune responses against a pathogen could be inserted into a suitable recipient organism (vector), such as a naturally or artificially attenuated virus or bacterium *(141)*. An advantage of this technique is that vectors are often capable of accepting multiple pieces of genetic information, each of which can be transcribed and expressed. Several examples of this approach are being studied in experimental vaccines. Vectors derived from a canarypoxvirus, containing genes from a variety of microorganisms, have reached clinical trials: rabies (G protein) *(142)*, HIV (*env, gag, pol*, and *nef* proteins) *(143)*, Japanese encephalitis (envelope, S1 and M proteins) *(144)*, and malaria (seven different proteins) *(145)*. Cytokines also may be inserted into vectors for expression of their adjuvant activity.

Another experimental technique that may have practical possibilities for combination vaccines is DNA or genetic immunization. Intramuscular or subcutaneous injections of DNA plasmids containing genes that encode antigenic proteins can induce immune responses. By mixing plasmids containing different genes, or using plasmids that contain more than one gene, it may be possible to immunize against several antigens with a single injection *(146,147)*.

The Effect of Combinations on Future Vaccine Development

Table 6 summarizes the combinations already being used and those in development. Most pediatricians and internists would be delighted to administer more vaccines with fewer injections, and one can expect that new vaccine combinations will gain rapid acceptance. Vaccination of children in most coun-

**Table 6. Combination Vaccines Licensed
in at Least One Country or Under Development**

Licensed	
Whole-cell pertussis based	
DTwP-Hib (PRP-T)	Pasteur Mérieux Connaught (PMC) (France, US, and Canada)
DTwP-Hib (HbOC)	Wyeth-Lederle (WL)
DTwP-eIPV	PMC (France), North American Vaccines (NAVA), RIVM
DTwP-HB	SmithKline Beecham Biologicals (SB)
DTwP-eIPV-Hib (PRP-T)	PMC (France and Canada)
Acellular pertussis based	
DTaP(3)-HB	SB
DTaP(3)-IPV	SB
DTaP(2)-IPV	PMC (France)
DTaP(5)-IPV	PMC (Canada)
DTaP(1)-IPV	NAVA
DTaP(2)-Hib (PRP-T)	PMC (US) (booster)
DTaP(2)-Hib (PRP-T)-IPV	PMC (France)
DTaP(3)-Hib (PRP-T)-IPV	SB (booster)
DTaP(5)-Hib (PRP-T)-IPV	PMC (Canada)
Combinations in development	
Whole-cell pertussis based or acellular pertussis based	
DTwP-HB-Hib (PRP-OMP)	Merck-CSL
DTaP(4)-Hib (HbOC)	WL
DTaP(3)-Hib (PRP-T)-HB	SB
DTaP(2)-Hib (PRP-T)-IPV-HB	PMC (France and US)[a]
DTaP(3)-Hib (PRP-T)-IPV-HB	SB

[a]In partnership with Merck.

tries is built around a schedule of three primary immunizations in the first year of life, followed by a booster in the second year. A hexavalent combination vaccine protecting against tetanus, diphtheria, pertussis, polio, Hib, and HB will fit in well with that schedule. However, as HB vaccine only requires two primary doses, use of such a combination will imply the administration of an extra dose of HB. Because there are no safety issues involved, such "overimmunization" is likely to be accepted for the sake of simplicity.

Importantly, pediatric combinations will facilitate the use of new vaccines. HA *(148)*, meningococcal conjugate *(149)*, and pneumococcal conjugate *(150)* vaccines are three likely additions to future pediatric vaccine schedules. Given a combination containing the six vaccines now recommended, these new vaccines could be given in association by separate injections. However, there is no doubt that an effort will be made to incorporate the new vaccines into the basic combination, or alternatively there will be a fission of the basic combination to create two new combinations containing, four and five vaccine components. Of course, this is not the end of the story, as other candidate vaccines, notably respiratory syncytial virus *(151)*, one day will need to be added to the combinations used.

References

1. Gupta, R. K., Relyveld, E. H., Lindblad, E. B., et al. (1993) Adjuvants—a balance between toxicity and adjuvanticity. *Vaccine* **11,** 293–306.
2. Claesson, B. A., Trollfors, B., Lagergard, T., Taranger, J., Bryla, D., Otterman, G., Cramton, T., Yang, Y., Reimer, C. B., Robbins, J. B., et al. (1988) Clinical and immunologic responses to the capsular polysaccharide of *Haemophilus influenzae* type *b* alone or conjugated to tetanus toxoid in 18- to 23-month-old children. *J. Pediatr.* **112,** 695–702.
3. Sawyer, L. A., McInnis, J., Patel, A., et al. (1994) Deleterious effect of thimerosal on the potency of inactivated poliovirus vaccine. *Vaccine* **12,** 851–855.
4. Insel, R. A. (1995) Potential alterations in immunogenicity by combining or simultaneously administering vaccine components. *Ann. NY Acad. Sci.* **754,** 35–47.
5. Ferreccio, C., Clemens, J., Avendano, A., Horwitz, I., Flores, C., Avila, L., Cayazzo, M., Fritzell, B., Cadoz, M., and Levine, M. (1991) The clinical and immunologic response of Chilean infants to *Haemophilus influenzae* type *b* polysaccharide-tetanus protein conjugate vaccine coadministered in the same syringe with diphtheria-tetanus toxoids-pertussis vaccine at two, four and six months of age. *Pediatr. Infect. Dis. J.* **10,** 764–771.
6. Watember, N., Dagan, R., Arbelli, Y., et al. (1992) Safety and immunogenicity of Haemophilus type b-tetanus protein conjugate vaccine, mixed in the same syringe with diphtheria-tetanus-pertussis vaccine in young infants. *Pediatr. Infect. Dis. J.* **10,** 758–763.
7. Eskola, J., Litmanen, L., Saarinen, L., and Kayhty, H. (1996) Responses at 24 months to a combined DTPa-Hib conjugate vaccine in children vaccinated with the same vaccines at 4 and 6 months. (Abst. G60) 36th ICAAC, Sept. 15–18, 1996, New Orleans, LA, p. 154.
8. Hoppenbrouwers, K., Kanra, G., Silier, T., Desmyter, J., Bande-Knops, J., Ceyhan, M., Yurdakök, K., Berut, F., Blondeau, C., and Pehlivan, T. (1997) Priming effect of the combined DTaP/Act-HIB vaccine. (Abst. 73) The 15th Annual Meeting of the European Society for Paediatric Infectious Diseases (ESPID); Paris 1997, p. 37.
9. Schmitt, H. J. (1998) Immunogenicity and reactogenicity of 2 Hib tetanus conjugate vaccines administered by reconstituting with DTPa or given as separate injections. (Abst. G63) 35th ICAAC 1998.
10. Mills, E. L., Russell, M., Cunning, L., Guasparini, R., Meekison, W., Thipphawong, J., Fox, M., and Barreto, L. (1997) A fully liquid acellular pertussis vaccine combined with IPV and Hib vaccines (DTaP-IPV-PRP-T) is safe and immunogenic without significant interaction. (Abst. G95) 37th ICAAC, Sept. 28–Oct. 1, 1997, Toronto, Canada, p. 209.
11. Decker, M. D. and Edwards, K. M. (1995) Issues in design of clinical trials of combination vaccines. *Ann. NY Acad. Sci.* **754,** 234–240.
12. Ramon, G. (1923) Sur le pouvoir floculant et sur les proprietes immunisantes d+une toxine diphterique rendue anatoxique (anatoxine). *Compt. Rend. Acad. Sci.* **177,** 1338,1339.

13. Ramon, G. (1949) Quatrième mémoire. Les vaccinations associées au moyen des "vaccins combinés". *Bases. Essor. Résultats.* Revue d'Immunologie **13**, 41–65.

14. DiSant Agnese, P. (1947) Combined immunization against diphtheria, tetanus, and pertussis in children over three months of ages; including an evaluation of the effectiveness of two immunizing agents. *J. Pediatr.* **31**, 251–265.

15. Miller, J. J. and Saito, T. (1942) Concurrent immunization against tetanus, diphtheria, and pertussis. *J. Pediatr.* **21**, 31–44.

16. Eskola, J., Kayhty, H., Gordon, L., Hovi, T., Stenvik, M., Ronnberg, P. R., Kela, E., and Peltola, H. (1988) Simultaneous administration of *Haemophilus influenzae* type b capsular polysaccharide-diphtheria toxoid conjugate vaccine with routine diphtheria-tetanus-pertussis and inactivated poliovirus vaccinations of childhood. *Pediatr. Infect. Dis. J.* **7**, 480–484.

17. Scheifele, D., Bjornson, G., Barreto, L., Meekison, W., and Guasparini, R. (1992) Controlled trial of *Haemophilus influenzae* type b diphtheria toxoid conjugate combined with diphtheria, tetanus and pertussis vaccines, in 18-month-old children, including comparison of arm versus thigh injection. *Vaccine* **10**, 455–460.

18. Barreto, L., Schelfele, D., Noseworthy, G., Stratton, F., Bjornson, G., and Schaart, W. (1993) A controlled comparison of *Haemophilus influenzae* type b diphtheria toxoid conjugate vaccine given concurrently or in combination with DPT-IPV vaccine to 18-month-old children. *Immunol. Infect. Dis.* **3**, 316–320.

19. Amir, J., Melamed, R., Bader, J., Ethevenaux, C., Fritzell, B., Cartier, J. R., Arminjon, F., and Dagan, R. (1997) Immunogenicity and safety of a liquid combination of DT-PRP-T vs lyophilized PRP-T reconstituted with DTP. *Vaccine* **15**, 149–154.

20. Avendano, A., Ferreccio, C., Lagos, R., Horwitz, I., Cayazzo, M., Fritzell, B., Meschievitz, C., and Levine, M. (1993) *Haemophilus influenzae* type b polysaccharide—tetanus protein conjugate vaccine does not depress serologic responses to diphtheria, tetanus or pertussis antigens when coadministered in the same syringe with diphtheria-tetanus-pertussis vaccine at two, four and six months of age. *Pediatr. Infect. Dis. J.* **12**, 638–643.

21. Miller, M. A., Meschievitz, C. K., Ballanco, G. A., and Daum, R. S. (1995) Safety and immunogenicity of PRP-T combined with DTP: Excretion of capsular polysaccharide and antibody response in the immediate post-vaccination period. *Pediatrics* **95**, 522–527.

22. Clemens, J. D., Ferreccio, C., Levine, M. M., Horwitz, I., Rao, M. R., Edwards, K. M., and Fritzell, B. (1992) Impact of *Haemophilus influenzae* type b polysaccharide-tetanus protein conjugate vaccine on responses to concurrently administered diphtheria-tetanus-pertussis vaccine. *JAMA* **267**, 673–678.

23. Mulholland, E. K., Hoestermann, A., Ward, J. I., Maine, N., Ethevenaux, C., and Greenwood, B. M. (1996) The use of *Haemophilus influenzae* type b-tetanus toxoid conjugate vaccine mixed with diphtheria-tetanus-pertussis vaccine in Gambian infants. *Vaccine* **14**, 905–909.

24. Jones, I. G., Tyrrell, H., Hill, A., Horobin, J. M., and Taylor, B. (1998) Randomised controlled trial of combined diphtheria, tetanus, whole-cell pertussis vaccine administered in the same syringe and separately with *Haemophilus influenzae* type b vaccine at two, three and four months of age. *Vaccine* **16**, 109–113.

25. Begg, N. T., Miller, E., Fairley, C. K., Chapel, H. M., Griffiths, H., Waight, P. A., and Ashworth, L. A. E. (1995) Antibody responses and symptoms after DTP and either tetanus or diphtheria *Haemophilus influenzae* type B conjugate vaccines given for primary immunisation by separate or mixed injection. *Vaccine* **13**, 1547–1550.

26. Black, S. B., Shinefield, H. R., Ray, P., Lewis, E. M., Fireman, B., Hiatt, R., Madore, D. V., Johnson, C. L., and Hackell, J. G. (1993) Safety of combined oligosaccharide conjugate *Haemophilus influenzae* type b (HbOC) and whole cell diphtheria-tetanus toxoids-pertussis vaccine in infancy. The Kaiser Permanente Pediatric VACCINE Study Group. *Pediatr. Infect. Dis. J.* **12**, 981–985.

27. Paradiso, P. R., Hogerman, D. A., Madore, D. V., Keyserling, H., King, J., Reisinger, K. S., Blatter, M. M., Rothstein, E., Bernstein, H. H., Pennridge Pediatric Associates, et al. (1993) Safety and immunogenicity of a combined diphtheria, tetanus, pertussis and *Haemophilus influenzae* type *b* vaccine in young infants. *Pediatrics* **92,** 827–832.

28. Scheifele, D., Barreto, L., Meekison, W., Guasparini, R., and Friesen, B. (1993) Can *Haemophilus influenzae* type *b*-tetanus toxoid conjugate vaccine be combined with diphtheria toxoid-pertussis vaccine-tetanus toxoid? *Can. Med. Assoc. J.* **149,** 1105–1112.

29. Unpublished Results, 1998.

30. Scheifele, D. W., Meekison, W., Guasparini, R., Roberts, A., Barreto, L., Thipphawong, J., and Wiltsey, S. (1995) Evaluation of booster doses of *Haemophilus influenzae* type *b*- tetanus toxoid conjugate vaccine in 18-month-old children. *Vaccine* 13, 104–108.

31. Scheifele, D., Law, B., Mitchell, L., and Ochnio, J. (1996) Study of booster doses of two *Haemophilus influenzae* type *b* conjugate vaccines including their interchangeability. *Vaccine* **14,** 1399–1406.

32. Papaevangelou, G., Karvelis, E., Alexiou, D., Kiossoglou, K., Roumeliotou, A., Safary, A., Collard, F., and Vandepapeliere, P. (1995) Evaluation of a combined tetravalent diphtheria, tetanus, whole-cell pertussis and hepatitis B candidate vaccine administered to healthy infants according to a three-dose vaccination schedule. *Vaccine* **13,** 175–178.

33. Aristegui, J., Garrote, E., Gonzalez, A., Arrate, J. P., Perez, A., and Vandepapeliere, P. (1997) Immune response to a combined hepatitis B, diphtheria, tetanus and whole-cell pertussis vaccine administered to infants at 2, 4 and 6 months of age. *Vaccine* **15,** 7–9.

34. Diez-Delgado, J., Dal-Ré, R., Llorente, M., Gonzales, A., and Lopez, J. (1997) Hepatitis B component does not interfere with the immune response to diphtheria, tetanus and whole-cell *Bordetella pertussis* components of a quadrivalent (DTPw-HB) vaccine: a controlled trial in healthy infants. *Vaccine* **15,** 1418–1422.

35. Usonis, V., Bakasenas, V., Taylor, D., and Vandepapeliere, P. (1996) Immunogenicity and reactogenicity of a combined DTPw-hepatitis B vaccine in Lithuanian infants. *Eur. J. Pediatr.* **155,** 189–193.

36. Nolan, T., Hogg, G., Darcy, M. A., et al. (1997) 18m booster immunogenicity and reactogenicity in infants immunised with a combination DTwP-Hib-Hepatitis B vaccine. Pediatr. Res. **41** (Abst. 751), 128A.

37. Nolan, T., Hogg, G., Darcy, M. A., Varigos, J., and Skeljo, M. (1996) Immunogenicity and reactogenicity in infants immunised with a new pentavalent (DTwP-Hib-HepB) vaccine. Pediatr. Res. **39** (Abst. 1071), 181A.

38. Murdin, A. D., Barreto, L., and Plotkin, S. A. (1996) Inactivated poliovirus vaccine: past and present experience. *Vaccine* **7,** 735–746.

39. Vidor, E., Caudrelier, P., and Plotkin, S. (1994) The place of DTP/eIPV vaccine in routine paediatric vaccination. *Rev. Med. Virol.* **4,** 261–277.

40. Halsey, N. A., Blatter, M., Bader, G., Thoms, M. L., Willingham, F. F., O.Donovan, J. C., Pakula, L., Berut, F., Reisinger, K. S., and Meschievitz, C. (1997) Inactivated poliovirus vaccine alone or sequential inactivated and oral poliovirus vaccine in two-, four- and six-month-old infants with combination *Haemophilus influenzae* type *b/* hepatitis B vaccine. *Pediatr. Infect. Dis. J.* **16,** 675–679.

41. Schatzmayr, H. G., Maurice, Y., Fujita, M., and Bispo de Fillipis, A. M. (1986) Serological evaluation of poliomyelitis oral and inactivated vaccines in an urban low-income population at Rio de Janeiro. *Vaccine* **4,** 111–114.

42. Qureshi, A. W., Zulfiqar, I., Raza, A., and Siddiqi, N. (1989) Comparison of immunogenicity of combined DTP-inactivated injectable polio vaccine (DTP-IPV) and association of DTP and attenuated oral polio vaccine (DTP+OPV) in Pakistani children. *JAMA* **39,** 31–35.

43. Drucker, J., Soula, G., Diallo, O., and Fabre, P. (1985) Evaluation of a new combined inactivated DTP-Polio vaccine. *Dev. Biol. Stand.* **65,** 145–151.

44. Coursaget, P., Bringer, L., Bourdil, C., et al. (1991) Simultaneous injection of hepatitis B and measles vaccines. *Trans. R. Soc. Trop. Med. Hygiene* **85,** 788.
45. Coursaget, P., Relyveld, E., Brizard, A., Frenkiel, M. P., Fritzell, B., Teulières, L., Bourdil, C., Yvonnet, B., Jeannée, E., Guindo, S., et al. (1992) Simultaneous injection of hepatitis B vaccine with BCG and killed poliovirus vaccine. *Vaccine* **10,** 319–321.
46. Gold, R., Scheifele, D., Barreto, L., Wiltsey, S., Bjornson, G., Meekison, W., Guasparini, R., and Medd, L. (1994) Safety and immunogenicity of *Haemophilus influenzae* vaccine (tetanus toxoid conjugate) administered concurrently or combined with diphtheria and tetanus toxoids, pertussis vaccine and inactivated poliomyelitis vaccine to healthy infants at two, four and six months of age. *Pediatr. Infect. Dis. J.* **13,** 348–355.
47. Dagan, R., Botujansky, C., Watemberg, N., Arbelli, Y., Belmaker, I., Ethevenaux, C., and Fritzell, B. (1994) Safety and immunogenicity in young infants of Haemophilus b-tetanus protein conjugate vaccine, mixed in the same syringe with diphtheria- tetanus-pertussis-enhanced inactivated poliovirus vaccine. *Pediatr. Infect. Dis. J.* **13,** 356–362.
48. Ethevenaux, C., Langue, J., Fritzell, B., et al. (1995) Safety and immunogenicity of Haemophilus b-tetanus protein conjugate vaccine (PRP-T) presented in a dual-chamber syringe with diphtheria tetanus pertussis and inactivated poliomyelitis vaccine (DTP-IPV). (Abstract) Soc. Pediatr. Res. Mtg, San Diego, May 11–13, 1995; 105A.
49. Boucher, J., Ethevenaux, C., Guyot, C., Leroux, M. C., Fritzell, B., Saliou, P., and Reinert, P. (1996) Essai de prévention des infections graves à *Haemophilus influenzae* type b et essai de tolérance, après vaccination PRP-T, dans le département du Val-de-Marne. *Arch Pédiatr.* **3,** 775–781.
50. Ethevenaux, C., Langue, J., Fritzell, B., et al. (1996) Immunogenicity of Haemophilus B-tetanus protein conjugate vaccine (PRP-T), presented in a dual-chamber syringe with diphtheria tetanus pertussis and inactivated poliomyelitis vaccine (DTP-IPV). (Abstract) 2nd European Paediatric Congress, Berlin, Germany 1996.
51. Ethevenaux, C., Hoppenbrouwers, K., Lagos, R., et al. (1996) Safety and immunogenicity of Haemophilus b-tetanus protein conjugate vaccine (PRP-T), presented in a dual-chamber syringe with diphtheria tetanus pertussis vaccine (DTP). (Abstract) 2nd European Paediatric Congress, Berlin, Germany 1996.
52. Carlsson, R. M., Claesson, B. A., Iwarson, S., and Selstam, U. (1995) Studies on a Hib conjugate vaccine (PRP-T): The effects of coadministered tetanus toxoid vaccine, combined administration with injectable polio vaccine, and administration route. 35th *ICAAC* (Abst. 674), **6,** San Francisco, CA.
53. Howson, C., Howe, C., and Fineberg, J. (1991) Adverse effects of pertussis and rubella vaccines: a report of the committee to review the adverse consequences of pertussis and rubella vaccines. National Academy of Sciences, Washington, DC, 1–186.
54. Fine, P. E. M. and Clarkson, J. A. (1987) Reflections on the efficacy of pertussis vaccines. *Rev. Infect. Dis.* **9,** 866–883.
55. Mortimer, E. A. (1994) Pertussis vaccine. *Vaccines*, 2nd ed. W.B. Saunders, Philadelphia; **5,** pp. 91–135.
56. Simondon, F., Yam, A., Gagnepain, J. Y., Wassilak, S., Danve, B., and Cadoz, M. (1996) Comparative safety and immunogenicity of an acellular versus whole- cell pertussis component of diphtheria-tetanus-pertussis vaccines in Senegalese infants. *Eur. J. Clin. Microb. Infect. Dis.* **15,** 927–932.
57. Madore, D. V. (1993) Progress and challenges for a new combination vaccine composed to diphtheria, tetanus, acellular pertussis, and Haemophilus b conjugate, in *Combined Vaccines and Simultaneous Administration: Current Issues and Perspectives* (Williams, J. C., ed.), Conference, Bethesda, Maryland, July 28–30, 1993, pp. 356–358.

58. Olin, P., Rasmussen, F., Gustafsson, L., Hallander, H. O., and Heijbel, H. (1997) Randomised controlled trial of two-component, three-component, and five-component acellular pertussis vaccines compared with whole-cell pertussis vaccine. *Lancet* **350,** 1569–1577.

59. Cherry, J. D., Heininger, U., Christenson, P. D., Eckhardt, T., Laussucq, S., Hackell, J. G., Mezzatesta, J. R., and Stehr, K. (1995) Surrogate serologic tests for the prediction of pertussis vaccine efficacy. *Ann. NY Acad. Sci.* 359–363.

60. Eskola, J., Ölander, R. M., Litmanen, L., Peltola, S., and Käyhty, H. (1996) Randomised trial of the effect of co-administration with acellular pertussis DTP vaccine on immunogenicity of *Haemophilus influenzae* type *b* conjugate vaccine. *Lancet* **348,** 1688–1692.

61. Liese, J. G., Harzer, E., Hosbach, P., Froeschle, J., and Meschievitz, C. (1996) Hib antibody response of a combined DTaP-PRP-T conjugate vaccine compared to separate injections in infants. (Abst. G105) 36th ICAAC, Sept. 15–18, 1998, **162,** New Orleans, LA.

62. Pichichero, M. E., Latiolais, T., Bernstein, D. I., Hosbach, P., Christian, E., Vidor, E., Meschievitz, C., and Daum, R. S. (1997) Vaccine antigen interactions after a combination diphtheria-tetanus toxoid-acellular pertussis/purified capsular polysaccharide of *Haemophilus influenzae* type *b*-tetanus toxoid vaccine in two-, four- and six-month-old infants. *Pediatr. Infect. Dis. J.* **16,** 863–870.

63. Lee, C. Y., Huang, L. M., Lee, P. I., Chiu, H. H., Lin, W., Thipphawong, J., Debois, H., Xie, F., and Harrison, D. (1997) An acellular pertussis DTacP combined with a lyophilized *Haemophilus influenzae* type *b* (PRP-T) vaccine is safe and immunogenic in Taiwanese infants. (Abst. G93) 37th ICAAC 1997.

64. Bell, F., Heath, P., Shackley, F., Maclennan, J., Shearstone, N., Diggle, L., Moxon, E. R., and Finn, A. (1997) Diphtheria and tetanus responses to whole-cell and acellular pertussis DTP/HIB combination vaccines. (Abst.) *The 15th Annual Meeting of the European Society for Paediatric Infectious Diseases (ESPID),* Paris 1997, (Abst. 71, p. 36).

65. Bell, F., Heath, P., Shackley, F., Maclennan, J., Shearstone, N., Diggle, L., Moxon, E. R., and Finn, A. (1997) Immunological memory to HIB following combined acellular pertussis diphtheria, tetanus/HIB vaccine. (Abst.) *The 15th Annual Meeting of the European Society for Paediatric Infectious Diseases (ESPID),* Paris 1997.

66. Liese, J. G., Harzer, E., Hosbach, P., et al. (1997) Immunogenicity of a combined DTaP-PRP-D conjugate vaccine compared to separate injections in infants. (Abst. G106) *2nd European Paediatric Congress,* Berlin, Germany 1997.

67. Rennels, M., Hohenboken, M., Clements, D., Reisinger, K., Nonenmacher, J., and Hackell, J. (1996) Antibodies to pertussis induced by DTaP and HbOC administered simultaneously versus combined in children < 15 months versus ≥ 15 months. (Abst. G101) *36th ICAAC 1996.*

68. Kovel, A., Wald, E., Guerra, N., Serdy, C., and Meschievitz, C. (1992) Safety and immunogenicity of acellular diphtheria-tetanus-pertussis and Haemophilus conjugate vaccines given in combination or at separate injection sites. *J. Pediatr.* **120,** 84–87.

69. Eskola, J., Takala, A., Käyhty, H., Peltola, H., and Mäkelä, P. H. (1991) Experience in Finland with *Haemophilus influenzae* type *b* vaccines. *Vaccine* **9,** S14–S16.

70. Black, S. B., Shinefield, H. R., Fireman, B., Hiatt, R., Polen, M., and Vittinghoff, E. (1991) Efficacy in infancy of oligosaccharide conjugate *Haemophilus influenzae* type b (HbOC) vaccine in a United States population of 61080 children. *Pediatr. Infect. Dis. J.* **10,** 97–104.

71. Eskola, J., Käyhty, H., Takala, A. K., Peltola, H., Rönnberg, P. R., Kela, E., Pekkanen, E., McVerry, P. H., and Mäkelä, H. (1990) A randomized, prospective field trial of a conjugate vaccine in the protection of infants and young children against invasive *Haemophilus Influenzae* type *b* disease. *N. Engl. J. Med.* **323,** 1381–1387.

72. Eskola, J., Peltola, H., Takala, A. K., Käyhty, H., Hakulinen, M., Karanko, V., Kela, E., Rekola, P., Rönnberg, P. R., Samuelson, J. S., et al. (1987) Efficacy of Haemophilus

98. Pichichero, M. E. and Passador, S. (1997) Administration of combined diphtheria and tetanus toxoids and pertussis vaccine, hepatitis B, and *Haemophilus influenzae* type *b* (Hib) vaccine to infants and response to a booster dose of Hib conjugate vaccine. *Clin. Infect. Dis.* **25,** 1378–1384.
99. Greenberg, D. P., Wong, V. K., Partridge, S., Chang, S. J., Howe, B. J., and Ward, J. I. (1996) Immunogenicity of a booster dose of Hib conjugate vaccine in children with impaired immune response following primary vaccination with DTaP-Hep B-PRP-T vaccine. (Abst. G61) *36th ICAAC 1996.*
100. Habermehl, P., Knuf, M., Mannhardt, W., Schuind, A., Rebsch, C., Schmidtke, P., Slaoui, M., Clemens, R., and Zepp, F. (1997) Safety and immunogenicity of a new DTaP-HBV-HIB combination vaccine for primary immunization of infants. *8th European Congress of Clinical Microbiology and Infectious Diseases 1997,* Paris, France.
101. Zepp, F., Schmitt, H. J., Kaufhold, A., Schuind, A., Knuf, M., Habermehl, P., Meyer, C., Bogaerts, H., Slaoui, M., and Clemens, R. (1997) Evidence for induction of polysaccharide specific B-cell-memory in the 1st year of life: plain *Haemophilus influenzae* type *b* - PRP (Hib) boosters children primed with a tetanus-conjugate Hib-DTPa-HBV combined vaccine. *Eur. J. Pediatr.* **156,** 18–24.
102. Fabre, P. and Mallet, E. (1996) Safety and immunogenicity of a fully liquid combination vaccine, with acellular pertussis diphtheria tetanus, inactivated poliovirus, *Haemophilus influenzae* serotype *b*, and hepatitis B when given in infants at 2, 3 and 4 months of age. (Abst. LB31) *36th ICAAC 1996.*
103. Fabre, P., Boslego, J., Wiens, B., Bailleux, F., Blondeau, C., and Mallet, E. (1998) Immunogenicity of the fourth dose of a hexavalent, fully liquid, acellular pertussis combination vaccine given to infants at 12 to 14 months of age. *The 16th Annual Meeting of the European Society for Paediatric Infectious Diseases (ESPID)*, Bled, Slovénie 1998.
104. West, D. J., Hesley, T. M., Jonas, L. C., Feeley, L. K., Bird, S. R., Burke, P., Sadoff, J. C., and HIB-HB Vaccine Study Group (1997) Safety and immunogenicity of a bivalent *Haemophilus influenzae* type b/hepatitis B vaccine in healthy infants. *Pediatr. Infect. Dis. J.* **16,** 593–599.
105. Bernstein, H. H., Rothstein, E. P., Reisinger, K. S., Blatter, M. M., Arbeter, A. M., Fontana, M. E., Jacobs, J. M., Long, S. S., Rathfon, H., Crayne, O., et al. (1994) Comparison of a three-component acellular pertussis vaccine with a whole-cell pertussis vaccine in 15- through 20-month-old infants. *Pediatrics* **93,** 656–659.
106. Heininger, H., Cherry, J. D., Christenson, P. D., Eckhardt, T., Göering, U., Jakob, P., Kasper, W., Schweingel, D., Laussucq, S., Hackell, J. G., et al. (1994) Comparative study of Lederle/Takeda acellular and Lederle whole-cell pertussis-component diphtheria-tetanus-pertussis vaccines in infants in Germany. *Vaccine* **12,** 81–86.
107. Merck & Co. (1997) I. Comvax *Haemophilus* b conjugate (meningococcal protein conjugate) and hepatitis R (recombinant) combined vaccine. *JAMA* **277,** 620,621.
108. Bruguera, M., Bayas, J. M., Vilella, A., Tural, C., Gonzalez, A., Vidal, J., Dal, R. R., and Salleras, L. (1996) Immunogenicity and reactogenicity of a combined hepatitis A and B vaccine in young adults. *Vaccine* **14(15),** 1407–1411.
109. Kallinowski, B., Bock, H. L., Clemens, R., and Theilmann, L. (1996) Immunogenicity and reactogenicity of a combined hepatitis A/B candidate vaccine: first results. *Liver* **16,** 271–273.
110. Leroux-Roels, G., Moreau, W., Desombere, I., and Safary, A. (1996) Safety and immunogenicity of a combined hepatitis A and hepatitis B vaccine in young healthy adults. *Scand. J. Gastroenterol.* **31,** 1027–1031.
111. Ambrosch, F., Wiedermann, G., André, F. E., Delem, A. D., Gregor, H., Hofmann, H., D'Hondt, E., Kundi, M., Wynen, J., and Kunz, C. (1994) Clinical and immunological investigation of a new combined hepatitis A and hepatitis B vaccine. *J. Med. Virol.* **44,** 452–456.

112. Ambrosch, F., André, F. E., Delem, A. D., D'Hondt, E., Jonas, S., Kunz, C., Safary, A., and Wiedermann, G. (1992) Simultaneous vaccination against hepatitis-A and hepatitis-B - results of a controlled study. *Vaccine* **10**, S142–S145.

113. Weibel, R. E., Carlson, A. J., Villarejos, V. M., Buynak, E. B., McLean, A. A., and Hilleman, M. R. (1980) Clinical and laboratory studies of combined live measles, mumps, and rubella vaccine using the RA 27/3 rubella virus (40979). *Proc. Soc. Exp. Biol. Med.* **165**, 323–326.

114. Lerman, S., Bollinger, M., and Brunken, J. (1981) Clinical and serologic evaluation of measles, mumps, and rubella (HPV-77:DE5 and RA27/3) virus vaccines, singly and in combination. *Pediatr* **68**, 18–22.

115. Brunell, P., Weigle, K., Murphy, D., et al. (1983) Antibody response following measles-mumps-rubella vaccine under conditions of customary use. *JAMA* **250**, 1409–1412.

116. White, C., Stinson, D., Staehle, B., et al. (1997) Measles, mumps, rubella, and varicella combination vaccine: safety and immunogenicity alone and in combination with other vaccines given to children. *Clin. Infect. Dis.* **24**, 925–931.

117. Englund, J., Suarez, C., Kelly, J., et al. (1989) Placebo-controlled trial of varicella vaccine given with or after measles-mumps-rubella vaccine. *J. Pediatr.* **114**, 37–44.

118. Kilboune, E. (1994) Inactivated influenza vaccines. *Vaccines*, 2nd ed. (Plotkin, S. and Mortimer, J. J., eds.), Philadelphia, Saunders, pp. 565–581.

119. Mostow, S., Schoenbaum, S., Dowdle, W., et al. (1970) Studies on inactivated influenza vaccines.II. Effect of increasing dosage on antibody response and adverse reactions in man. *Am. J. Epidemiol.* **92**, 248–256.

120. Keitel, W., Couch, R., and Quarles, J. (1993) Trivalent attenuated cold-adapted influenza virus vaccine: reduced viral shedding and serum antibody responses in susceptible adults. *J. Infect. Dis.* **167**, 305–311.

121. Nelshe, D., Iacuzioi, D., Mendelman, P., et al. (1997) Efficacy of a trivalent live attenuated intranasal influenza vaccine in children. [Abstract] *Inf. Dis. Soc.* **9**, 13–16.

122. Sabin, A. (1960) Polio vaccine, oral: testing and standardizaton of live polio vaccines. 6th International Congress on Microbiological Standardization. Wisbaden: H. Hoffman Verlag, Berlin Zehlendorf.

123. Plotkin, S., Koprowski, H., and Stokes, J. (1998) Clinical trials in infants of orally administered attenuated poliomyelitis viruses. *Pediatrics* **23**, 1041–1062.

124. Perkins, F., Yetts, R., and Gaisford, W. (1963) Response of 3-month-old infants to 3 doses of trivalent oral poliomyelitis in Brazil. *Br. Med. J.* **1**, 1573,1574.

125. Patriarca, P., Laender, F., Palmeira, G., et al. (1988) Randomized trial of alternative formulations of oral poliovaccine in Brazil. *Lancet* **1**, 429–433.

126. Kapikian, A., Hoshino, Y., Chanok, R., et al. (1996) Efficacy of a quadrivalent rhesus rotavirus-based human rotavirus aimed at preventing severe rotavirus diarrhea in infants and young children. *J. Infect. Dis.* **174(Suppl)**, S65–S72.

127. Rennels, M., Glass, R., Dennehy, P., et al. (1996) Safety and efficacy of high-dose rhesus-human reassortant rotavirus vaccines:report of the national multicenter trial. *Pediatrics* **97**, 7–13.

128. Ward, J., Lieberman, J., and Cochi, S. (1994) Haemophilus influenzae vaccines, *Vaccines*, 2nd ed. (Plotkin, S. and Mortimer, E., eds.), Philadelphia, Saunders, pp. 337–386.

129. Lepow, M. (1994) Meningococcal vaccines, *Vaccines*, 2nd ed. (Plotkin, S. and Mortimer, E., eds.), Philadelphia, Saunders, pp. 503–515.

130. Fedson, D. and Musher, D. (1994) Pneumococcal vaccine, *Vaccines*, 2nd ed. (Plotkin, S. and Mortimer, E., eds.), Philadelphia, Saunders, pp. 517–564.

131. Björkholm, B., Granström, M., Taranger, J., Wahl, M., and Hagberg, L. (1995) Influence of high titers of maternal antibody on the serologic response of infants to diphtheria vaccination at three, five and twelve months of age. *Pediatr. Infect. Dis. J.* **14**, 846–850.

132. Boughton, C. R. (1996) Pertussis vaccines: acellular versus whole-cell. *Med J. Aust.* **164**, 564–566.

133. Ramsay, M. E. B., Rao, M., Begg, N. T., Redhead, K., and Attwell, A. M. (1993) Antibody response to accelerated immunisation with diphtheria, tetanus, pertussis vaccine. *Lancet* **342,** 203–205.
134. Booy, R., Aitken, S. J. M., Taylor, S., Tudor-Williams, G., Macfarlane, J. A., Moxon, E. R., Ashworth, L. A. E., Mayon-White, R. T., Griffiths, H., and Chapel, H. M. (1992) Immunogenicity of combined diphtheria, tetanus, and pertussis vaccine given at 2, 3, and 4 months versus 3, 5, and 9 months of age. *Lancet* **339,** 507–510.
135. Ramsay, M. E. B., Corbel, M. J., Redhead, K., Ashworth, L. A. E., and Begg, N. T. (1991) Persistence of antibody after accelerated immunisation with diphtheria/tetanus/pertussis vaccine. *BMJ* **302,** 1489–1491.
136. West, D. J., Calandra, G. B., Hesley, T. M., Ioli, V., and Miller, W. J. (1993) Control of hepatitis B through routine immunization of infants: the need for flexible schedules and new combination vaccine formulations. *Vaccine* **11,** S21–S27.
137. Jilg, W., Schmidt, M., and Deinhardt, F. (1989) Vaccination against Hepatitis B: comparison of three different vaccination schedules. *J. Infect. Dis.* **160,** 766–769.
138. West, D. J. and Calandra, G. B. (1996) Vaccine induced immunologic memory for hepatitis B surface antigen: implications for policy on booster vaccination. *Vaccine* **14,** 1019–1027.
139. West, D. J., Watson, B., Lichtman, J., Hesley, T. M., and Hedberg, K. (1994) Persistence of immunologic memory for twelve years in children given hepatitis B vaccine in infancy. *Pediatr. Infect. Dis. J.* **13,** 745–747.
140. Da Villa, G., Pelliccia, M. G., Peluso, F., Ricciardi, E., and Sepe, A. (1997) Anti-HBs responses in children vaccinated with different schedules of either plasma-derived or HBV DNA recombinant vaccine. *Res. Virol.* **148,** 109–114.
141. Plotkin, S. A. (1993) Vaccination in the 21st Century. *J. Infect. Dis.* **168,** 29–37.
142. Cadoz, M., Strady, A., Meignier, B., et al. (1992) Immunization with canarypox virus expressing rabies glycoprotein. *Lancet* **339,** 1429–1432.
143. Excler, J. and Plotkin, S. (1997) The prime-boost concept applied to HIB preventive vaccines. *AIDS* **11(A)(Suppl.),** S127–S137.
144. Konishi, E., Kuraine, I., Mason, P. W., et al. (1998) Induction of Japanese encephalitis virus-specific cytotoxic T lymphocytes in humans by poxvirus-based JE vaccine candidates. *Vaccine* **16,** 842–849.
145. Ockenhouse, C., Sun, P., Lanar, D., et al. (1998) Phase I/IIa safety, immunogenicity and efficacy of NYVAC-Pf7, a pox-vectored, multiantigen, multistage vaccine candidate for *Plasmodium falciparum* malaria. *J. Infect. Dis.* **177,** 1664–1673.
146. Wolff, J., Malone, R., Williams, P., et al. (1990) Direct gene transfer into mouse muscle in vivo. *Science* **247,** 1465–1468.
147. Ulmer, J. B., Sadoff, J. C., and Liu, M. A. (1996) DNA vaccines. *Curr. Opin. Immunol.* **8,** 531–536.
148. Jilg, W., Deinhardt, F., and Hilleman, M. (1994) Hepatitis A vaccine, *Vaccines,* 2nd ed. (Plotkin, S. and Mortimer, E., eds.), Philadelphia, Saunders, pp. 583–595.
149. Leach, A., Twumasi, P., Kumah, S., et al. (1997) Induction of immunologic memory in Gambian children by vaccination in infancy with a Group A plus Group C meningococcal polysaccharide-protein conjugate vaccine. *J. Infect. Dis.* **175,** 200–204.
150. Siber, G. (1994) Pneumococcal disease: prospects for a new generation of vaccines. *Science* **265,** 1385–1387.
151. Crowe, J. J. (1995) Current approaches to the development of vaccines against disease caused by respiratory syncytial virus (RSV) and parainfluenza virus (PIV). *Vaccine* **13(4),** 415–421.
152. Lerman, S., Bollinger, M., and Brunken, J. (1991) Clinical and serological. *Pediatrics* **48,** 18–22.

2 Combination Vaccines in Adolescents and Adults

Peter A. Gross

Introduction

Immunization of adults does not receive the same priority as immunization of children *(1)*. The low priority shown toward adult immunizations is not consistent with the fact that yearly in the United States, 50,000–70,000 deaths are estimated to occur from vaccine-preventable diseases, namely, influenza, pneumococcal disease, and hepatitis B (HB). These numbers far exceed the annual deaths from automobile accidents or acquired immunodeficiency syndrome (AIDS). Deaths in childhood from diseases prevented by immunizations amount to fewer than 500.

Recent data released from the Centers for Disease Control and Prevention (CDC) *(2)* show that in adults over 65 years, a target group for pneumococcal and influenza vaccine, only 59% receive influenza vaccine (range among states from 44–70%) and only 36% receive pneumococcal vaccine (range among states from 11–47%). The Year 2000 goals are 80% for influenza vaccine and pneumococcal vaccine for institutionalized chronically ill or older people and 60% for both vaccines in noninstitutionalized, high-risk populations, as defined by the Advisory Committee on Immunization Practices (ACIP) *(3)*.

As new vaccines become licensed and are recommended for children, more consideration should be focused on adults who may not be immune to those same diseases. Recent examples include the varicella-zoster virus (VZV), HB, and hepatitis A (HA) virus. Many adults would benefit by vaccination against these three infectious diseases.

Some of the factors responsible for the inadequate approach to adult immunization are lingering doubts of the public as well as healthcare providers about the safety and efficacy of vaccines; ineffectiveness of selecting target groups for immunization instead of recommending universal immunization for adults; liability concerns; poor or no reimbursement for immunizations; lack of an accepted delivery system for adult immunization; unacknowledged fear of

From: *Combination Vaccines: From Clinical Research to Approval*
Edited by: R. W. Ellis © Humana Press Inc., Totowa, NJ

Table 1. Recommended Immunization Schedule for Adults

Age	Recommended schedule
Teenagers/young adults	Completion of all childhood primary immunizations
	HB for those not immunized in childhood
	Td booster[a]
50 years	Completion of all primary immunizations[b]
	Td booster[a]
	Assessment of risk factors indicating need for pneumococcal vaccine and annual influenza immunization
65 years or older	Completion of all primary immunizations[b]
	Yearly influenza vaccine
	Pneumococcal vaccine[c]

[a]Td = Tetanus and diptheria toxoids. The Task Force Adult Immunization endorses two strategies as equivalent: the traditional recommendation of Td boosters every 10 years throughout life; and special emphasis on completion of the primary immunization series followed by a single midlife booster at age 50 years for individuals who have completed the full pediatric series including the teenage/young adult booster.

[b]Mainly Td. Individuals born before 1957 are not targeted for primary immunization for MMR. Similarly, poliomyelitis has become such a rare disease that the primary immunization of older adults is not cost-effective.

[c]Individuals who first receive pneumococcal vaccine five or more years before this age should be considered for reimmunization at age 65 years, although data are incomplete.

needles; and patients who are unaccustomed to regular physician office visits *(1)*. A collaborative effort by the public, the government, and the medical community is necessary. The National Vaccine Program is attempting to provide the lead in this effort.

Excellent sources for adult immunization information are the *American College of Physician's Guide for Adult Immunization*, third ed. and the CDC's *Update on Adult Immunization (Table 1) (1,4)*. An excellent source for adolescent immunization information are the combined recommendations of the ACIP, the American Academy of Pediatrics, the American Academy of Family Physicians and the American Medical Association published in at least two journals *(Table 2) (5)*.

The importance of adolescent immunization was re-emphasized when it was realized that immunity from measles vaccination in childhood waned in the adolescent years. Therefore, a recommendation was made to give a second measles, mumps, and rubella (MMR) vaccine to adolescents on entrance to college. This time period should be a time to re-examine the need for other immunizations that might not have been given in infancy such as HB vaccine, or that might require a booster dose such as the tetanus-diphtheria vaccine for adults (adult Td) vaccine.

The emphasis in this chapter will be on the use of combination vaccines in adolescents and adults *(6,7)*. A major review of combination vaccines was written in 1993 *(8)*. At that time, the points were made that the term "combination vaccine" can refer to: a physically mixed preparation of two or more vaccine immunogens and two or more immunogens expressed in the host following administration of vectored vaccines or nucleic acid vaccines *(9,10)*. The combination may consist of multiple antigens of the same infectious organism such as the 23 serotypes of pneumococcus and the three types of poliovirus (multivalent) or multiple antigens of different infectious organisms such as MMR or Td (multidisease). The simultaneous administration of two or more single strain vaccines given at the same time at separate sites will not be considered a combination vaccine.

The purpose of combination vaccines is to increase compliance with vaccine recommendations by reducing the number of needlesticks and reducing the number of visits to healthcare providers. Vaccine storage and shipping would become easier with combination as opposed to separate vaccines. The worldwide need to create combination vaccines is great. Geographic, socioeconomic, and behavioral factors make many populations around the world relatively inaccessible for repeated immunization visits. The ideal vaccine would provide lifetime immunity for all childhood and adult infectious diseases after the administration of one dose of an oral vaccine given in infancy. Unfortunately, we are not even near that realization at this time. Nevertheless, currently available combination vaccines and others being developed bring us closer to our goal than was appreciated just a few decades ago.

Potential adverse consequences may occur from combining vaccines such as reduced immunogenicity and/or efficacy and increase side effects. These are the factors that should be monitored when vaccines are combined into a single dosage format or given simultaneously. Protective effects should be comparable to when the vaccines are given individually. Adverse effects should be no more than additive *(10)*. Although the literature suggests that adverse reactions are more common with combinations or simultaneous administration, it would be inappropriate to make any generalizations about the lack of adverse reactions or the maintenance of efficacy when vaccines are administered simultaneously or in combination. Consequently, each combination or simultaneous administration needs to be tested. Finally, it is necessary to examine if we will only look for the common, self-limited, local and systemic side effects or if we will also try to measure neurological and other rare adverse events that often become apparent after the vaccine is licensed and used in larger numbers of patients.

Determination of the efficacy of new combinations of existing vaccines is a particularly vexing problem *(11)*. The diseases in the new combination may have been eliminated or at least brought under control. Consequently, efficacy

Table 2. Recommended Schedule of Vaccinations for Adolescents Ages 11–12 Years

Immunobiologic	Indications	Name	Dose	Frequency	Route
Hepatitis A vaccine	Adolescents who are at increased risk of HA infection or its complications	HAVRIX[a]	720 EL.U[b]/0.5 mL[c]	A total of two doses at 0, 6–12 mo[d]	IM[e]
		VAQTA[®a]	25 U/0.5 mL	A total of two doses at 0, 6–18 mo	IM
Hepatitis B vaccine	Adolescents not vaccinated previously for HB	Recombivax HB[®a]	5 µg/0.5 mL	A total of three doses at 0, 1–2, 4–6 mo	IM
		Engerix-B[®a]	10 µg/0.5 mL	A total of three doses at 0, 1–2, 4–6 mo	IM
Influenza vaccine	Adolescents who are at increased risk for complications caused by influenza or who have contact with persons at increased risk for these complications	Influenza virus vaccine[f]	0.5 mL	Annually (Sept.–Dec.)	IM
MMR	Adolescents not vaccinated previously with two doses of measles vaccine at ≥12 mo of age	MMR[®a]	0.5 mL	One dose	SC[g]
Pneumococcal polysaccharide vaccine	Adolescents who are at increased risk for pneumococcal disease or its complications	Pneumococcal vaccine polyvalent[f]	0.5 mL	One dose	IM or SC

Td	Adolescents not vaccinated within the previous 5 yr	Tetanus and diptheria toxoids, adsorbed (for adult use)^f	0.5 mL	Every 10 yr	IM
Varicella virus vaccine	Adolescents not vaccinated previously and who have no reliable history of chickenpox	VARIVAX®^{a}	0.5 mL	One dose^h	SC

^{a}Manufacturer's product name.
^{b}Enzyme-linked immunosorbent assay (ELISA) unit.
^{c}Alternative dosage and schedule of 360 EL.U/0.5 mL and a total of three doses administered at 0, 1, and 6–12 months.
^{d}Zero months represents timing of the initial dose, and subsequent numbers represent months after the initial dose.
^{e}Intramuscular injection.
^{f}Generic name.
^{g}Subcutaneous injection.
^{h}Adolescents ≥13 years of age should be administered a total of two doses (0.5 mL/dose) subcutaneously at 0 and 4–8 weeks.

trials in an immune population are impossible. Surrogate markers such as immunogenicity become the new standard to determine comparability of combination versus single vaccine effects. The unpredictability of combination effects are illustrated by comparing different diphtheria-tetanus-whole cell pertussis vaccine combined with a *Haemophilus influenzae* type *b* vaccine conjugate vaccine (DTP$_w$-Hib) vaccines. Administration to children of a combination of Lederle-Praxis' DTP$_w$ and the mutant toxin (CRM197) isolated from Corynebacterium diphtheriae (HbOC) conjugated to *H. influenzae* type *b* (Hib) resulted in an enhanced immune response to all antigens, while administration of the combination of Merieux's DTP$_w$ and polyribosylribitol phosphate-tetanus (PRP-T) Hib conjugate vaccine suppressed the immune response to all antigens significantly. Additionally, when DTP$_w$ and PRP-T Hib were given simultaneously but at separate sites, depression of the immune response to the pertussis agglutinin depended on which DTP$_w$-adjuvant vaccine was used *(12)*. Vaccine lot-to-lot variations may also effect immunogenicity. As a result, we need to consider how physical and chemical interactions, immunological interference, interactions between live viruses, the effects of buffers and adjuvants, and other factors will ultimately effect the immune response, safety, and efficacy of combination vaccines *(13)*.

Optimizing the immunogenicity of the components in combination vaccines can be accomplished in a number of ways. The most basic concept is that polysaccharides can be made more potent when combined with protein. This was demonstrated as far back as the 1920s and 1930s by Landsteiner, Goebel, and Avery *(14)*. Without a protein conjugate, a polysaccharide is usually not immunogenic in infants, children, and immunodeficient persons. Also, the addition of adjuvants, conjugating protein to a carrier, immunizing in the presence of cytokines, using alternate routes of administration, and using different forms and doses of antigens may enhance the immune response *(15)*. Which of these vaccine supplements is chosen depends on which type of T helper subset (i.e., TH1 or TH2) is protective for the particular antigen.

Adjuvants in particular have been extensively studied *(16)*. They have two major effects. First, they increase the biological and immunological half-life of an antigen through its depot effect. Second, they enhance antigen presentation that affects MHC I and II and secretory antibody responses. Several types of adjuvants are being used or tested: gel-type adjuvants (e.g., alum), bacterial adjuvants (e.g., muramyl peptides), particulate adjuvants (e.g., liposomes, immunostimulatory complexes [ISCOMS], biodegradable microspheres), oil-emulsion and emulsifier-based adjuvants (saponins, squalene, incomplete Freund's adjuvant), and synthetic adjuvants (e.g., synthetic lipid A, nonionic block copolymers). Aluminum salts, such as alum, are the only currently licensed adjuvants.

Microorganisms themselves may be carriers of vaccine antigens. Utilizing genetic fusion, the core antigen of HB (HBcAg) virus has been used to immunize experimental animals against malaria, salmonella, and various viruses *(17)*. Vaccinia virus, tobacco mosaic virus, yeast, and live recombinant BCG vaccine are other examples of carriers. Finally, DNA vaccines promise to be important vaccine vectors in the future *(18)*.

Adult and Adolescent Combinations

Vaccine Combinations in the Developed World

Most of the following vaccines are used for booster immunizations in adults and adolescents when they have received a primary series with the same vaccine in childhood. If not, the vaccines can be used for primary immunization with the exception of OPV. Pneumococcal vaccine is currently only given to persons at high risk of complications of pneumococcal disease and to all persons over 65 years of age regardless of their underlying disease. An earlier immunization age of 50 years would allow a better antibody response to develop *(1)*.

Immunization of immunosuppressed adolescents and adults, although more difficult, still should be attempted. Allogeneic bone marrow transplant patients often lose immunity to many vaccine-preventable diseases and should be re-immunized when they are likely to respond *(19)*.

Healthcare workers are another special target for immunization because of the diseases they can transmit or be the recipients of while working in the healthcare setting *(20)*.

ADULT TD VACCINE

Diphtheria toxoid was first licensed in 1926 and tetanus toxoid in 1933, but it was not until 1955 that the Adult Td combination was licensed *(10)*. Its pediatric counterpart, DTP_w, was actually the first licensed combination vaccine. It was licensed by the Food and Drug Administration (FDA) in 1949 *(21)*.

MMR VACCINE

Live measles vaccine was licensed in 1963, live mumps vaccine in 1967, and live rubella vaccine in 1969. The MMR combination was approved in 1971 *(10)*.

The original Edmonton B strain in the measles vaccine may have interfered with the response to the mumps vaccine; although the numbers in the study were small *(22,23)*. The mumps vaccine was reported to interfere with the rubella vaccine in a combination vaccine produced by Biken (Osaka, Japan) *(24)*. It should be noted that adolescents are more likely to have vaccine side effects from MMR *(25)*.

A combination of MMR with varicella-zoster virus vaccine (MMRV) would combine protection against the major childhood exanthems into one vaccine. Studies to document enhancement or inhibition of immunity are being conducted. Given simultaneously, MMR and varicella vaccines are equally immunogenic as when given six weeks apart *(26,27)*. Whether they will be as immunogenic when given in the same syringe is under study. If they are equally immunogenic, then one of the two VZV vaccine doses given to susceptible adolescents could be given as MMRV when the same adolescents require a booster dose of the MMR vaccine.

PNEUMOCOCCAL VACCINE

A hexavalent vaccine was licensed in 1946, but was abandoned shortly thereafter with the widespread use of penicillin. It was incorrectly thought that penicillin would solve the problem of pneumococcal disease, so a vaccine was no longer necessary. Now, of course, the problem of penicillin resistance has emerged making the need for preventing pneumococcal disease even more urgent. The 14-valent vaccine was licensed in 1977 and the 23-valent vaccine was approved for use in 1983 *(10)*—the latter being the most ambitious multivalent vaccine to date *(21)*.

INFLUENZA VACCINE

Influenza vaccine was first licensed in 1945 *(10)*. It was a bivalent product for many years with a type A and a type B strain present in the vaccine. Since the late 1970s, it has routinely become a trivalent vaccine with two type A strains (subtype H3N2 and subtype H1N1) and a type B strain present.

Influenza vaccine and pneumococcal vaccine can be given simultaneously at separate sites producing comparable immunity to giving the vaccines one month apart *(28)*.

A multistrain, live respiratory virus vaccine is under investigation that would incorporate influenza A (H1N1), influenza A (H3N2), influenza B, respiratory syncytial virus, and parainfluenza viruses. While the initial targets for the vaccine are children, all of these viruses cause significant disease in adolescent and adult hosts with respiratory compromise and would be useful in these older age groups *(29)*.

INACTIVATED POLIOVIRUS VACCINE

The trivalent inactivated poliovirus vaccine (IPV) was licensed in 1955. It was introduced as a mixture from the beginning and was the first multivalent killed virus vaccine licensed *(21)*. The current enhanced potency IPV (E-IPV) is more immunogenic than the earlier Salk IPV (S-IPV) *(30)*. E-IPV is immunogenic in fewer doses than S-IPV. It is now used for the initial doses in a combined IPV-oral poliovirus (OPV) primary immunization schedule. Theoretically, the

IPV-OPV sequential immunization schedule should reduce the incidence of vaccine-associated polio in the vaccine recipient, although it would not be expected to do the same in susceptible contacts of the vaccinee. No difference is expected in vaccine-associated polio among susceptible contacts as the frequency and duration of OPV virus shedding is the same whether IPV is given initially or not.

OPV

The three strains in the oral poliovirus vaccine were licensed individually in 1961 and 1962 and then combined into a trivalent vaccine in 1963 *(10)*. Interestingly, type 2 poliovirus grows preferentially in the human host, so six times as much type 3 and ten times as much type 1 poliovirus are included in the trivalent OPV *(31)*. Three doses are required in part because the three poliovirus types interfere with each other and compete for the development of immunity. Only after multiple doses are given is the immune response adequate against all three virus types *(32)*. OPV has three disadvantages: vaccine-associated paralytic polio (VAPP) in vaccine recipients as well as contacts, low immunogenicity in children in developing countries, and relative thermolability *(31)*. The concern for VAPP has prevented OPV from being used for primary and booster immunization in adults *(33)*.

A live, combined oral enteric vaccine against polioviruses and rotaviruses is under investigation. The new oral rotavirus vaccines, however, may interfere with the replication of live poliovirus vaccines and alter the immunogenicity of both vaccines. But this combination should be pursued for the developing world. Separately, both vaccines facilitate the development of local mucosal immunity which may interrupt transmission of the virus from person-to-person.

HA AND HB VACCINES

A combination of HA and HB vaccines would be desirable. A new recommendation for universal immunization of infants against HA would be required. Then, given the current recommendation for universal immunization of infants against HB, testing of a combination HA and HB vaccine would be appropriate. A HA-HB combination is licensed in Europe and may soon be licensed in the United States. It would be appropriate for routine immunization of adolescents and adults since HA and HB are common diseases in both groups.

The HB vaccine has been combined with a conjugated *H. influenzae* type *b* vaccine *(34)*. Increased antibody levels were observed in healthy adults who were previously exposed to these two antigens.

PERTUSSIS VACCINE

This vaccine is not currently recommended for use in adolescents and adults. Because of the increasingly recognized occurrence of pertussis in adolescents and adults, and the low reactogenicity of the acellular vaccine compared with the whole cell pertussis vaccine, the acellular vaccine may be recommended as a booster for these groups in the future *(35)*. Also, it could be combined with Adult Td, E-IPV, and HB as an adult "super combination" vaccine.

Travelers Vaccines

Administration of yellow fever vaccine and cholera vaccine simultaneously or one to three weeks apart elicited lower than normal antibody responses to both vaccines *(36,37)*. So, if both vaccines have to be given, they should be administered at least four weeks apart. Alternatively, cholera vaccine can be omitted entirely for foreign travel as the efficacy against *Vibrio cholerae* O1 infection is 50% at best and the risk to United States travelers is low. No country in the world requires cholera vaccination for entry. When the new, more efficacious oral cholera vaccine is licensed, it may be worthwhile considering for travel to certain high risk areas of the world *(38)*.

The potential for interference when yellow fever vaccine is given simultaneously with vaccines against typhoid, paratyphoid, typhus, plague, rabies, or Japanese encephalitis is unknown *(38)*. In the United States, when yellow fever vaccine is given with commercially available immune globulin, no alteration of the immunological response to yellow fever occurs because there is no antibody to yellow fever in the commercial immune globulin preparations.

Yellow fever vaccine can be given simultaneously with measles, Bacille Calmette-Guérin (BCG), and hepatitis vaccines without a reduction in immunogenicity or an increase in side effects. In general, however, when live virus vaccines are not given simultaneously, they should be given four weeks apart.

An ideal combination travelers vaccine would be a typhoid-HA vaccine. It would be appropriate for travel to all developing areas of the world. A second dose of a lone HA vaccine would be necessary for the development of complete, long-lasting HA immunity.

Meningococcal Vaccine

A bivalent vaccine against types A and C was licensed in 1975, followed by the tetravalent vaccine against serotypes A, C, Y, and W-135 in 1981 *(10)*. A vaccine incorporating type B is not available in the United States, but it is available elsewhere. Meningococcal vaccine has been mixed in the same syringe with typhoid vaccine. The combination produced antibody responses and side effects comparable to administration with separate syringes *(39)*.

Dengue Vaccine

The incidence of dengue is increasing in South America, Central America, and the Caribbean. A four strain dengue vaccine is being studied but is not available *(40)*.

Additional Vaccine Combinations in the Developing World

Tuberculosis Vaccine

BCG vaccine is a live attenuated vaccine. It currently is the most widely used vaccine in the world. Approximately three billion people have received it. It was originally designed to protect against tuberculosis. For this purpose, it has received mixed reviews.

Now BCG is being considered as a vaccine vector candidate. Recombinant BCG (rBCG) has served as a carrier for the infectious agents of Lyme borreliosis, tetanus, *Streptococcus pneumoniae* bacteremia, *H. influenzae* disease, and Leishmaniasis *(41)*. Its advantages are that it can be given at any age after birth, it is unaffected by maternal antibody, it can sensitize to tuberculoproteins for 5–50 years, it is a potent adjuvant, it is low cost, it can be given orally, and it is known for inducing long-lasting cellular immunity.

Vaccine Combinations No Longer Used

Although smallpox vaccine is no longer being given with other vaccines, the members of the orthopox genus, such as vaccinia virus and various avipox viruses, are being studied as vaccine vectors. Further attenuation of the vaccinia virus vaccine is necessary to avoid the rare but serious complications associated with the vaccinia virus vaccines used for smallpox eradication. These newer recombinant vaccines have been used as carriers for HB virus, Epstein-Barr virus, *Plasmodium falciparum*, influenza, and herpes simplex virus.

New Multivalent Vaccines Being Tested

Group B Streptococcus (GBS) Vaccine

GBS is a common cause of morbidity and mortality in the gestational period. While six GBS capsular polysaccharides have been identified, Types Ia, Ib, II, and III account for most newborn cases. Protein conjugate technology has been applied here too. A more difficult question is who should be immunized to reduce the incidence of disease. Should pregnant women be immunized in the last trimester? Should women of child-bearing age be immunized? Should infants and children be immunized? These questions will be debated until vaccine trials are conducted and may not be resolved even then *(42)*.

Staphylococcus aureus *Vaccine*

Infections with *S. aureus* are common and can be serious, particularly in immunocompromised hosts. Two of the eleven known capsular polysaccharides are responsible for about 80% of bacteremic cases. A capsular polysaccharide-protein conjugate vaccine is being pursued.

Human Immunodeficiency Virus (HIV) Vaccine

Immunizing the host against the surface proteins of HIV is unlikely to result in an effective vaccine because like hepatitis C and Herpes simplex virus, antibody to the surface proteins does not neutralize the virus. In addition, there are innumerable antigenic strains of HIV, so the standard methods of inducing humoral immunity against the surface proteins of the virus will not work with HIV *(43)*. The yeast retrotransposon Ty protein self-assembles virus-like particles for the core protein p24 of HIV which can induce antibody and T-cell proliferative responses *(44)*. These more broadly reactive responses may result in a more effective vaccine to combat HIV. But any HIV vaccine would probably require a combination vaccine containing at least several serotypes of the surface proteins in addition to other critical proteins.

Diarrheagenic Escherichia coli Vaccines

Several candidate vaccines are being investigated for protection against the various types of *E. coli* that cause enteric infections, primarily strains of enterotoxigenic *E. coli* (ETEC) and enteropathogenic *E. coli* (EPEC) *(45)*. An oral vaccine is undergoing study that contains inactivated ETEC strains with different fimbrial colonizing factor antigens attached to the B subunit of cholera toxin. EPEC strains are being studied that contain a plasmid which encodes for bundle-forming pili, an adherence factor, and regulation of the expression of intimin, a protein required for intimate attachment to enterocytes. EPEC vaccines are being investigated that are attenuated EPEC strains, wherein these proteins are altered to a nonvirulent, but immunogenic state or are attached to nonvirulent *S. typhi* or *E. coli* vectors.

Summary

In summary, combination vaccines for adolescents and adults hold the promise of a reduced number of injections to deliver protection against a multitude of diseases. Before this promise can be realized, the problem of vaccine interference has to be adequately tested. Serological surrogates or correlates of protection have to be established as the incidence of many of these vaccine preventable diseases have already been reduced significantly, making efficacy trials difficult to conduct. Licensure of vaccines is possible using serological surrogates and has, in fact, already occurred. Finally, the issue of adverse reactions with multiple antigens in the combination has to be determined in randomized, double-blind, placebo controlled trials *(46)*.

References

1. American College of Physicians Task Force on Adult Immunization and Infectious Diseases Society of America. (1994) *Guide for Adult Immunization,* 3rd ed., American College of Physicians, Philadelphia, PA, 218 pp.
2. Centers for Disease Control and Prevention (1997) Pneumococcal and influenza vaccination levels among adults aged >65 years—United States, 1995. *MMWR* **46,** 913–919.
3. Healthy People 2000: National Health Promotion and Disease Prevention Objectives. U.S. Department of Health and Human Services, Public Health Service, Jones & Bartlett Publishers, Boston, MA, p. 521.
4. Centers for Disease Control and Prevention (1991) Update on adult immunization. Recommendations of the Immunization Practices Advisory Committee (ACIP). *MMWR* **40,** 1–94.
5. Centers for Disease Control and Prevention (1996) Immunization of Adolescents. Recommendations of the Advisory Committee on Immunization Practices (ACIP), the American Academy of Pediatrics (AAP), the American Academy of Family Physicians (AAFP) and the American Medical Association (AMA). *MMWR* **45(No RR-13),** and *JAMA* (1997) **227,** 202–207.
6. Ellis, R. W. and Douglas, R. G. (1994) New vaccine technologies. *JAMA* **271,** 929–931.
7. Ellis, R. W. and Brown, K. R. (1997) Combination vaccines. *Adv. Pharmacol.* **39,** 393–423.
8. Williams, J. C., Goldenthal, K. L., Burns, D. L., and Lewis, B. P., eds. (1995) *Combined Vaccines and Simultaneous Administration: Current Issues and Perspectives.* Annals of New York Academy of Sciences, New York, NY, 404 pp.
9. Williams, J. C., Goldenthal, K. L., Burns, D. L., and Lewis, B. P. (1995) Overview—combination vaccines and simultaneous administration: past, present and future, in *Combined Vaccines and Simultaneous Administration: Current Issues and Perspectives* (Williams, J. C., Goldenthal, K. L., Burns, D. L., and Lewis, B. P., eds.), Annals of New York Academy of Sciences, New York, pp. xi–xv.
10. Parkman, P. D. (1995) Combined and simultaneously administered vaccines: a brief history, in *Combined Vaccines and Simultaneous Administration: Current Issues and Perspectives* (Williams, J. C., Goldenthal, K. L., Burns, D. L., and Lewis, B. P., eds.) Annals of New York Academy of Sciences, New York, pp. 1–9.
11. McClintock, D. K. (1995) Combination vaccines: regulatory issues, in *Combined Vaccines and Simultaneous Administration: Current Issues and Perspectives* (Williams, J. C., Goldenthal, K. L., Burns, D. L., and Lewis, B. P., eds.) Annals of New York Academy of Sciences, New York, pp. 27–34.
12. Clemens, J., Brenner, R., and Rao, M. (1995) Interactions between PRP-T vaccine against *Haemophilus influenzae* Type b and conventional infant vaccines: lessons for future studies of simultaneous immunization and combined vaccines, in *Combined Vaccines and Simultaneous Administration: Current Issues and Perspectives* (Williams, J. C., Goldenthal, K. L., Burns, D. L., and Lewis, B. P., eds.) Annals of New York Academy of Sciences, New York, pp. 255–266.
13. Insel, R. A. (1995) Potential alterations in immunogenicity by combining or simultaneously administering vaccine components, in *Combined Vaccines and Simultaneous Administration: Current Issues and Perspectives* (Williams, J. C., Goldenthal, K. L., Burns, D. L., and Lewis, B. P., eds.) Annals of New York Academy of Sciences, New York, pp. 35–47.
14. Robbins, J. R. and Schneerson, R. (1990) Polysaccharide-protein conjugates: a new generation of vaccines. *J. Infect. Dis.* **161,** 821–832.
15. Golding, B. and Scott, D. E. (1995) Vaccine strategies: targeting helper T Cell responses, in *Combined Vaccines and Simultaneous Administration: Current Issues and Perspectives* (Williams, J. C., Goldenthal, K. L., Burns, D. L., and Lewis, B. P., eds.) Annals of New York Academy of Sciences, New York, pp. 126–137.

16. Vogel, F. R. (1995) Immunologic adjuvants for modern vaccine formulations, in *Combined Vaccines and Simultaneous Administration: Current Issues and Perspectives* (Williams, J. C., Goldenthal, K. L., Burns, D. L., and Lewis, B. P., eds.) Annals of New York Academy of Sciences, New York, pp. 153–160.

17. Milich, D. R., Peterson, D. L., Zheng, J., Hughes, J. L., Wirtz, R., and Schodel, F. (1995) The hepatitis nucleocapsid as a vaccine carrier moiety, in *Combined Vaccines and Simultaneous Administration: Current Issues and Perspectives* (Williams, J. C., Goldenthal, K. L., Burns, D. L., and Lewis, B. P., eds.) Annals of New York Academy of Sciences, New York, pp. 187–201.

18. Pisetsky, D. S. (1998) Antibody responses to DNA in normal immunity and aberrant immunity. *Clin. Diagn. Lab. Immunol.* **5,** 1–6.

19. Henning, K. J., White, M. H., Sepkowitz, K. A., and Armstrong, D. (1997) A national survey of immunization practices following allogeneic bone marrow transplantation. *JAMA* **277,** 1148–1151.

20. Centers for Disease Control and Prevention (1997) Immunization of health-care workers: recommendations of the Advisory Committee on Immunization Practices (ACIP) and the Hospital Infection Control Practices Advisory Committee (HICPAC). *MMWR* **46(No. RR-18),** 1–44.

21. Elliott, A. Y. (1995) Manufacturing issues for multivalent vaccines, in *Combined Vaccines and Simultaneous Administration: Current Issues and Perspectives* (Williams, J. C., Goldenthal, K. L., Burns, D. L., and Lewis, B. P., eds.) Annals of New York Academy of Sciences, New York, pp. 23–26.

22. Buynak, E., Weibel, R. E., Whitman, J. E., Stokes, J., and Hilleman, M. R. (1969) Combined live measles, mumps and rubella virus vaccines. *JAMA* **207,** 2259–2262.

23. Hilleman, M. R., Buynak, E. B., Weibel, R. E., and Villarejos, V. M. (1973) Immune responses and duration of immunity following combined live virus vaccines. International Symposium on Vaccination against Communicable Diseases, Monaco 1973. *Symp. Ser. Immunobiol. Stand.* **22,** 145–158.

24. Minekawa, Y., Ueda, S., Yamanishi, K., Ogino, T., Takahashi, M., and Okuno, Y. (1974) Studies on live rubella vaccine. V. Quantitative aspects of interference between rubella, measles and mumps viruses in their trivalent vaccine. *Biken J.* **17,** 161–167.

25. Davis, R. L., Marcuse, E., Black, S., et al. (1997) MMR2 immunization at 4 to 5 years and 10 to 12 years of age: a comparison of adverse clinical events after immunization in the Vaccine Safety Datalink Project. *Pediatrics* **100,** 767–771.

26. Brown, K. R. (1995) Industry perspective on clinical trial issues for combination vaccines, in *Combined Vaccines and Simultaneous Administration: Current Issues and Perspectives* (Williams, J. C., Goldenthal, K. L., Burns, D. L., and Lewis, B. P., eds.) Annals of New York Academy of Sciences, New York, pp. 241–249.

27. Johnson, C. E., Stancin, T., Fattlar, D., et al. (1997) A long-term prospective study of varicella vaccine in healthy children. *Pediatrics* **100,** 761–766.

28. Fletcher, T. J., Tunnicliffe, W. S., Hammond, K., Roberts, K., and Ayres, J. G. (1997) Simultaneous immunisation with influenza vaccine and pneumococcal polysaccharide vaccine in patients with chronic respiratory disease. *Br. Med. J.* **314,** 1663–1665.

29. Clements, M. L. (1995) Combination live respiratory virus vaccines, in *Combined Vaccines and Simultaneous Administration: Current Issues and Perspectives* (Williams, J. C., Goldenthal, K. L., Burns, D. L., and Lewis, B. P., eds.) Annals of New York Academy of Sciences, New York, pp. 351–355.

30. Ogra, P. L. (1995) Comparative evaluation of immunization with live attenuated and inactivated poliovirus vaccines, in *Combined Vaccines and Simultaneous Administration: Current Issues and Perspectives* (Williams, J. C., Goldenthal, K. L., Burns, D. L., and Lewis, B. P., eds.) Annals of New York Academy of Sciences, New York, pp. 97–107.

31. Katz, S. L. (1995) Combination live enteric virus vaccines, in *Combined Vaccines and Simultaneous Administration: Current Issues and Perspectives* (Williams, J. C., Goldenthal, K. L., Burns, D. L., and Lewis, B. P., eds.) Annals of New York Academy of Sciences, New York, pp. 347–355.
32. Sabin, A. B. (1959) Recent studies and field tests with a live attenuated poliovirus vaccine, in *Live Poliovirus Vaccines: Papers Presented and Discussions Held at the First International Conference on Live Poliovirus Vaccines.* Pan American Sanitary Bureau (Special Publication No. 44). Washington, DC.
33. Sutter, R. W., Pallansch, M. A., Sawyer, L. A., Cochi, S. L., and Hadler, S. C. (1995) Defining surrogate serologic tests with respect to predicting protective vaccine efficacy: poliovirus vaccination, in *Combined Vaccines and Simultaneous Administration: Current Issues and Perspectives* (Williams, J. C., Goldenthal, K. L., Burns, D. L., and Lewis, B. P., eds.) Annals of New York Academy of Sciences, New York, pp. 289–299.
34. Bulkow, L. R., McMahon, B. J., Wainright, R. B., et al. (1993) Safety and immunogenicity of a combined hepatitis B virus—*Haemophilus influenzae* type B vaccine formulation in healthy adults. *Arctic Med. Res.* **52,** 118–126.
35. Pichichero, M. E., Deloria, M. A., Rennels, M. B., et al. (1997) A safety and immunogenicity comparison of 12 acellular pertussis vaccines and one whole-cell pertussis vaccine given as a fourth dose in 15- to 20-month-old children. *Pediatrics* **100,** 772–788.
36. Felsenfeld, O., Wolff, R. H., Gyr, K., Grant, S., and Dutta, K. (1973) Simultaneous vaccination against cholera and yellow fever. *Lancet* **1,** 457,458.
37. Gateff, P. C., LeGonidec, G., Boche, R., Sarrat, P., Lemarinier, G., Monchicourt, D., and Labusquiere, R. (1973) Influence de la vaccination anticholérique sur l'immunisation antiamarile associée. *Bull. Soc. Pathol. Exot.* **66,** 258–266.
38. Centers for Disease Control and Prevention (1996) *Health Information for International Travel 1996–97.* U.S. Public Health Service, Atlanta, GA, 210 pp.
39. Khoo, S. H., St. Clair Roberts, J., and Mandal, B. K. (1995) Safety and efficacy of combined meningococcal and typhoid vaccine. *Br. Med. J.* **310,** 908,909.
40. Rigau-Perez, J. G. (1995) Dengue in travelers-prevention, diagnosis and treatment, in *Abstracts of the Fourth International Conference on Travel Medicine* 1995. The International Society of Travel Medicine, abstr. 268, p. 158.
41. Hanson, M. S., Vigil Lapcevich, C., and Haun, S. L. (1995) Progress on development of the live BCG recombinant vaccine vehicle for combined vaccine delivery, in *Combined Vaccines and Simultaneous Administration: Current Issues and Perspectives* (Williams, J. C., Goldenthal, K. L., Burns, D. L., and Lewis, B. P., eds.) Annals of New York Academy of Sciences, New York, pp. 214–221.
42. Robbins, J. B., Schneerson, R., Vann, W. F., Bryla, D. A., and Fattom, A. (1995) Prevention of systemic infections caused by group B streptococcus and *Staphylococcus aureus* by multivalent polysaccharide-protein conjugate vaccines, in *Combined Vaccines and Simultaneous Administration: Current Issues and Perspectives* (Williams, J. C., Goldenthal, K. L., Burns, D. L., and Lewis, B. P., eds.) Annals of New York Academy of Sciences, New York, pp. 68–82.
43. Berzofsky, J. A. (1995) Designing peptide vaccines to broaden recognition and enhance potency, in *Combined Vaccines and Simultaneous Administration: Current Issues and Perspectives* (Williams, J. C., Goldenthal, K. L., Burns, D. L., and Lewis, B. P., eds.) Annals of New York Academy of Sciences, New York, pp. 161–168.
44. Kingsman, A. J., Burns, N. R., Layton, G. T., and Adams, S. E. (1995) Yeast retrotransposon particles as antigen delivery systems, in *Combined Vaccines and Simultaneous Administration: Current Issues and Perspectives* (Williams, J. C., Goldenthal, K. L., Burns, D. L., and Lewis, B. P., eds.) Annals of New York Academy of Sciences, New York, pp. 202–213.

45. Levine, M. M. and Noriega, F. (1993) Vaccines to prevent bacterial enteric infections in children. *Ped. Annals.* **22,** 719–725.
46. Decker, M. D. and Edwards, K. M. (1995) Issues in design of clinical trials of combination vaccines, in *Combined Vaccines and Simultaneous Administration: Current Issues and Perspectives* (Williams, J. C., Goldenthal, K. L., Burns, D. L., and Lewis, B. P., eds.) Annals of New York Academy of Sciences, New York, pp. 234–240.

3

Pharmaceutical Aspects of Combination Vaccines

Dennis M. Katkocin and Chia-Lung Hsieh

Rationale and Benefits for Combining Vaccines

In 1990, the Children's Vaccine Initiative (CVI) issued a challenge to vaccine developers and manufacturers *(1)*. The challenge was to combine all childhood vaccines into a single dose, preferably oral, and to formulate the *multidisease* combination to be stable at ambient temperature. Heroic efforts will be required to accomplish this objective, but this is a task well worth pursuing.

From a health delivery viewpoint, the reason for desiring a complex, multidisease vaccine is simple: this is the best way to ensure that the maximum number of children will be vaccinated with the maximum number of antigens at any one medical visit. Underimmunization, even in well-developed countries, remains a problem and is a logical explanation for the sporadic outbreak of disease where effective vaccines exist and are affordable. Complicated immunization schedules that require multiple visits are a major reason for less than desirable compliance rates. By combining different antigens and administering them in a simplified well-baby visit schedule, the vaccination rate in developed as well as developing countries will improve substantially.

Unprecedented advances in technology and in vaccine development also have contributed to the realization that vaccines should be combined. The coupling of new technology and a greater understanding of the microbial factors required for virulence and the immune response to infection have resulted in a multitude of new approaches and clinical leads *(2)*. The sheer number of licensed and soon-to-be licensed stand-alone vaccines, estimated at 27 by the end of 1997, can be effectively delivered only if the individual antigens are combined. *Table 1* shows the current recommendation of Advisory Committee on Immunization Practices (ACIP) for United States children *(3)*. With current licensed vaccines, a child will receive three or four shots at the 2-month visit, depending on how polio vaccine is administered. Within the next few years, additional childhood

From: *Combination Vaccines: Development, Clinical Research, and Approval*
Edited by: R. W. Ellis © Humana Press Inc., Totowa, NJ

Table 1. A Generalized Immunization Schedule in US[a]

Vaccines	Birth	2 mo	4 mo	6 mo	12–18 mo	4–6 yr
Hepatitis B	•	•	•			
Diphtheria-tetanus pertussis (DTP or DTaP)		•	•	•	•	•
Haemophilus influenzae type *b*		•	•	•	•	
Polio		•	•		•	•
Measles-mumps-rubella					•	•
Varicella					•	•

[a]Source: Ref. *3*.

vaccines such as pneumococcal and meningococcal conjugates will be licensed. A very effective way to implement the immunization program is through the development of combination vaccines.

Other reasons for combining vaccines are humanitarian in nature and relate to the desire to minimize discomfort for the vaccinee—particularly in the case of infants. Equally important, and often overlooked, is the anguish endured by the parent or guardian of the child during the vaccination process. The discomfort felt by the child is disproportionate to the response following immunization; however, this unpleasant memory may persist with the adult and actually result in the delay or missing altogether of the remaining scheduled immunizations. Combining vaccines will be more convenient for both the guardian and the health care provider alike. The latter will enjoy additional benefits resulting from a distribution and record-keeping viewpoint.

Types of Combination Vaccines

Bacterial

Individual vaccines designed to protect against bacterial pathogens are numerous. A list of these vaccines and the corresponding pathogen are detailed on *Table 2*. A number of these vaccines already are delivered as combination vaccines. For example, the first multidisease combination vaccine provided protection against diphtheria, tetanus, and pertussis (DTP). This vaccine was first licensed in 1949. However, the highest number of antigens combined to date in a single vaccine to protect against any bacterial disease remains the 23-valent pneumococcal polysaccharide vaccine.

Protection against a number of bacterial pathogens is now available through immunization. Those pathogens whose proliferation in the human is not under control by vaccination are at least partially susceptible to various therapeutic

Table 2. Licensed Vaccines to Protect Against Bacterial Disease

Agent or vaccine	Genus of bacterium	No. of serotypes in multivalent combinations
Anthrax	Bacillus anthracis	1
Bacille Calmette-Guerin	Mycobacterium bovis	1
Cholera	Vibrio cholera	1
Diphtheria toxoid	Corynebacterium diphtheriae	1
Pertussis	Bordetella pertussis	$\geq 1^a$
Hib	Haemophilus influenzae type b	1
Lyme	Borrelia burgdorferi	1
Meningococcal polysaccharide	Neisseria meningitidis	4
Plague	Pasteurella pestis	1
Pneumococcal polysaccharide	Streptococcal pneumoniae	23
Tetanus toxoid	Clostridium tetani	1
Typhoid	Salmonella typhi	1

[a]May contain more than one isolate of B. pertussis.

strategies including antibiotic treatment. Included in this category are microorganisms associated with venereal disease, e.g., *Neisseria gonorrhea* and the spirochete *Treponema palladium*. Bacteria associated with inner-ear infections, such as nontypable *Haemophilus influenzae* and *Moraxella catarrhalis*, can be controlled with appropriate antibiotics. However, reinfection is likely to occur once antibiotic therapy is discontinued as a result of the anatomical structure of the infant's ear and to the emergence of antibiotic-resistant strains of streptococci and other bacterial pathogens.

Viral

Significant progress has been made in controlling viral disease by the development of vaccines. Most notable of these prophylactic approaches are vaccines to control smallpox, polio, measles, mumps, rubella, hepatitis A and B, tick-borne encephalitis, and most recently varicella (*see Table 3* for a more complete listing of vaccines by virus type). Individually, a number of these vaccines also are multivalent combination vaccines because they are formulated with multiple serotypes. Vaccines against different viruses also have been combined. For example, measles–mumps–rubella vaccine (MMR) is a multidisease combination vaccine first licensed in 1970. MMR vaccine recently was combined with varicella; this new combination is in Phase III clinical trials *(20)*. In February, 1998, the ACIP recommended to the Food and Drug Administration (FDA) that

Table 3. Licensed Vaccines to Protect Against Viral Disease

Agent or vaccine	Family/genus of virus	No. of serotypes in multivalent combinations
Adenovirus	Adenoviridae/Mastadenovirus	2–3
Hepatitis A	Picornaviridae/Hepatovirus	1
Hepatitis B	Hepadnaviridae/Orthohepadnavirus	1
Influenza	Orthomyxoviridae/Influenza virus A, B	3
Japanese encephalitis	Flaviviridae/Flavivirus	1
Measles	Paramyxoviridae/Morbillivirus	1
Mumps	Paramyxoviridae/Rubulavirus	1
Polio	Picornaviridae/Enterovirus	3
Rabies	Rhabdoviridae/Lyssavirus	1
Rotavirus	Reoviridae/Rotavirus	4
Rubella	Togaviridae/Rubivirus	1
Vaccinia[a]	Poxviridae/Orthopoxvirus	1
Varicella-zoster	Herpesviridae/Varicellovirus	1
Yellow fever	Flaviviridae/Flavivirus	1

[a]Due to the eradication of smallpox, this vaccine is no longer commercially available.

a new tetravalent rotavirus vaccine be adopted for routine use in the infant population.

The control of other viral diseases has proven to be more of a challenge. Included in this category are human immunodeficiency virus (HIV), respiratory syncytial virus, parainfluenza virus, cytomegalovirus, and herpes simplex virus.

Bacterial and Viral Combinations

Bacterial and viral antigens were first admixed during development of a diphtheria (D)-tetanus (T)-whole-cell pertussis (wP)-inactivated polio (IPV) combination vaccine (DTP-IPV). The driving force for this combination was a desire to formulate the IPV, which was developed as an injectable, with the liquid DTwP. Mixing of the antigens had the benefit of reducing the number of injections during the primary series. This strategy was proven to be effective and is being expanded to include vaccines designed to protect against hepatitis B (HB). It is likely that a licensed product protecting against the bacterial pathogens responsible for diphtheria, tetanus, pertussis, and *Haemophilus influenzae* type *b* (Hib) diseases will be formulated successfully with vaccines to protect against polio and HB. Just how far the formulation of complex combination vaccines can proceed, and the obstacles that must be overcome to succeed, will be explored in detail in the remaining sections of this review.

Table 4. Combination Vaccines Licensed and Under Development

Vaccine	Status	Reference
DTaP-Hib	Approved in United States (toddler)	4–7
	Approved in Germany (infants)	
DTaP-HB	Approved in EU countries	8–11
DTaP-IPV	Approved in Canada, Denmark and France	12–13
DTaP-IPV-Hib	Approved in Canada and France (toddler)	14–15
DTaP-HB-Hib	Clinical	16
DTaP-IPV-Hib-HB	Clinical	17
Hib-HB	Approved in United States (infants)	18
HA-HB	Approved in UK (infants)	19
MMR-V[a]	Clinical	20
DTP-IPV-rabies	Clinical	21

[a]MMR itself is licensed in essentially all developed countries.

Table 4 shows a brief summary of new combination vaccines that are recently licensed or are under development at the present time. In the United States, individual combinations of DTwP and Hib conjugate, and HB and Hib vaccines, were approved for the primary series. Additional combination vaccines based on the acellular pertussis component (aP), DTaP+Hib and DTaP+Hib+IPV, were approved in a few countries, but in certain cases only for a booster indication. Global approval for all these combination vaccines is not anticipated in the immediate future.

A major difficulty in combination vaccine development is the reduction of immunogenicity in infants for a number of antigens, most noticeably against Hib. The most recent example of this latter phenomenon was observed following the reconstitution of TriPedia (DTaP) vaccine with ActHIB (Hib) vaccine *(22)*. Because of the absence of a suitable animal model for Hib and other antigens, it was not possible to predict a reduced response in infants prior to the clinical trials.

General Concerns and Issues

Regulatory Issues

The development of new combination vaccines also presents a new challenge for regulatory agencies. In 1993, the Center for Biologic Evaluation and Research (CBER) sponsored a symposium *(23)* to explore issues related to combination vaccines. This was followed by the release of guidelines in 1997 *(24)*. A similar workshop was held earlier during the 2nd European Conference on Vaccinology in 1994 and was sponsored by European Vaccine Manufacturers *(25)*. This meeting also resulted in a draft guideline *(26)* produced by the Biotechnology

Working Party of the European Agency for the Evaluation of Medicinal Products. This guideline may be adopted for use in the near future.

Both guidelines provide the basic framework for vaccine manufacturers to follow in developing combination vaccines. However, the evaluation of a combination vaccine is a rather complex issue, and the guideline will not cover every aspect of every problem encountered by the vaccine developer. For example, the guideline does not address the issue of combining a new vaccine with a licensed vaccine. The definition of consistency batches is also a complicated issue, especially if it involves multiple antigens from different suppliers. Finally, the issue of release testing for a combined vaccine also needs to be considered almost on a case-by-case basis. Consequently, a vaccine manufacturer must work very closely with regulatory agencies in order to meet their requirements and thus expedite licensure of new combination vaccines.

The documentation associated with the filing of a new combination vaccine will be substantial and certainly will be no less than the sum of the individual vaccines. Each component must be addressed as a separate entity in terms of how the product is manufactured, tested, released and stored. If the individual components are also to be marketed as stand-alone vaccines, the intended indication must be defined. Once all these requirement are fulfilled, the new combination vaccine then can be addressed as a new entity with its own manufacturing criteria, stability profile, and target population.

Safety Concerns

Safety is the single most important issue in the design and formulation of combination vaccines. The safety profile of a new combination vaccine will be held to very rigid standards (24), and reactogenicity will be closely scrutinized. The reactogenicity profile of the new combination vaccine will be compared directly with the profile following separate administration of the individual components. Large numbers of vaccinees will be required from the target population to demonstrate safety. It is possible that responses such as tenderness at the injection site, redness, increased irritability, etc., may be accentuated by the simple act of mixing individual antigen components and/or different adjuvants. However, some regulatory agencies may have the opinion that any increased reactogenicity of a new combination vaccine is unacceptable, despite the benefits and advantages of combining individual antigens.

Potential causes of increased reactogenicity of a combined vaccine were outlined in a previous publication (27). The increase in endotoxin load as a result of combining different vaccines is a relatively minor problem since endotoxin can be accurately measured. For any new vaccine, it is highly desirable to reduce the endotoxin level in each of the components to the minimum level prior to formulation. This is a particular concern for new combination vaccines because the endotoxin level in the formulated bulk will represent the sum of the individual components.

Overloading with toxoid is another possible source of reactogenicity. This problem may be encountered when a toxoid is used as a carrier protein for a conjugate vaccine. Since all toxoids may contain trace levels of residual toxin, the total level of toxoid in the multiple conjugate vaccine added to the toxoid from the original formulated vaccine may generate an undesirable immunological reaction.

The effect of adjuvant requires special attention, especially if a nonadjuvanted antigen is added to an adjuvanted vaccine. The adjuvant may affect the immunological profile of the nonadjuvanted antigen. Also, as in the case of an aluminum adjuvant, the new antigen may affect the adsorption of other antigens, which also can result in a change in the immunogenic response and, in some cases, the reactogenicity. Similarly, a new antigen may replace an adsorbed toxic factor on the aluminum gel during the formulation process, resulting in a heightened adverse response.

Preclinical toxicology studies should be implemented to assess the safety of new combination vaccines. For a licensed component, safety data already exists and the requirements for further toxicity studies will be relatively minor. For a new vaccine component, detailed testing will be required in order to meet the requirements of regulatory agencies. With the implementation of the International Conference on Harmonization Guidelines (ICH) *(28)*, toxicity studies for new combination vaccines will be more extensive as part of the preclinical characterization program

Variable Immunization Schedules

All major vaccine manufacturers have as a goal to develop new vaccines for the global market. From a formulation viewpoint, it is highly desirable to a develop a single formulation. However, this may not always be possible based on regional requirements for release testing. Regional differences also exist in immunization schedules. For example, in the United States, the primary immunization series is given at two, four, and six months of age. In the UK, two, three, and four months of age represent the norm. The situation is different in Germany where three, four, and five months of age represent standard practice *(29)*. Local practice will dictate that to obtain licensure, the combination vaccine must be tested using local conditions. With new combination vaccines, subtle variation in antibody titer based on regional immunization schedules is not unexpected. However, this problem may be accentuated by the increased number of antigens and may lead to difficulties in the interpretation of data. One possible outcome may be difficulty in licensing new combination vaccines with a singular formulation.

Table 5. A Proposal for Harmonization
of Immunization Schedule for European Children[a]

	Birth	2 mo	4 mo	6 mo	15–18 mo	5–6 yr
DTP	•	•	•		•	•
Hib	•	•	•	•	•	
OPV/IPV	•	•	•	•	•	•
HB	•	•	•	•	•	•
MMR					•	•

[a]Source: Ref. 30.

Within the EU countries, efforts to harmonize vaccination schedules are being pursued (30). A proposed immunization schedule is shown in Table 5. This harmonization effort will reduce confusion associated with vaccine schedules. However, children will continue to receive multiple shots. An appropriate way to add new vaccines to this schedule is to combine different antigens. According to the World Health Organization (WHO), the Expanded Program on Immunization (EPI) requires fewer injections (31) than other programs where Hib and Meningococcal vaccines are routinely administered. A new multidisease combination vaccine is thus less urgent an issue until a decision is made to include these vaccines in the immunization program.

The Number of Different Formulations and Combinations

In the past, most vaccines were generic. For example, D and T toxoids were semipurified proteins which were detoxified, usually with formaldehyde. Likewise, P vaccine was a whole-cell product which was inactivated by heat or by chemical treatment. All three antigens were adsorbed to an aluminum salt, either the phosphate or the hydroxide species. In general, these products were similar and shared a number of common traits. New vaccine development now is accomplished with an impressive array of technological tools resulting in greater diversity of the final product. A prime example is the Hib conjugate vaccine. Manufacturers have elected to activate the haptene (in this case Poly-Ribosylribitol Phosphate [PRP]) differently, to use different conjugation chemistries, and to use different carrier proteins to make their glycoconjugate vaccines. Clinical results suggest qualitative and quantitative differences in the immune response in infants following the use of different Hib conjugate vaccines (32). Consequently, interchangeability should be a consideration when combining similar vaccines from different manufacturers. In addition to differences in immunogenicity, vaccines from different manufacturers may exhibit different reactogenicity profiles and chemical properties.

In certain cases, it is desirable to concurrently administer live viral vaccines with the standard childhood vaccines such as DTP *(33)*. This is done to maximize immunization coverage but presents difficulty in evaluating overall effectiveness of the different vaccines. For example, the onset of fever may be a result of incomplete attenuation of the live vaccine component or to the P component. A rise in body temperature, for whatever reason, may be restrictive for replication of a temperature-sensitive virus, and thus makes interpretation of the results extremely difficult.

The Number of Vaccine Manufacturers

There are four major global vaccine manufacturers: Wyeth-Lederle, SmithKline-Beecham, Pasteur-Mérieux-Connaught, and Merck. A number of other companies produce vaccines for the global market but offer a limited product line, e.g., North American Vaccine, Chiron, Swiss Serum & Vaccine Institute, and Medeva-Evans, to name a few. In addition, many countries produce vaccine exclusively for domestic or regional use. Most of the vaccines produced by this latter group protect against diseases that have been under control for some time; the prime example of a combination vaccine in this category is the DTP vaccine. Combining the new generation of high-technology vaccines, such as Hib conjugate and HB vaccines, with the many different DTPs available will require considerable amount of effort in formulation development and clinical studies. Based on experience, it is anticipated that a variable degree of success will be realized but some combinations will be problematic. This is a result of the subtle differences in the composition of the individual components and is a further reflection of how the vaccines are formulated. Vaccine manufacturers now anticipate that reformulation of the individual components will be required for new combination products.

Combination of Licensed and Unlicensed Vaccines

Demonstrating efficacy of a new antigen is a requirement for licensure. Blinded and randomized clinical trials must be performed. In the case of a replacement vaccine, e.g., one containing a new D toxoid, it is acceptable to generate immunogenicity data to show equivalence. This is possible based on an established antibody correlate for protection; e.g., ≥ 0.01 IU of anti-D antibody per milliliter of serum. For other diseases such as pertussis, a serological correlate in not well established *(34)*. The lack of an accepted antibody correlate for any antigen can be an impediment to further vaccine development, particularly in the case of new combination vaccines.

The addition of an unlicensed antigen to a licensed vaccine most likely will reflect the formulation of the licensed product since the new antigen is likely to be highly purified and concentrated. In some cases, reformulation may be required in order to increase the compatibility of the different antigens. Reformulation also may be needed to improve the stability of the new vaccine, e.g., the new antigen may not be stable at the pH of the licensed vaccine. In other instances, a change in formulation may be the unintentional consequence of mixing different antigens. This will occur when a nonadjuvanted antigen is mixed with an adjuvanted antigen. The new vaccine component may be adsorbed and may replace a previously bound antigen on the adjuvant. This may result in a different reactogenicity profile or an altered immunological response to either the displaced antigen or to those antigens that remain bound.

Cost of Combination Vaccine Development

Developing new combination vaccines is an expensive undertaking. The process begins in the formulation laboratories where effort is expended to identify a milieu that is compatible for all the active components including the adjuvant. Assays need to be developed or modified to quantify each of the components in the complex mixture and to document real-time stability in final containers. Effort is expended to design preclinical studies to identify possible interactions among the different antigens. Additional studies to demonstrate safety and immunogenicity have to be performed. In some instances, these studies require the use of multiple animal models. Once this is established, the vaccine mixture is ready for clinical testing, at which point the response to each component is measured and compared to separate administration and to historical values.

Clinical testing is the most expensive part of vaccine development. The greater the number of components or variables in a new combination vaccine, the greater the "statistical power" of the required study. Efficacy of a new vaccine is one issue; how that vaccine performs in combination with other antigens is a second issue. The latter requires a comparison of the immune response of vaccinees to both the combined product and to separate administration of the individual components. Since many of these vaccines are intended for the pediatric population, extensive interaction studies need to be performed to ensure that the response to other licensed vaccines administered with the same immunization schedule is not significantly altered.

In certain cases, a reduction in manufacturing cost may be realized as a consequence of combining vaccines. This is possible since a substantial portion of a vaccine's cost is associated with release testing and with packaging. Controlling cost is highly desirable from both the manufacturing and the consumer view. This may be especially important for the long-term success WHO's EPI.

Another major cost associated with immunization is the administration cost. Combining vaccines will substantially reduce the cost for delivering multiple antigens, which will further reduce the overall cost of the program. Although

new vaccines produced by breakthroughs in technology undoubtedly will aug-
ment the cost of vaccines, the end result for society will be beneficial since these
developments will lower the burden of disease *(35)*.

However, combining different antigens dose not necessarily result in cost
reduction. For example, currently licensed multidisease vaccines can contain
antigens such as P, IPV, HB, D and T toxoids, or Hib conjugate. A potency test
for each component antigen is performed on the formulated bulk combination
vaccine. As a result of the sheer number of tests involved and the biological
variability of animal tests, a certain number of batches may be rejected. Rejection of the combined vaccine at this late stage in the formulation is costly, a factor
which must be considered in the overall cost of vaccine manufacture.

Compatibility of Vaccine Components

The combination of antigens in a new combination vaccine may result in an
enhancement of the immune response to one or more components *(36)*. However, not all vaccine components will be compatible. This incompatibility may
surface as a stability problem or it may be reflected in a suboptimal immunogenic response. When DTwP and IPV were combined and tested in infants, a
reduction in the immune response to the P antigens was detected *(13)*. For
example, following two doses, the antibody level to a number of antigens were
reduced, including filamentous hemagglutinin and fimbriae; after three
doses, the response to pertussis toxin was also impaired relative to separate administration of the two vaccines. In other studies, a similar reduction
in the response to P was observed when DTwP vaccine was formulated with a
Hib conjugate *(37)*. These results underscore and emphasize the inherent differences between component vaccines made by manufacturers using diverse technologies and formulated into combination vaccines.

Interference also can exist in live attenuated vaccines. When the trivalent oral
polio vaccine was first studied, it was apparent that the three serotypes
were competing with one another *(38)*. Three doses were required for
>90% seroconversion. Since each serotype replicated at different rates in the
host, different levels of each serotype had to be added to the final formulation.

Assay Issues

Assay and characterization of a combination vaccine are the most challenging
aspects of the preclinical study. Typical methods for assaying a combination
vaccine are physical—chemical analysis, immunochemical analysis, and
immunological assays with suitable animal models. Assays developed to quantify purified components may need to be modified to quantify that same component in a complex mixture. This can be a result of chemical interference and/or
inability to separate the active component from other components including the

adjuvant. Interference can be observed with HPLC assays where two different components may coelute as a single or overlapping peak. However, this problem often can be solved by selection of an alternative solvent system or by modifying column height. Both approaches, either singularly or in combination, may result in an improved and acceptable baseline resolution. Assays based on gas chromatography where derivitization procedures are often unsatisfactory as a result of trace levels of contaminating components or to the presence of excipients in one of the components are more problematic. For example, excipients such as lactose and sucrose, when added as a stabilizer to vaccines during lyophilization, interfere in the quantification of the specific carbohydrate. Obstacles such as this can be overcome; however, they require heroic efforts in assay modification and subsequent validation. This latter issue is particularly important. The more processing steps required to prepare an antigen for assay, the greater the risk of under-recovery and the more difficult the validation program.

Immunochemical assays such as an enzyme-linked immunosorbent assay (ELISA) and nephelometry *(39)*, can be powerful tools for characterizing combination vaccines. These assays have the advantage of being highly sensitive and specific and allow for the detection of a small quantify of antigen in a mixture of many proteins and carbohydrates.

Immunological studies with one or more animal models should be pursued during combination vaccine development. For the older licensed vaccine components such as DTwP, animal potency tests will continue to be required as release tests. For other vaccines such as HB, animal immunogenicity results correlate with protection, making the assay very useful during formulation development. On the other hand, animal immunogenicity results do not always correlate with clinical results. In these cases, animal immunogenicity results can be considered as a qualitative evaluation of the vaccine. In designing stability assays for new combination vaccines, it also is recognized that individual antigens and/or adjuvant may have an impact on the immunogenicity but not on antigenicity of other antigens *(40)*.

Demonstrating Equivalence

Demonstrating equivalence of a combination vaccine to the separately administered individual vaccines in a clinical trial requires a careful statistical design. Ideally, the design of the clinical plan would show rates of reactogenicity, antibody levels, and disease attack *(41)*. Blackwelder also noted that the clinical trial is designed to show that the combined vaccine is similar to the separately administered vaccines, not necessarily identical, and that small differences may not be clinically relevant *(41)*. If this premise is not established and accepted by regulatory authorities, it will be very difficult to obtain approval for new combination vaccines because of natural biological variability.

86. Hoffenbach, A., Langue, J., Mallet, E., Roussel, F., David, T., Pines, E., and Salomon, H. (1997) Influence of combining DTaP-IPV and Act-HIB vaccines and of changing the primary vaccination schedule on the antibody response to *Haemophilus influenzae* type b. (Abst. 80) *The 15th Annual Meeting of the European Society for Paediatric Infectious Diseases (ESPID)*, Paris 1997.

87. Mills, E., Russell, M., Cunning, L., Gasparini, R., Meekison, W., Thippawong, J., Fox, M., and Barreto, L. (1996) Comparative immunogenicity of an acellular pertussis-inactivated polio (DTaP-IPV) vaccine used to reconstitute lyophilized *H. influenzae b* (PRP-T) or licensed DTwP-IPV-PRP-T vaccine in infants. (Abst. 703) *Pediatr. Res.* **39**.

88. Mallet, E., Hoffenbach, A., Salomon, H., Blondeau, C., and Fritzell, B. (1996) Primary immunization with combined acellular DTaP-IPV-Act-HIB vaccine given at 2-3-4 or 2-4-6 months of age. (Abst. 19) *The 14th Annual Meeting of the European Society for Paediatric Infectious Diseases (ESPID)*, Elsinore, Denmark 1996.

89. Siler, T., Langue, J., Blondeau, C., and Fritzell, B. (1996) Simultaneous administration of DTaP-IPV-Act-HIB and MMR vaccines at 14 to 16 months (Abst. 22) *ESPID 1996*.

90. Mallet, E., Hoffenbach, A., Pines, E., Salomon, H., and Seine Maritime Paediatricians (1997) Immunogenicity of the fourth dose of a combined DTaP-IPV/Act-HIB vaccine administered at 15 months of age to children primed either at 2, 3, and 4 or at 2, 4, and 6 months of age. (Abst. 81) *The 15th Annual Meeting of the European Society for Paediatric Infectious Diseases (ESPID)*, Paris 1997.

91. Langue, J., Mallet, E., David, T., Roussel, F., Pines, E., Salomon, H., and Hoffenbach, A. (1997) Safety of the fourth dose of a DTaP-IPV vaccine administered in combination with an *Haemophilus influenzae* type b vaccine (Act-HIB) at 12 to 16 months of age. (Abst.) *The 15th Annual Meeting of the European Society for Paediatric Infectious Diseases (ESPID)*, Paris 1997.

92. Kanra, G., Siler, T., Yurdakök, K., Baskan, S., Yavuz, T., Ceyhan, M., Bulut, B., Özmert, E., and Pehlivan, T. (1997) Simultaneous administration of the combined DTaP-IPV/Act-HIB vaccine and a Hepatitis B vaccine at 2-3-4 months. (Abst.) *The 15th Annual Meeting of the European Society for Paediatric Infectious Diseases (ESPID)*, Paris 1997.

93. Carlsson, R. M., Claesson, B., Selstam, U., Fagerlund, E., Granström, M., Blondeau, C., and Hoffenbach, A. (1997) Safety and immunogenicity of a combined DTaP-IPV/PRP-T vaccine, administered either at 3,5 and 12 months or at 2,4,6 and 13 months. (Abst. 78) *The 15th Annual Meeting of the European Society for Paediatric Infectious Diseases (ESPID)*, Paris 1997.

94. Begue, P., Stagnara, J., Vie-le-Sage, F., Bernard, J. C., Xerri, B., and Abitbol, V. (1997) Immunogenicity and reactogenicity of a booster dose of diphtheria, tetanus, acellular pertussis and inactivated poliomyelitis vaccines given concurrently with *Haemophilus* type b conjugate vaccine or as pentavalent vaccine. *Pediatr. Infect. Dis. J.* **16**, 787–794.

95. Dagan, R., Agbaria, K., Piglansky, L., Melamed, R., Willems, P., and Grossi, A. (1996) Immunogenicity of a combined diphtheria, tetanus, acellular pertussis, inactivated poliovirus and *h. influenzae* type b- tetanus conjugate vaccine (DTPa-IPV-Hib) in infants. (Abst. G59) *36th ICAAC 1996*.

96. Dagan, R., Igbaria, K., Piglansky, L., Melamed, R., Willems, P., Grossi, A., and Kaufhold, A. (1997) Safety and immunogenicity of a combined pentavalent diphtheria, tetanus, acellular pertussis, inactivated poliovirus and *Haemophilus influenzae* type b-tetanus conjugate vaccine in infants, compared with a whole cell pertussis pentavalent vaccine. *Pediatr. Infect. Dis. J.* **16**, 1113–1121.

97. Bell, F., Heath, P., Shackley, F., Maclennan, J., Shearstone, N., Diggle, L., Griffiths, H., Moxon, E. R., and Finn, A. (1997) Effect of reconstitution with an acellular pertussis, diphtheria, tetanus vaccine on antibody response to HIB vaccine (PRP-T). (Abst. 69) *The 15th Annual Meeting of the European Society for Paediatric Infectious Diseases (ESPID)*, Paris 1997.

influenzae type *b* polysaccharide-diphtheria toxoid conjugate vaccine in infancy. *N. Engl. J. Med.* **317,** 717–722.

73. Committee for Proprietary Medicinal Products (1997) The European Agency for Evaluation of Medicinal Products, ed. European public assessment report (EPAR): Infanrix HepB. London. p. 1.

74. Usonis, V., Bakasenas, V., Willems, P., and Clemens, R. (1997) Feasibility study of a combined diphtheria-tetanus-acellular pertussis-hepatitis B (DTTa-HBV) vaccine and comparison of clinical reactions and immune responses with diphtheria-tetanus-acellular pertussis (DTPa) and hepatitis B vaccines applied as mixed or injected into separate limbs. *Vaccine* **15,** 1680–1686.

75. Greenberg, D. P., Wong, V. K., Partridge, S., Howe, B. J., and Ward, J. I. (1997) Safety and immunogenicity of a combination DTPa-Hepatitis B vaccine (DTPa-HepB) administered to infants at 2, 4 and 6 months of age. (Abst. 602) *IDSA.*

76. Kanra, G., Ceyhan, M., Ecevit, Z., Bogaerts, H., De Grave, D., Hauser, P., and Desmons, P. (1995) Primary vaccination of infants with a combined diphtheria-tetanus- acellular pertussis-hepatitis B vaccine. *Pediatr. Infect. Dis. J.* **14,** 998–1000.

77. Greenberg, D., Vadheim, C. M., MArcy, M., Partridge, J., Chiu, C. Y., Greene, T., Margolis, H. S., Ward, J. I., and The Kaiser-UCLA Vaccine Study Group (1996) Safety and immunogenicity of a recombinant hepatitis B vaccine administered to infants at 2, 4 and 6 months of age. *Vaccine* **14,** 811–816.

78. Greenberg, D. P., Vadheim, C. M., Wong, V. K., MArcy, M., Partridge, S., Greene, T., Chiu, C. Y., Margolis, H. S., and Ward, J. I. (1996) Comparative safety and immunogenicity of two recombinant hepatitis B vaccines given to infants at two, four and six months of age. *Pediatr. Infect. Dis. J.* **15,** 590–596.

79. Black, S., Shinefield, H., Lewis, N., Ray, P., Ensor, K., and Adelman, T. (1996) Safety and immunogenicity of a combined aPDT-hepatitis B vaccine in infancy. (Abst. G99) *36th ICAAC.*

80. Halperin, S. A., Davies, H. D., Barreto, L., Guasparini, R., Meekison, W., Humphreys, G., and Eastwood, B. J. (1997) Safety and immunogenicity of two inactivated poliovirus vaccines in combination with an acellular pertussis vaccine and diphtheria and tetanus toxoids in seventeen-to nineteen-month-old infants. *J. Pediatr.* **130,** 525–531.

81. Auzerie, J., Danjou, G., Siller, T., and Dupuy, M. (1997) Comparison of DTAP-IPV and D.T. Polio vaccines as a second booster at 8 to 12 years. (Abst.) *The 15th Annual Meeting of the European Society for Paediatric Infectious Diseases (ESPID),* Paris 1997.

82. Danjou, G., Siller, T., and Dupuy, M. (1997) Association Française de Pédiatrie Ambulatoire. Comparison of DTAP-IPV vaccine with DTP-IPV (TETRACOQ) vaccine administered as a second booster at 4 to 7 years of age. (Abst.) *The 15th Annual Meeting of the European Society for Paediatric Infectious Diseases (ESPID),* Paris 1997.

83. Lagos, R., Koloff, A., Hoffenbach, O., San Martin, O., Abarego, P., Ureta, A. M., Pines, E., and Levine, M. (1997) Clinical response to pentavalent parenteral diphtheria, tetanus, acellular pertussis (DTaP), inactivated polio (eIPV) and *Haemophilus influenzae b* (Hib) conjugate vaccine in 2, 4 & 6 month-old Chilean infants. (Abst. 609) *IDSA 1997.*

84. Reinert, P., Boucher, J., Pines, E., Leroux, M. C., Hoffenbach, A., and Salomon, H. (1997) Primary or booster immunization with DTaP-IPV vaccine administered either in combination or in association with a *Haemophilus influenzae* type *b* vaccine (Act-HIB): a large-scale safety study. (Abst.) *The 15th Annual Meeting of the European Society for Paediatric Infectious Diseases (ESPID),* Paris 1997.

85. Langue, J., David, T., Roussel, F., Pines, E., Hoffenbach, A., and Association Française de Pédiatrie Ambulatoire (1997) Safety and immunogenicity of DTaP-IPV and Act-HIB vaccines administered either combined or separately to infants at 2, 3, and 4 months of age. (Abst. 79) *The 15th Annual Meeting of the European Society for Paediatric Infectious Diseases (ESPID),* Paris 1997.

Preclinical Testing of Combination Vaccines

Preclinical data are used to demonstrate safety and immunogenicity and to justify evaluation of the combination vaccine in the target population. An important aspect of preclinical testing is to demonstrate that the individual vaccine components retain their chemical and immunological integrity following formulation into a combination vaccine.

Toxicology

Toxicological studies are required prior to the clinical testing of new biological products. Reformulation of existing licensed vaccines to permit their combination into a new product historically has not required new toxicology testing. However, this situation is subject to change as the regulatory climate in general has become more conservative. As discussed previously, the ICH guidelines suggest that comprehensive toxicological analyses be performed prior to initiation of clinical studies.

Chemical Interactions

An individual vaccine may be quite crude in nature, e.g., wP vaccine. This vaccine contains all the cellular components of the *Bordetella pertussis* organism, spent growth medium not removed during the clarification process, and chemical agents added to inactivate the live cells or to preserve the vaccine. Conversely, modern-day vaccines made with state-of-the-art technology can be highly purified proteins and glycoconjugates. The latter consist of a purified protein component covalently linked to a purified oligosaccharide or polysaccharide. Simply combining these vaccines will invariably result in chemical interaction as chemically different milieu are blended. Some of these interactions may be deleterious to the chemical stability or immunogenicity of one or more components. Results of early efforts to combine DTwP components with crude IPV resulted in a reduced response to the bacterial components *(42)*. Chemical interference was suspected and follow-up studies showed that one or more factors in the lysed kidney cells were responsible for the reduced response. In anticipation of such interactions, formulation studies seek to determine if an antigenic component has retained its stability and immunogenicity in a complex mixture by utilizing highly specific methodology.

ASSAY ISSUES

The formulation of complex antigens into new combination vaccines creates a challenge for the analytical chemist to quantify all of the individual components. The formulation of combination vaccines may alter the secondary and tertiary structure of antigens. In some cases, the functional groups on proteins or carbohydrates may be less stable within a complex milieu. Efforts to evaluate these changes by physicochemical means are not always successful. Methodology to document this type of change may involve both in vitro and in vivo immunological testing.

Preservative Compatibility

The two most common preservatives used in biological products are thimerosal and 2-phenoxyethanol. Thimerosal is added at 0.01% final concentration while 2-phenoxyethanol is added at 0.5%; the latter is usually fortified with 75 ppm formalin in order to satisfy requirements for all preservative effectiveness testing. Some vaccines may contain both preservatives (43) but this is the exception. Many vaccines are unpreserved in a single-dose presentation but are usually preserved when filled into a multidose vial to provide an additional level of protection against multiple re-entry.

Combining vaccines with different preservatives raises the issue of which preservative to choose for the new combination. If an old vaccine is preserved with thimerosal, it is tempting to eliminate thimerosal from the formulation given the preference for nonmercury-containing preservatives, particularly abroad. However, this may be difficult to accomplish if the thimerosal is associated with stabilizing one or more proteins in the vaccine, or if the thimerosal is added during component processing, as is done to inactivate live *B. pertussis* cells. In the former example, long-term studies would be required to demonstrate stability of the protein components following removal of thimerosal. In the latter example, a new method of inactivating the cells would need to be identified and validated. Modification of the wP manufacturing process is not a practical alternative given the recent approval of a number of aP-containing vaccines for use in the infant population. It is anticipated that aP vaccines will gradually replace wP vaccines in most developing countries.

Initial efforts to combine DTwP and IPV surfaced two examples of a detrimental affect of preservative on antigen. Benzethonium chloride was used as a preservative in IPV, and its presence in a combined vaccine compromised the effectiveness of the DTP components (44). The preservative used in the DTwP vaccine, thimerosal, was found to adversely effect the poliovirus (45). Subsequent studies of a combined DTwP and an enhanced IPV (eIPV) combination vaccine (46) showed that the preservative (thimerosal) reduced the antigenicity of at least one of the serotypes in the eIPV vaccine. One method of addressing this issue is to fill both vaccines into separate chambers of a dual-barrel syringe and then to concurrently administer both vaccines with a single injection.

The suitability of 2-phenoxyethanol/formalin preservative must be assessed on a case-by-case basis for a number of reasons. The acidic phenoxy group tends to lower the pH of the vaccine formulation, particularly in nonbuffered systems. The effect of formalin on vaccine components also must be addressed. Formalin (even at 75 ppm) can act as a cross-linking agent, particularly following prolonged storage. Before adopting a new preservative, stability studies are initiated to demonstrate compatibility with all vaccine components.

Biochemical Interaction and/or Modification

The formulation of two different vaccines into a new combined vaccine may have an adverse effect on the stability and/or immunological response of one or more components. An example of this phenomenon was observed during the clinical testing of an aP vaccine with D and T toxoids and Hib conjugate vaccine *(47)*. The immune response in infants to all components, except the Hib conjugate vaccine, was similar in the combined vaccine when compared with separate administration. The response to the Hib component was significantly reduced. It is tempting to speculate that the reduced response was a result of some form of biochemical interaction, but no data exist to support this view.

An unexpected biochemical interaction thwarted early efforts to formulate a stable multivalent meningococcal polysaccharide vaccine. The instability problem was attributed to trace levels of ferrous iron in the mannitol stabilizer *(48)*, that resulted in depolymerization of the polysaccharide, particularly for type A. This problem was overcome by the use of highly purified lactose.

Adjuvant Compatibility

In designing combination vaccines, there may be a desire to combine an adjuvanted vaccine with one which has no adjuvant. Alternatively, different vaccines may be formulated with different adjuvants. The question of antigen compatibility must be addressed, as does the impact of the use of a new adjuvant or an adjuvant mixture on the immune response. In addition, it is established that adjuvants act through a variety of different and well-defined immunological mechanisms *(49)*, and some or all of these mechanisms may be required in order to ensure an optimized immune response for new combination vaccines.

Some vaccines contain a mixture of aluminum hydroxide and aluminum phosphate. To meet the requirement of manufacturing consistency, the ratio of the two aluminum species must be uniform from batch to batch. The amount and ratio of aluminum species is empirically determined as part of formulation development and is designed to maximize the immune response. Formulation of a vaccine of this type with a second vaccine containing phosphate buffer can alter this ratio as hydroxyl ions are exchanged by phosphate ions. This can result in a shift in the equilibrium of the gel, thus altering the phosphate:hydroxyl ratio. The impact of this type of change on immunogenicity and stability of the component antigens must be assessed on a case-by-case basis.

Adjuvant compatibility may become a larger issue as new adjuvants, such monophosphoryl lipid A (MPL) and the saponin QS-21, are licensed for use in humans. Both of these adjuvants stimulate a cell-mediated response in addition to a humoral response and are particularly exciting for weakly antigenic protein vaccine candidates, or where there is a need to modulate the immune response in a direction different from that induced by use of aluminum-type adjuvants. The question will be: Which immune response will predominate when the two different types of adjuvants are used concurrently in a combined vaccine? In addition, particular attention will need to be focused on formulation of the combined vaccine given the pH sensitivity of both MPL and QS-21.

ANTIGEN ADSORPTION

It is generally recognized that the antigen must be bound to the aluminum adjuvant to observe an enhancement in the immune response. Formulation protocols are designed to ensure maximum adsorption, e.g. , antigen is incubated with the aluminum gel, often at temperatures of 30–35°C, to optimize binding. The pH of the formulation also may be altered to enhance binding. Both pH and ionic strength are known to affect antigen binding by altering the net charge on the gel and on the antigen *(50)*. However, alteration of pH is only possible if there is no adverse effect on the stability of the antigen. The species of aluminum adjuvant also affects binding. Basic proteins bind preferentially to aluminum phosphate, which has an isoelectric point <7.4, whereas acidic proteins favor binding to aluminum hydroxide; the isoelectric point of the latter is >11.1 *(51)*.

Combining two vaccines, one with and one normally without adjuvant, raises the issue of the effect on the previously unadjuvanted antigen. The antigen may bind or remain unbound. This is irrelevant as long as immunogenicity or stability are unaffected. However, it is possible that the antigen may exhibit variable levels of binding on a lot-to-lot basis. This situation can raise the issue of consistency of manufacture. Regulatory authorities have taken the posture that antigens must bind to a consistent level and then remain bound through the shelf-life of the product.

pH AND BUFFER COMPATIBILITY

Formulating multiple antigens with nonoverlapping pH stability profiles into a single combination vaccine represents a real challenge, which can be met with one of two approaches. The first approach is to select an intermediate pH with respect to the stability of the two antigens. To be acceptable, sufficient antigen activity must remain to meet potency requirements throughout the stability program. This may require the addition of excess antigen during formulation in order to compensate for antigen that is destabilized during the shelf-life of the product.

The second approach is to select the formulation pH that is compatible with the most labile antigen. Efforts then can be focused on maintaining the stability of the second antigen by utilizing a number of proven procedures including chemical modification.

VISUAL APPEARANCE

It is important for a formulated vaccine to appear homogeneous and to retain normal visual appearance throughout the shelf life of the product. Combining new antigens has the potential to adversely impact the appearance of the formulated product without impacting immunogenicity or stability. Inquiries from the field are often in response to the appearance of the vaccine, e.g., precipitates, stringlike aggregates in clear products, discoloration, or unusual difficulty in resuspending adjuvanted products. It has been suggested that failure to achieve a uniform suspension suitable for immediate use by the medical practitioner may result in a reluctance to use the product for aesthetic reasons *(52)*. Judicious selection of buffer or choice of ions in the formulation design are acceptable methods to preclude or address aggregate formation *(53)*. The mechanism by which buffer or ion addition precludes or reverses aggregation is presumed to be disruption of electrostatic attraction between the different components.

It is standard practice to incorporate a terminal filtration step for bulk formulated vaccine, provided that the formulation is clear and homogeneous. The tendency of certain formulations to aggregate may cause difficulty in filtration. This can result in rejection of the batch if potency analyses suggest selective binding or retention on the filters. The more vaccines that are combined, the greater the likelihood of aggregation and subsequent rejection of the product.

Aggregation also can create difficulty in filling of the final product. Adjuvanted vaccines will settle out of suspension at a rate inversely proportional to their particle size. An extremely rapid settling rate can require a manufacturer to use high-speed pumps with a recirculation loop in order to ensure maintenance of a homogeneous suspension. However, this is only possible if the antigens retain their stability during the filling process. High-speed recirculation and rapid mixing have the potential to destabilize labile antigens as a result of increased shear and turbulence in the filling apparatus.

Immunological Interactions

For a combination vaccine to work, the antigens must be stable in the formulation and must evoke the desired immune response in the target population. There are a number of documented reports where new combination vaccines do not elicit the required immune response to one or more antigens suggesting some form of immunological incompatibility. As previously mentioned, a formulation of DTwP and IPV produced a reduced immune response to pertussis antigens in infants *(13)*. Similarly, DTaP combined with Hib resulted in a reduced response to the Hib component *(37)*. Earlier efforts to combine viral and bacterial antigens were equally unsuccessful. For example, measles vaccine formulated with meningococcal polysaccharide types A and C resulted in reduced seroconversion for both vaccines *(54)*. However, the clinical relevance of these observations are in question. Some researchers *(16)* have concluded that the reduced antibody response is not clinically relevant since vaccinees were primed and exhibited an anamnestic response. Manifestations of interference are not limited to inactivated products and are more likely to be seen in live viral products *(55)*. For example, a one-way interference was observed when live measles and mumps vaccines were initially formulated, resulting in reduced immunogenicity toward the mumps vaccine *(56)*. A mixture of yellow fever, smallpox, and measles vaccines showed a suboptimal seroconversion rate compared to separate administration of these antigens in different parts of the body *(57)*. The theoretical possibilities by which immunization with combination vaccines could lead to immunological interactions between vaccine components were reviewed elsewhere *(58)*. Conclusive evidence does not exist yet to explain interference, but a number of explanations, namely epitopic suppression and antigenic overload, appear to dominate the current thinking.

EPITOPIC SUPPRESSION

Carrier-mediated epitopic suppression may be a mechanism to account for the reduced immune response to one or more antigens in new combination vaccines. For this to occur, there must be a very close antigenic similarity between two antigens in the combination vaccine. In one hypothetical example, the immune response to the hapten component of a glycoconjugate vaccine may be suppressed because of competition for the recruitment of T-cells between the carrier protein and other components in the combination vaccine.

ANTIGENIC OVERLOAD OR COMPETITION

Efforts to combine new antigens into a single vaccine dose may be thwarted by limitations of the immune system to concurrently process multiple antigens. At what point antigenic overload will be observed is not known. However, it is generally accepted that it will be crucial in formulating new combination vaccines to ensure that the load of distinct antigens does not exceed the capacity of the presentation system *(59)*.

ANTIBODY SUBCLASS RESPONSE

For diseases where an antibody correlate is known, the immunogenicity of new vaccines are assessed by measuring the quantitative and qualitative antibody response. It is possible that one or another response of the immune system may be altered by combining new antigens. Measurement of the total IgG response to a new combination vaccine, followed by a direct comparison with separate administration of individual vaccines, may be insufficient in support of the preclinical characterization program. Measurement of individual antibody subclass response is preferred, since qualitative information will be collected. In addition, comparisons of relative bactericidal and opsonic activities would be highly desirable if not absolutely required. New combinations of antigens, particularly with adjuvants such as MPL, may alter the type of immune response. The degree of benefit for this type of immune modulation must be assessed on a case-by-case basis.

ANIMAL MODEL SELECTION

Ideally, a complete preclinical characterization package for a new vaccine would include demonstration of activity in vivo, i.e., provide protection against the disease entity in a suitable animal host. Often this is impractical for lack of a validated challenge model. The problem is further compounded when one wishes to test new combination vaccines. Under these circumstances, demonstration of immunogenicity in animals is an acceptable alternative.

Another permutation of this dilemma is the choice of animal species if one wishes to demonstrate immunogenicity of a multicomponent vaccine. For example, guinea pigs are traditionally used to assess the response to D toxoid, mice for Hib conjugate, and chinchilla for nontypable *H. influenzae* vaccine candidates. The question is, does one utilize a nonoptimized animal system (for one or more antigens) to assess immune responses to all the antigens in the combination vaccine, or does one use separately optimized animal systems for each antigen?

Stability

A major concern in formulating new combination vaccines is the maintenance of stability of each of the individual components. If the vaccine is a protein, polysaccharide, glycoconjugate, nucleic acid, or a live viral or bacterial preparation, preclinical characterization efforts must focus on documenting the integrity of each component, including the adjuvant (if applicable), throughout the expiry period. This can be a heroic task, particularly for a complex combination vaccine. Nonetheless, success has been realized by reformulation studies, e.g., the stability of oral, attenuated live polio vaccine (OPV) was dramatically improved by the inclusion of 1.0 M MgCl$_2$ in the vaccine formulation *(60)*.

STABILITY-INDICATING ASSAY

The first step in initiating a stability program is to identify and/or develop a suitable stability-indicating assay or assay profile for each component in the vaccine mixture. Ideally, the stability-indicating assay should be an in vitro assay and would require little, if any, sample manipulation prior to performing the analysis. Also, the assay should directly quantify the active component of the antigen or a breakdown product that is known to correlate with immunogenicity in the target population or in a surrogate animal model.

A simple example of a stability-indicating assay is the measurement of viability of a live attenuated viral or bacterial vaccine. In the case of a viral vaccine, this measurement can be made on a suitable cell substrate. For a bacterial vaccine, the measurement can be made on an agar surface. The results are unambiguous and straightforward. In fact, if one can demonstrate that inactivation kinetics are first-order, as has been done for rotavirus (61), elevated temperatures can be used to estimate potency loss at low temperatures, thus providing an opportunity to rapidly evaluate different formulations.

The more complex the antigen, the more difficulty associated with demonstrating stability. An example of a stability-indicating assay for a glycoconjugate is the measurement of free or unconjugated saccharide in the vaccine mixture. The net amount of free saccharide can be expressed on a percent basis following correction for free saccharide introduced from the bulk vaccine concentrate. However, this latter assay only partly addresses the issue of the saccharide component. A second and equally important issue is that of epitope stability. In the case of a polysaccharide, side groups, such as acetyl or pyruvyl moieties, may contribute to the protective immunogenic response. These groups, as a result of their lability, may be lost following formulation or slowly throughout the course of the stability study. It is more difficult and problematic to quantitatively measure these epitopes. A method of dealing with this situation is to incorporate an antigenicity assay into the stability program, i.e., to develop an assay using antibody reagents. Examples of these assays are ELISA and nephelometric assays; the latter measures the rate at which the antigen reacts with type-specific antibody. Finally, there is the issue of stability of the carrier protein. This may be the most difficult component to assess, either by in vitro or in vivo methodology. A number of techniques have been developed to characterize the carrier protein following conjugation. One such technique involves removal of the saccharide component. This permits analysis of the protein moiety by well established procedures, e.g., sodium dodecyl sulfate polyacrylamide gel electrophoresis (SDS-PAGE) and immunoblot. The data gathered in support of stability of the glycoconjugate are derived from a host of different assays. The outcome is a stability profile resulting from a cadre of stability-indicating assays.

Increasingly more complex vaccines will be developed and formulated together, and the challenge for testing these complex mixtures will be increased. For example, it is conceivable that multivalent pneumococcal conjugate vaccines will be combined and tested in clinical trials. The scenario described above for demonstrating stability of a single glycoconjugate vaccine with a battery of stability-indicating assays must then be multiplied by the number of different serotypes in the conjugate mixture. The situation is compounded by the presence of adjuvant. Many of the antigens may be adsorbed to the adjuvant. Thus, the first step in demonstrating stability is to desorb the antigen(s). This can be accomplished by any number of proven methods, e.g., treatment with high salt, or incubation of the vaccine at elevated temperature in the presence of sodium citrate. A major disadvantage of this type of processing step is the potential to alter the integrity of one or more of the active components. Sample processing artifacts can lead to misinformation with respect to the stability of the antigen and, if antigen recovery is not optimized, to under-reporting of total antigen content. The need to analyze and understand the chemistry of increasingly more complex vaccine mixtures will require the use of high-resolution analytical tools such as laser desorption time-of-flight mass spectrometry *(61)*.

FREQUENCY OF TESTING

For a new combination vaccine, it is desirable to test as many of the active components as practical at regular intervals. Following formulation of the bulk vaccine, all the active components are tested by potency assay. These assays may be in vitro or in vivo tests. For the first stability study, it is not uncommon to test within three months of formulation. Testing then is performed at six-month intervals unless instability of one or more antigens is suspected. In the latter case, more frequent testing is performed. Often, efforts are expended at developing accelerated stability tests which are designed to be predictive of long-term, real-time stability. Accelerated testing is normally performed at an elevated temperature over a short period of time in order to simulate what might happen in real time under ordinary storage temperature. However, accelerated testing is of limited value unless a correlation is shown between the accelerated conditions and real-time results.

Matrix Testing

The most conservative design of a stability program is to test every component at each time interval. This is very expensive and at times impractical, particularly in the case of animal testing where up to six weeks may be required to complete the test. In the case of very complex combination vaccines, the shear number of individual tests may become prohibitive. An alternative to testing at each time point is to develop a matrix testing scheme, which usually is based on a statistical analysis of stability programs of similar formulations. This approach reduces the cost of testing and the expenditure of animals.

ICH Guidelines

Regulatory bodies have worked together in an effort to develop stability testing guidelines *(28)* for vaccine manufacturers. Uniform guidelines have the advantage that vaccines from different manufacturers will be subjected to the same criteria. This will make it easier to compare different products and will insure that all products are tested in a similar fashion.

STABILITY OF FORMULATED BULK

From a planning perspective, vaccine manufacturers must be able to demonstrate stability of the formulated bulk vaccine for at least one year. This is necessary because of the length of time to test and release vaccines and must allow for retesting of vaccine in the event of an invalid test or an unsatisfactory result. This time frame is additionally lengthened if there is a requirement that a regulatory agency also test the formulated bulk. As a result of cost considerations, formulated vaccine is rarely filled until release of the bulk is obtained.

STABILITY IN FILLED CONTAINERS

Shelf life of the formulated vaccine in the final container has important economic considerations and must be maximized to ensure competitiveness and profitability. Three-year dating in the final container is the objective of all manufacturers. The stability of the formulated product will be dependent on the most labile component. It follows that the greater number of the antigens in a combination vaccine, the greater the likelihood that the instability of a single antigen will make it difficult to meet this objective. For reasons discussed elsewhere in this review, the overall stability of the combination vaccine is never greater than the stability of the individual components.

Container Compatibility

It is not uncommon that individual vaccines made by the same manufacturer may be filled in different types of containers, e.g., molded or tubing vials. This situation may reflect the era during which the vaccines were developed where one type of container was preferred to all others. Furthermore, consolidation of vaccine manufacturers and merger of their respective product portfolios resulted in a combined product line filled into a variety of different types of containers.

Efforts to combine vaccines raises the issue of which container to use to fill the formulated product. In general terms, tubing vials are preferred to molded vials based on machinability and on a lower reject rate following inspection of the filled product. However, stability of the product remains the overriding issue, and the choice of vial must be determined based on empirical results. One additional consideration is the pH stability of the vaccine formulation and whether or not the vaccine contains sufficient buffering capacity to resist the leaching of alkaline ions from the surface of the glass. Over time, the leaching of alkaline ions, especially from tubing vials, will increase the pH to the level where some antigens will become unstable. This issue can also be addressed by selecting vials which are specially processed to reduce or totally eliminate leaching of alkaline ions.

Closure Compatibility

Closely related to container selection is the choice of stopper. Most stoppers are siliconized to facilitate seating of the closure on the filled vial. However, there are exceptions, e.g., the Purcoat™ stopper. A variety of silicon formulations exist as do different siliconization processes. This issue also must be resolved by a stability study to ensure compatibility of the silicon formula with the components of the vaccine. Different vaccine components, such as proteins or carbohydrates, may exhibit different sensitivities to silicone formulations and will need to be evaluated on a case-by-case basis. One manifestation of an undesirable interaction is reflected by precipitation or aggregation of the component antigen. Extreme care must be made in making an assessment of compatibility, particularly if the vaccine formulation contains insoluble components such as adjuvants. In this type of formulation one would not normally observe the interaction, but that in itself does not preclude that the interaction did not occur.

Latex Issue

Over the past several years, sporadic reports have surfaced linking allergic reactions to natural rubber latex. This type of reaction can have severe consequence for the individual and can cause death in rare instances. In response to this concern, regulatory agencies have considered restrictions on the use of latex in all pharmaceutical products, including biologicals. This restriction would apply to the latex used in some container closures and in syringe gaskets. If implemented, this restriction has profound consequence for manufacturers of biologicals, particularly if the restrictions were imposed within the next several years. For example, new stability programs would need to be initiated to demonstrate stability with latex-free stoppers and syringes. Since real-time stability programs for filled products normally run 36–48 months, there could be a substantial delay in the appearance of mature vaccines products filled into the new presentation. As far as new vaccine combinations are concerned, manufacturers are making every effort to place these new products on stability study with closures that comply with the proposed new restrictions. Pending a final decision, the FDA recently issued a directive requiring that a warning label be affixed to the packaging of all pharmaceuticals and biologicals that have the potential to come in contact with natural rubber latex during dispensing of the product (62).

Manufacturing Concerns

Formulation

"Batching" is a dated manufacturing term used to describe how vaccine concentrates are diluted and blended with aluminum adjuvant prior to filling. This term is slowly being replaced with the word "formulation." The latter encompasses much more than blending and reflects the realization that true process technology is involved and that this technology is an integral part of the larger vaccine development process. Each step in the process must be defined empirically and optimized in order to ensure consistency and uniformity of final product. The magnitude of the formulation challenge has increased as the need to combine new and different antigens has unfolded. This effort will be further complicated by the desire to use the next generation of adjuvants, e.g., MPL or QS-21, as a critical component of new combination vaccines.

SCALE

The manufacturing scale of final formulations may range from 50 to more than 1000 L. The volume and timing of the batch will be determined by the materials-management function and will reflect the projected market requirements. Smaller batches usually are made to reflect a relatively small market demand where additional specialty testing or high-purity components may be required. For convenience, smaller batches may be made in glass vessels. The use of glass is not practical at full-scale operation where formulation is performed in 316 stainless steel vessels that are cleaned-in-place (CIP) and steamed-in-place (SIP). The use of glass vessels in the early development process is an important consideration for new combination vaccines. For example, it is very important to be able to observe the mixing of the components during the formulation process in order to be cognizant of physical interactions.

It is the responsibility of the manufacturer to ensure that the vaccine produced at the smallest scale is identical to the vaccine produced at the largest scale. In all cases, components used in these formulations, including the adjuvant, are themselves manufactured at full production scale. Testing and release of vaccine is independent of the scale at which the vaccine is manufactured. From a economic viewpoint, the formulation of large scale batches is favored.

MIXING ISSUES

Consistent formulation at manufacturing scale is dependent on the selection and validation of a suitable method of mixing in the batching vessel. Mixing at small scale, i.e., 50 L, can be satisfactorily achieved by use of a magnetic stir bar. At larger scale, i.e., ≥200 L, more vigorous mixing is required; this is accomplished by using a turbine impeller or a marine impeller. Both impeller types permit thorough mixing but have the disadvantage of creating a vortex. If mixing is too vigorous, frothing will occur which may lead to the degradation of labile protein components. A more desirable alternative is to mix the components using a plate mixer that will vibrate within a defined amplitude. The commercial name for this devise is a VIBROmixer (R&S Rutten, GmbH, Switzerland). The plate in this device has from 8–16 holes depending on plate size. This design permits the formulated product to be expelled through the plate as the plate vibrates. Vibration of the plate is controlled by a rheostat, the amplitude of which can be closely monitored within narrow limits using a number of electronic instruments. This method is more accurate than use of the more conventional tachometer.

The primary purpose of mixing during formulation is to ensure a homogeneous vaccine suspension. Of equal concern is the need to maintain the integrity of the vaccine components during the mixing process. Some vaccine components, particularly those containing protein moieties, are very sensitive to shear forces. Excessive shear can be a problem with marine impellers if the rpm are too high. The problem of shear may also be observed with a VIBROmixer. The vibromixer in fact has been used by manufacturers to reduce the size of aluminum gels. In this latter case, prolonged mixing at high speed is required. During the formulation process, constant vigilance must be applied to ensure that stability of the components is maintained. Mixing strategy must be defined to ensure stability of the most labile component in a combination vaccine. Gross stability of an adjuvanted vaccine can be assessed by monitoring particle size where a direct correlation is seen between particle size and the length of mixing. Particle size may be more than a stability issue, since reports have surfaced that relate particle size to immunogenicity. Mixing dynamics are important for new combination vaccines if only to ensure that the antigens are thoroughly dispersed throughout the batching vessel and in the final product.

PROCESS DEVELOPMENT

Formulation process development for combination vaccines is often pursued on a trial-and-error basis. The process begins with a careful analysis and understanding of each of the vaccine components, including the adjuvant. Of particular interest are factors impacting the stability and immunogenicity of each component.

A target formulation is identified with respect to pH, antigen level, and adjuvant level. The order of addition for each of the components of the combination vaccine is empirically determined. Previous results have shown that the order of addition of antigens can influence immunogenicity (63). All possible permutations are explored and effect on the final formulation assessed. This is done to provide flexibility and information to formulation personnel responsible for the manufacturing process. The relationship between time and temperature also is established for the formulation process, since temperature can impact binding and stability of each of the antigens. A range for each of the above is documented as part of the validation process. If an aluminum gel is formed *in situ* as part of the formulation process, the rate of addition of each of the components contributing to the gel is carefully measured to ensure the proper phosphate:hydroxide ratio. This is critical to ensure batch-to-batch reproducibility. In extreme cases, it may be necessary to bind each of the antigens separately, and then to combine them under conditions where the uniformity of the formulated batch can be controlled more rigidly. The pH is monitored throughout the process and precautions taken to ensure that pH adjustments do not contribute to instability or desorption of the formulated vaccine. Minimal mixing times are established at each process step and the effect of prolonged mixing documented (if possible). These steps are performed initially at bench-process scale and then are repeated at 10- to 20-fold increases in volume. Each batch is characterized by physico-chemical means to ensure formulation consistency prior to continuing scale up to the next larger volume.

PROCESS VALIDATION

Validation of the formulation process for combination vaccines is required by regulatory agencies and is the only way to ensure consistency of manufacture. Process validation can be accomplished as a result of careful analysis of each step in the manufacturing process, followed by design and selection of a series of in-process tests that document process reproducibility. The final step of in-process validation usually involves full characterization of the formulated product and demonstration of lot-to-lot consistency.

Examples of in-process tests for combination vaccines include measurement of the degree of adsorption of each component (in the case of an adjuvanted vaccine), demonstration of a uniform pH profile and maintenance of its stability, demonstration of a uniform hydroxide:phosphate ratio for an aluminum gel formed *in situ*, achieving a similar mean particle size of the formulated vaccine and definition of the acceptable range, maintenance of a homogeneous suspension throughout the mixing phase, defining the relationship between time and temperature for antigen adsorption, documentation of a standard settling rate for the adjuvanted product, and achievement of a sterile product. This list is not all-inclusive; there are many more tests that can be performed. However, each of the above in-process tests has the advantage that the measurements can be performed rapidly and with standard laboratory instrumentation. The single exception is the sterility test, which requires 14 days to complete.

The final step in process validation involves complete characterization of the product. This aspect of process validation will involve both in vivo and in vitro assays. Given the nature of animal testing, a long lead time for completion of testing and tabulation of results is required.

CONSISTENCY LOTS

For a combination vaccine, consistency in production of the final formulation is the goal of the manufacturer. Consistency is documented by the accumulation of in-process data that demonstrate process control and final bulk test results that confirm process reproducibility. Regulatory agencies may require the preparation of 3–5 consistency lots in support of a new license application. A further requirement may be that the lots are consecutively manufactured, but this is the exception and, when enforced, is product-specific. An important issue with combination vaccines, as it relates to consistency of manufacturer, is how many different bulk intermediates are required to fulfill the requirement for three or more unique lots. Historically, for a new single component vaccine, manufacturers would prepare a minimum of three different lots. For a new combination vaccine, particularly where one or more components may already be licensed as stand-alone vaccines, manufacturers have rationalized with just cause that the requirement for up to five unique combinations may be too restrictive and is unwarranted in all cases. An extreme example of this situation is the 23-valent pneumococcal polysaccharide vaccine. If the requirement were imposed that three or more separate fermentations and purifications of each of the 23 serotypes be prepared at manufacturing scale, the cost of development would become prohibitive. A compromise acceptable to regulatory agencies and to manufacturers alike is to establish the requirement to demonstrate consistency of manufacture during the formulation process. With this alternative, it may acceptable to produce only two unique sets of the 23 polysaccharides and to formulate each of these two sets into two unique consistency lots. The third lot could be a unique combination of 12 serotypes from the first set and 11 serotypes from the second set. A recent review *(64)* details the industrial perspective of consistency lots.

CLEANING VALIDATION

The greater the number of components in a combination vaccine, the greater the challenge to demonstrate a validated cleaning procedure. Acceptable methodology for documenting a validated cleaning procedure is to perform total organic carbon (TOC) analysis on swabs of surfaces coming in contact with product prior to, during, and after cleaning. In exceptional cases or where changeover documentation is required, this program may be complemented with special testing that is peculiar to the antigen, e.g., this may involve the use of highly specific tests such as ELISA. In the event these latter tests are preferred or even required, an effort would be made to identify the one component of the combination vaccine that is the most difficult to remove. Removal of this particularly difficult component can be used to validate the cleaning program for the formulated product.

REWORK PROCEDURES

Rework procedures are routinely developed for monocomponent and multicomponent vaccines. For example, a rework may be proposed to address issues regarding pH, aluminum level, or potency of a component. In the above examples, the rework itself may involve a pH adjustment after the formulation process or the addition of supplemental adjuvant or antigen. Another approach is to formulate a second batch, and then blend this second batch with the first batch. In all cases, scientific data must be generated to support the rework proposal, and the reworked vaccine must pass all standard release testing. In certain cases, validation of a rework protocol may require that the vaccine be placed on real-time stability study to ensure that the shelf-life of the product is unaltered as a consequence of the rework process.

In the case of new combination vaccines, it will become increasingly more difficult to develop rework procedures due to the complexity of the mixture. The greater the number of antigens, the greater the likelihood of antigen interaction. This situation likely will preclude the development of simple rework procedures, since small changes are apt to have a large impact on the formulated product. From a manufacturing perspective, this is very disconcerting since the greater the number of antigens committed to a batch, the more expensive it is to reject a batch because of an inability to meet product release specifications.

EXPIRY DATING

For a monocomponent vaccine, expiry dating is assigned based on manufacturing date and on real-time stability data. Individual components in a combination vaccine will have very different manufacturing and expiry dates. Once vaccines are combined, the expiry date becomes a reflection of the most labile and/or oldest component in the formulation. It is possible that combining two or more vaccines may destabilize one of the components. Conversely, it is unlikely that the stability of a component in a combined vaccine would increase simply as the result of mixing with a second vaccine. Careful and thoughtful reformulation is required to ensure that the new combined vaccine has at least a similar shelf life as do the individual components. Analogous to the above, the more antigens formulated into a single vaccine, the greater the challenge to develop a product that possesses the required stability.

Filling

A clear solution of a monocomponent vaccine is the easiest product to fill. Mixing issues do not present a challenge, nor due practical issues of stopping the fill line for shift change or lunch break. However, once a vaccine is adjuvanted, maintaining a homogeneous suspension and preventing settling-out in the lines during the filling process becomes a serious concern. In-process testing is scrupulously adhered to and results monitored to ensure consistency. Test methodology can be as simple as measuring percent transmittance on a spectrophotometer. Samples are routinely taken prior to, during, and at the end of the fill. The data are reviewed by Quality Assurance, and deviation from the expected range are grounds for rejection of the fill.

New combination vaccines may present unforeseen challenges in this area. For example, a new formulation may have unusually rapid settling characteristics which may require modification of the filling apparatus. Similarly, formulations may be developed containing high levels of aluminum adjuvant to meet rigorous testing requirements, particularly animal potency tests. Higher aluminum-containing vaccines will settle out at a faster rate. Both of the above situations may require the purchase of new equipment, and/or require additional monitoring, thus adding to the cost of the final product.

Labeling and Package Insert

There are strict regulatory requirements that must be met in the labeling and packaging of a licensed vaccine. Both the trade name and the generic name must be approved prior to distribution and must not bear close resemblance to any currently licensed vaccine. This restriction is enforced in order to minimize confusion among health-care practitioners.

The package insert also is scrutinized by regulatory agencies for accuracy and for technical content. A great deal of information is required in the package insert, including detailed results of safety studies, adverse reactions and contraindications, detailed results of clinical trials in terms of efficacy and/or immunogenicity levels, the target population and details of vaccines approved for concurrent administration, vaccine formulation, and a brief description of the manufacturing process. For a monocomponent vaccine, this information can be captured on a single-page package insert. From a practical viewpoint, multicomponent vaccines present a real challenge to condense all the required information onto a single page and still adhere to the requirement that the font is readable by a person with average vision. Manufacturers have explored using larger page sizes for multicomponent vaccines but are confounded by the limitation of folding the package insert to fit into standard single-dose packaging.

Release Testing

In general, release test requirements for a combination vaccine may be a compilation of the release test requirements for each of the individual components. Obvious exceptions to this statement are that the formulated combination vaccine will only require one sterility test, one general safety test, and so forth. Assay interference issues may preclude performing all the testing on the formulated product that is required of the stand-alone product. In this situation, it may be possible to report potency by calculation once consistency of manufacture of the combined product is documented. Furthermore, it is conceivable that under specialized circumstances, a requirement may be imposed for one or more tests that are peculiar to the combination product, i.e., are not required for any of the stand-alone products.

The greater the number of antigens in a combination vaccine, the greater the likelihood that a release test result may fail to meet specification. This outcome may reflect an error in formulation or the inadvertent use of a subpotent intermediate. In a number of cases, a test result may be found to be unsatisfactory, but a subsequent investigation may reveal that the test was invalid. A typical example of an invalid test would be nonparallel lines between the test sample and the standard. A retest can be initiated under these conditions. Product can be released only if the investigation identifies the reason for the failure, and the retest result meets product specification.

Cost of Manufacture

The average estimated cost for vaccines produced and used in the United States range from approx $0.50–$2.50/dose *(65)*. A significant percent of this cost, perhaps as high as 50%, is related to filling and packaging. This is particularly true if the vaccine is filled into a syringe for ease of delivery. For this reason, formulating antigens into new combination vaccines has the potential to reduce the overall cost of manufacture due to savings realized in reduced packaging. However, this savings will be realized only if the cost of testing the combination does not exceed the test costs of the individual components. Furthermore, the rejection rate of combination vaccines also must be less than the individual products. This appears to be an absolute requirement because rejection of a multi-component vaccine for one unsatisfactory test result will increase the overhead for the other components (that must be discarded with the formulated vaccine).

Manufacturing for the Global Market

Vaccine manufacturers target the development of a single formulation for any given antigen. To accomplish this objective, the vaccine must be formulated to meet different regional test requirements and also must meet the stability requirements of the different geographic areas. This objective can be a real challenge, particularly for more mature vaccines such as DTwP. However, the incentives to successfully meet this challenge justify the efforts. A vaccine formulated to meet global demand reduces the complexity of the manufacturing process and minimizes the possibility of formulation error. For example, multiple formulations of the same vaccine require the existence of multiple sets of batch records and Standard Operating Procedures (SOP). Additionally, two or more inventories of the same antigen concentrates may need to be maintained if regional requirements specify the use of antigen with different levels of purity. The acceptance of preservatives also reflects regional preferences. Thimerosal is accepted in North America, although pressure is mounting to eliminate this mercury-based preservative from parenteral products. In Europe, there is strong objection to the use of thimerosal as a preservative. Because single-dose containers are the preferred way of delivering vaccine, preservatives are not needed or used. When preservative is added, a combination of 2-phenoxyethanol and formalin is preferred over mercury derivatives.

With respect to stability, different issues are involved. In the United States, vaccines are routinely held in the physician's office at refrigerated temperatures, e.g., 2–8°C. In other cases, facilities exist to store the vaccine frozen at –20°C. These storage conditions are impractical in certain geographic areas, particularly in third-world countries. Economic concerns in these areas dictate that vaccines be formulated to have greater stability at ambient temperature. Facilities for storage of vaccine under frozen conditions are rarely seen, even in Europe. Furthermore, certain vaccines, particularly those containing aluminum adjuvant, cannot be frozen since the gel structure is destroyed by freezing *(66)*.

Formulation of new combination vaccines for global use may not be practical or economical under all circumstances. For example, there are 85 known serotypes of *Streptococcus pneumoniae* responsible for systemic pneumococcal disease. Certain serotypes are devastating in confined geographic areas, while little or no disease attributable to these serotypes are known elsewhere. For a multivalent polysaccharide vaccine, this is a mute issue since it is common practice to add the 23 most prevalent serotypes to provide maximum protection even though inclusion of a number of these serotypes will provide little or no benefit. This is not a straightforward issue in the case of conjugate vaccines since two additional factors are involved, e.g., the cost of manufacture and the possibility of carrier protein overload.

The manufacture of glycoconjugate vaccines is cost-intensive relative to the polysaccharides. For example, consider the following theoretical consideration: activation of the polysaccharide and subsequent downstream processing steps, such as purification and lyophilization, may result in a type-specific variable yield ranging from 50–90%. It is not inconceivable that the conjugation reaction and subsequent purification may further result in a 15–50% stepwise yield. The overall yield for this type of multistep process may range from 8–45%. A second major contribution to cost is the carrier protein. This protein requires a separate fermentation, purification, and stabilization. Furthermore, both the protein component and the conjugate vaccine itself require a significant amount of very expensive qualification testing.

One additional confounding issue impacting the desire for a single formulation is that different formulations actually may be required to trigger an optimal immune response. For example, studies with the HIV gp160 *(67)* have shown that priming with a recombinant live vector followed by boosting with a subunit vaccine is preferred to all other presentations.

Inventory Control

A single global formulation makes inventory management and control easier to maintain. This situation results in maximum flexibility and permits the manufacturer to respond to changing market needs. This is particularly important in countries where the vaccine business involves the awarding of tenders, which may be awarded anywhere from a quarterly to a year-to-year basis.

Inventory control is also a concern for the medical practitioner. Combination vaccines in themselves will not reduce the inventory of vaccines in the physician's office but rather have the potential to require the physician to maintain a supply of each of the components as well (68). This is necessary since the combination vaccine may not be suitable for all vaccinees. Record keeping is also seen as a major challenge.

Vaccine Presentations

Presentation

The presentation of a vaccine is influenced by a number of factors, the most important being the stability of the formulated product and the nature of the disease entity.

Stability is an overriding concern in determining how a vaccine is delivered. For example, some antigens are unstable as liquid formulations and must be lyophilized to preserve their integrity. Other vaccines are stable only in the frozen state and must be kept at $-20°C$ or even lower to ensure potency. Most vaccines are stable as liquid formulations at $2–8°C$ and are injected.

The method of vaccine presentation also is influenced by the desired type of immune response and by the site of entry or colonization of the pathogen. If protection against the disease entity is the result of a strong humoral response, then parental injection is a suitable mechanism for delivery of the antigen. Similarly, for infection of the upper respiratory tract, intranasal administration of the antigen is desirable. In the case of oral vaccines, the antigens must be stable in the acidic environment of the gut. If viral replication is required, as with polio, the latter method of administration increases the likelihood of the more desirable cell mediated response.

LIQUID

A stable liquid formulation is without exception the preferred vaccine presentation. The liquid presentation is the most flexible; the vaccine can be delivered as an injectable, as an oral vaccine, or intranasally by drop or spray. Combined vaccines administered by the parenteral route will be limited by the volume of material that can be injected, particularly if infants are the target population. Greater volumes of vaccines can be administered by mucosal routes. It is not uncommon for a vaccine to be introduced in a form other than as a liquid in order to reduce the time required to launch the product. A recent example was Merck's (Whitehouse Station, NJ) Hib conjugate vaccine (PedvaxHIB). This vaccine was launched as a lyophilized product, and once technical difficulties were resolved, a stable liquid formulation was introduced as a second-generation product.

LYOPHILIZED

Lyophilization of vaccines is pursued primarily because of stability concerns. For a new vaccine, the length of time required to develop a liquid formulation is usually longer than the time required to develop a lyophilization cycle. This is particularly true if the target is to combine antigens that have incompatible stability requirements, e.g., antigens with different and nonoverlapping pH stability profiles. However, lyophilization in itself does not guarantee product stability. For example, viral vaccines are lyophilized to maintain viability, antigenicity, and structural rigidity. Careful attention must be addressed to maintaining a low but defined level of moisture. Stabilizers are added to the viral vaccine formulation individually or as a crafted mixture of sucrose, polyalcohols, L-glutamate, gelatin hydrolysate, or human albumin *(69)*. Initial studies to lyophilize measles virus vaccine *(70)* were only marginally successful. The lyophilized product was inherently unstable and required considerable effort for cycle optimization and identification of the proper proportion of chemical stabilizers to meet product stability specifications.

Once a vaccine is lyophilized, a strategy to resuspend the product must be developed. Two options exist: resuspend the vaccine with diluent or resuspend with another vaccine. The latter alternative is being actively pursued by vaccine manufacturers since it is an opportunity to increase the number of antigens while minimizing the number of injections.

ADVANTAGES/DISADVANTAGES

From a manufacturing perspective, a liquid combination vaccine is the easiest to implement and is the most cost-effective to produce since all component vaccines must be formulated as liquids. A liquid presentation also is preferred from a marketing perspective since it affords maximum convenience for the health care provider and allows for the possibility of a prefilled syringe, seen by some as the preferred way to make an injectable vaccine available.

A lyophilized vaccine also has certain advantages, the most important being the opportunity to rapidly address stability issues since most antigens are stabilized following lyophilization. From a combination vaccine viewpoint, lyophilizing multiple antigens allows for the possibility of delivering a maximum number of antigens with a minimum number of formulation studies. The major disadvantage of lyophilization is the cost of manufacturing. Lyophilizers are capital-intensive and are expensive to maintain. Depending on the length of the lyophilization cycle, it is not unreasonable to assume that lyophilization could add from $0.50–$1.00/dose of vaccine. There is also cost associated with the diluent, not only in the formulation, but in the most expensive step, i.e., filling of the container. Lastly, there is the issue of physician preference where it is assumed that resuspending a lyophilized vaccine is less convenient than direct use of a liquid product.

Alternative Delivery Devices

Once it is determined how a vaccine is to be presented, either as a liquid or a lyophilized powder, there are a number of options that can be explored to maximize convenience for the physician or nurse and to minimize discomfort for the vaccinee. The range of delivery devices that are available also provide the manufacturer with additional options for combining new vaccines into a single injection. The classical methods for distributing vaccines are filled vials and pre-filled syringes. Other delivery devices are available for marketing combination vaccines where the antigens are not compatible.

Compartmentalized and Dual-Barrel Syringes

A compartmentalized syringe system, also referred to as a sequential or bypass syringe, consists of a single barrel separated into two compartments with a septum. Depression of the plunger forces admixing of the two components, one of which may be a lyophilized powder. This type of delivery system has the potential to permit the concurrent delivery of two or more otherwise incompatible antigens by allowing for their mixing at the time of immunization. Another method of accomplishing this objective is the use of a dual-barrel syringe, which was designed for the simultaneous mixing of two liquid vaccines, also at the time of injection. The two components feed into a single needle and comix as the plunger is depressed.

Air Gun and Needleless Injectors

Airgun and needleless injectors were envisioned to deliver antigens as part of mass immunization procedures and have enjoyed some success. The long-term acceptance of the liquid-based needleless injector is problematic since some discomfort is associated with the immunization process. A powder-based gas-driven needleless injector is in Phase I studies with HB vaccine and reportedly has less pain associated with vaccine delivery *(71)*. It is not anticipated at this time that any of these devices will play a major role in resolving issues related to compatibility of new combination vaccines unless a device is developed that permits the simultaneous injection of multiple antigens through multiple injection ports.

Multiple Vials

Under certain circumstances, e.g., when the incompatibility of two vaccines cannot be resolved by reformulation, it may be practical to comarket two vaccines in separate containers but under single packaging. At the time of immunization, one vaccine is drawn into a syringe and mixed with the second vaccine. The same syringe could be used to withdraw a 1-mL dose of the new combined vaccine. Preclinical and clinical studies would be required in support of a license application. Recent regulatory decisions suggest that once the license is granted, matched lots of the vaccines would need to be paired in order to meet the requirements of regulatory authorities. If implemented, this decision will reduce the flexibility of vaccine manufacturers in terms of inventory management, particularly as it relates to the pairing of separate products with different manufacturing dates and expiry dating.

INTRANASAL SPRAY

The delivery of antigens by the intranasal route is an attractive alternative to parenteral injection. Foremost is the potential to present antigens against certain diseases that may best be prevented by induction of a cell-mediated immune response, e.g., nontypable *H. influenzae*, respiratory syncytial virus, or any other upper respiratory tract pathogen. Preliminary indications suggest that Aviron has had success inducing a strong mucosal immune response toward its cold-adapted trivalent influenzae vaccine which was delivered by intranasal spray *(72)*. However, this concept needs to be proven through exhaustive clinical studies before it is recommended for widespread use.

Stability of the target antigen and the ability to combine different antigens for delivery with an intranasal device remain to be evaluated. The mechanics of filling and cost of the final product will also impact the rate and the extent to which this alternative can be commercially exploited.

ADVANTAGES/DISADVANTAGES

The development of mechanical devices to deliver antigens that have stability or incompatibility limitations offer an opportunity to launch new combination vaccines without having to resolve difficult incompatibility issues by reformulation. These devices depend on a physical barrier to keep the antigens separated prior to immunization. Even though individual vaccines may be licensed, clinical trials are required to show that concurrent administration produces the same immune response as separate administration of the antigens. However, there are a number of potential disadvantages to this approach. Foremost is the additional expense associated with the syringe; secondary, but equally important, is the additional cost associated with filling the vaccines. In the latter case, it is projected that a significant amount of development work is required to satisfactorily address all mechanical issues. Because the technology for these highly versatile syringes is relatively new, there are validation issues surrounding the ability of the system to routinely deliver the advertised dose. Mixing issues related to ability to uniformly resuspend a lyophilized powder with a second vaccine or diluent also may be problematic.

Safety

Interchangeability Issues

Advances in biotechnology have resulted in a broad spectrum of approaches to provide protection against disease caused by pathogenic organisms. A prime example are the new generation of combination vaccines. Effectiveness of a vaccine against a particular disease-causing organism is demonstrated by either of two mechanisms: an efficacy trial, where protection is shown in the field against a placebo vaccine, or by inducing an immune response known to be protective against the disease entity. This latter situation is referred to as the "immunological correlate of protection."

In the case of pertussis, efforts have focused on the development of an aP vaccine to replace the wP vaccine. These efforts were initiated in an attempt to produce a vaccine with reduced reactogenicity compared to the wP vaccine. A series of clinical trails recently were completed which show that different formulations of aP vaccine are efficacious against pertussis. The formulation of the aP vaccines differ in the number and quantity of the antigens (ranging from a single antigen to as many as five antigens) and also in the aluminum adjuvant. The situation is complicated further by the routine combination of D and T toxoids from different manufacturers with the new aP vaccines. Interchangeability among these different combination vaccines has not been fully resolved.

Even with all the clinical data that is now available, a true immunological correlate against pertussis disease has not been established by the scientific community. This situation has important implications for developers of new combination vaccines. For example, protection against pertussis may be formulation-specific and may reflect the selection of specific antigens presented in a specific formulation. Since protection against pertussis disease begins with a primary series of immunizations in infancy, followed by boosters at 12–18 mo, and at 5 years of age, the question of interchangeability of the different formulations has become an issue. This issue will actually extend into the adolescent and adult populations given the desire to provide protection against pertussis disease throughout life. Severe pertussis disease is rarely seen in adults; however, the diagnosis of pertussis in adults in increasing, and adults do serve as a reservoir for disease for the nonimmunized population, particularly infants.

The issue of interchangeability of P vaccines (formulated with D and T toxoids) will become a larger issue as additional antigens are combined into more complex mixtures, e.g., with HB and Hib conjugate vaccines. Extensive clinical testing will be required to show immunogenicity for all antigens, and equally important, the absence of interference. These new combinations will help to meet the larger objective of reducing the number of immunizations but will not reduce the requirement that the manufacturer develop and maintain an inventory of all different combinations in order to meet the needs of the population. As a result of personal, physician, and regional preference and/or requirements, it is unlikely that all potential vaccinees will receive all possible antigens as a single immunization. Catch-up doses and missed immunizations will need to be addressed, and the appropriate vaccine supplies made available by the manufacturer.

General Safety Considerations

Safety and antigen compatibility remain the two most important issues facing vaccine manufacturers. A safety profile must be established for each new antigen and for use of that new antigen following formulation with a previously licensed vaccine. Prior to initiating clinical studies with a new antigen, toxicological studies are required in animals. As with new drugs, it is possible that reproductive toxicological studies may be required at some point in time for new biologicals. This will become a particular concern as efforts intensity to evaluate and license vaccines intended for administration during the third trimester of pregnancy.

Once a new vaccine candidate is found to be safe following preclinical characterization, and is well tolerated by animals, new vaccines are routinely tested in descending age groups. For example, initiation of safety studies begins in adults and slowly makes it way down to adolescents and then toddlers, and finally infants if that is the target population. New combination vaccines must be concurrently administered with the standard range of childhood vaccines in order to look for evidence of interference. Even if a new vaccine is shown to be safe and efficacious by itself, its administration must be compatible with the other childhood immunizations from a safety perspective.

Potential for Enhanced Reactogenicity

The greater the number of antigens that are combined or administered at a single office visit, the increased likelihood of an adverse reaction, however minor. Under most circumstances, the adverse reaction will be minor and appear as a slightly elevated temperature or increased tenderness or redness at the site of injection. The safety profile of new combination vaccines will be monitored closely during clinical trials and analyzed prior to granting of licensure. Regulatory agencies will question reactogenicity rates of combined vaccines and will compare these rates with separate administration of the individual antigens. It may be difficult to meet an objective of similar reactogenicity for a combined vaccine compared to separate administration of the individual components since a negative synergistic interaction may occur as a simple consequence of mixing two or more of the components. Each combination vaccine must be examined on a case-by-case basis. Adverse effects have been reported following parenteral administration of whole-cell vaccines, such as with typhoid and pertussis vaccines. Problems associated with systemic delivery may be overcome with an appropriate mucosal delivery system containing lipopolysaccharide or inactivated cholera toxin *(73)*.

Summary and Future Prospects

Efforts to combine new antigens and to reformulate previously licensed vaccines will intensify as new approaches to prevent disease are identified. This activity will be required of vaccine manufacturers in order to deliver the more than 25 vaccines that will be available by the end of 1997. Within a few years, the immunization of infants is likely to be expanded to include pneumococcal and meningococcal conjugate vaccines. A plausible immunization schedule for United States children is shown in *Table 6*. Without combination vaccines, an infant will receive up to six injections during the two- and four-month visits. The goal of CVI is to combine all these antigens in one shot. However, the goal will not be realized in the near future. Alternatively, it may be possible to divide these antigens into two different combinations. Based on the number of antigens, 16 possible presentations for delivering a two-shot combination for infants exists. Obviously, no single vaccine manufacturer has the resources to evaluate all these combination vaccines in both preclinical and clinical studies. To further confound this already complex situation, no single vaccine manufacturer possesses all the antigens to prepare the different combinations. In the absence of established partnerships or joint ventures for the development of new combination vaccines, each vaccine manufacturer must select a combination vaccine strategy which is based on their product portfolio and global marketing plan. The manufacturer will have to define the best combination vaccine to develop based on physical-chemical characterization, the interaction of different antigens, current practice and immunization schedules, and finally on the availability of antigens.

Other schemes were proposed to combine different vaccines. For example, one system favors four combination vaccines *(74)*: one vaccine to contain all protein antigens, a second vaccine to contain all conjugate vaccines, a third vaccine to combine all live viral vaccines, and a fourth combination vaccine for adolescents; the latter vaccine would contain antigens to protect against cytomegalovirus, herpes simplex viruses, *Chlamydia trachomatis, N. gonorrhea,* and Group B *Streptococci.*

Significant resources will be required to address the many issues surrounding the developmental aspects of new combination vaccines. Formulation of the

Table 6. Future Immunization Schedule for United States Children

	0 mo	2 mo	4 mo	6 mo	12–18 mo	4–6 yr
HB	•	•	•			
DTaP		•	•	•	•	•
Hib		•	•	•	•	
Polio		•	•		•	•
Pn conjugate[a]		•	•	•	•	
Nm conjugate[a]		•	•	•	•	
MMR					•	•
Varicella					•	•
Rotavirus		•	•	•		

[a]Pn, Pneumococcal; Nm, Meningococcal.

product to ensure safety, stability, and compatibility of the antigens will be the primary concern. This effort will be followed by clinical studies to document that the combined vaccine maintains the safety profile and immune response associated with the individual vaccines. Vaccine manufacturers will be faced with the challenge of marketing combination vaccines in a way that will promote maximum uptake of the new vaccines for the benefit of mankind, but to minimize the confusion that will certainly result, at least initially, from the plethora of new biological products. During the next few years, it will be particularly important for regulatory agencies to work closely with the manufacturers to help expedite the approval process for new combination vaccines thus helping to fulfill the challenge of the CVI.

References

1. Mitchell, V. S., Philipose, N. M., and Sanford, J. P., eds. (1993) *Children's Vaccine Initiative, Achieving the Vision.* National Academy Press, Washington, DC.
2. Rabinovich, N. R., McInnes, P., Klein, D. L., and Hall, B. F. (1994) Vaccine technologies: view to the future. *Science* **265,** 1401–1404.
3. Centers for Disease Control and Prevention (1995) Recommended Childhood Immunization Schedule, United States, *MMWR* **44,** 2.
4. Centers for Disease Control and Prevention (1997) FDA approval of a *Haemophilus b* conjugate combined by reconstitution with an acellular pertussis vaccine. *JAMA* **277(1),** 13.
5. Eskola, J. (1996) Analysis of *Haemophilus influenzae* type b conjugate and diphtheria-tetanus-pertussis combination vaccines. *J. Infect. Dis.* **174(Suppl 3),** S302–305.
6. Eskola, J., Olander, R. M., Hovi, T., Litmanen, L., Peltola, S., and Kayhty, H. (1996) Randomised trial of the effect of co-administration with acellular pertussis DTP vaccine on immunogenicity of *Haemophilus influenzae* type b conjugate vaccines. *Lancet* **348(9043),** 1688–1692.
7. Halperin, S. A., Barreto, L., Eastwood, B. J., Medd, L., Guasparini, R., and Mills, E. (1997) Safety and immunogenicity of an acellular pertussis diphtheria-tetanus vaccine given as a single injection with *Haemophilus influenzae b* conjugate vaccine. *Vaccine* **15,** 295–300.

8. Greenberg, D. P., Wong, V. K., Partridge, S., Howe, B. J., and Ward, J. L. (1997) Safety and immunogenicity of a combination DTPa-hepatitis b vaccine administered to infants at 2, 4, and 6 months of age. *Clin. Infec. Dis.* **25,** 467.

9. Faldella, G., Alessandroni, R., Fantini, M. P., and Salvioli, G. P. (1996) Clinical development of a combined diphtheria, tetanus acelluar pertussis and hepatitis B vaccine in Italy. *J. Infect. Dis.* **174(Suppl 3),** S298–S301.

10. Usonis, V., Bakasenas, V., Willens, P., and Clemens, R. (1997) Feasibility study of a combined diphtheria-tetanus-acellular pertussis-hepatitis b (DTPa-HBV) vaccine, and comparison of clinical reactions and immune response with diphtheria-tetanus-acelluar pertussis (DTPa) and hepatitis b vaccines applied as mixed or injected into separate limbs. *Vaccine* **15,** 1680–1686.

11. Lee, C. Y., Lee, P. I., Huang, L. M., Chen, J. M., and Chang, M. H. (1997) A simplified schedule to integrate the hepatitis B vaccine into an expanded program of immunization in epidemic countries. *J. Pediatrics* **130,** 981–986.

12. Halperin, S. A., Davis, H. D., Barrelo, L., Guasparini, R., Meckison, W., Humphreys, G., and Eastwood, B. J. (1977) Safety and immunogenicity of two inactivated poliovirus vaccines in combination with an acellular pertussis vaccine and diphtheria and tetanus toxoids in seventeen to nineteen-month-old infants. *J. Pediatrics* **130,** 525–531.

13. Halperin, S. A., Langley, J. M., and Eastwood, B. J. (1996) Effect of inactivated poliovirus vaccine in the antibody response to bordetella pertussis antigens when combined with diphtheria-pertussis-tetanus vaccine. *Clin. Infect. Dis.* **22,** 59–62.

14. Begue, P., Stagnara, J., Vie-Le-Sage, F., Bernard, J. C., Zerri, B., and Abitol, V. (1997) Immunogenicity and reactogenicity of a booster dose of diphtheria, tetanus, acelluar pertussis and inactivated poliomyelitis vaccines given concurrently with haemophilus type b conjugate vaccine or as pentavalent vaccine. *Ped. Infect. Dis. J.* **16,** 787–794.

15. Schneerson, R. (1997) Immunogenicity and safety of mixed DTP/IPV/Hib vaccine. *Lancet* **349,** 881,882.

16. Zepp, F., Schmitt, H. J., Kaufhold, A., Schuind, A., Knuf, M., Hubermehl, P., Meyer, C., Bogarts, H., Slavoui, M., and Clemens, R. (1997) Evidence for induction of polysaccharide specific B-cell-memory in the first year of life: plain *Haemophilus influenzae* type b-PRP (Hib) boosters children primed with a tetanus-conjugate Hib-DTPa-HBV combined vaccine. *Eur. J. Ped.* **156,** 18–24.

17. Marketing agreement signed for pediatric product line. *Vaccine Weekly*, October 28, 1996 (D. J. DeNoon, Sr. Ed.). p. 12.

18. West, P. J., Hesley, T. M., Joans, L. C., Feeley, L. K., Bird, S. R., Burke, P., and Sadoff, J. C. (1997) Safety and immunogenicity of a bivalent *Haemophilus influenzae* Type b/hepatitis b vaccine in healthy infants. Hib-HB vaccine study group. *Ped. Infect. Dis. J.* **16,** 593–599.

19. Fessard, C. and Keystone, J. S. (1997) A role for combined vaccination against hepatitis A and B? *Int. J. Infect. Dis.* **1,** 226–232.

20. White, C. J., Stinson, D., Steahle, B., Cho, I., Matthews, H., Ngai, A., Keller, P., Eiden, J., and Kuter, B. (1997) Measles, mumps, rubella and varicella combination vaccine: safety and immunogenicity alone and in combination with other vaccines given to children. measles, mumps, rubella, varicella vaccine study group. *Clin. Infect. Dis.* **24,** 925–931.

21. Lang, J., Duong, G. H., Nguyen, V. G., Le, T. T., Nguyen, C. V., Kesmedjian, V., and Plotkin, S. A. (1997). Randomized feasibility trial of pre-exposure rabies vaccination with DTP-IPV in infants. *Lancet* **349,** 1663–1665.

22. FDC Reports, Connaught TriHIBit additional *Haemophilus* antibody data submitted to FDA for analysis to adress unresolved question concerning suppression. *The Pink Sheet*, June 16, 1997, pp. 13–14.

23. Williams, J. C., Goldenthal, K. L., Burns, D. R., and Lewis, Jr., B. P., eds., (1995) Combined vaccines and simultaneous administration: current issues and perspectives from conference sponsored by CBER, USFDA, NIH, CDC, WHO in Bethesda, MD July 28–30, 1993. *Ann. NY Acad. Sci.* **754**, xi–xv.

24. Center for Biologic Evaluation and Research (1997) Guidance for industry for the evaluation of combination vaccines for preventable diseases: production, testing and clinical studies. April. *Federal Register* **62**, 17,624–17,625.

25. European Vaccines Manufacturers (1994) Combined vaccines for Europe; pharmaceutical, egulatory and policy-making aspects. *Biologicals* **22**, 297–436.

26. Committee for Proprietary Medicinal Products (1997) Pharmaceutical, pre-clinical and regulatory aspects of combined vaccines. Draft #6. March 26, 1997. Presented at Biotechnology Working Party Meeting on May 6–7, 1997.

27. Corbel, M. J. (1994) Control testing of combined vaccines: a consideration of potential problems and approaches. *Biologicals* **22**, 353–360.

28. International Conference on Harmonization Guidelines. *Guidance on Non-Clinical Safety Studies for the Conduct of Human Clinical Trials for Pharmaceuticals. Federal Register* November 25, 1997, 62,922.

29. Plotkin, S. A. (1994) Problems in the choice of combined vaccines for Europe. *Biologicals* **22**, 411–414.

30. Schaack, J-C. (1997) Harmonization of vaccination policy. *Biologicals* **25**, 243–245.

31. World Health Organization (1996) State of the world's vaccine and immunization, WHO, Geneva, Switzerland, p. 29.

32. Schlesinger, Y., Granoff, D. M., and the Vaccine Study Group (1992). Avidity and bactericidal activity of antibody elicited by different *Haemophilus influenzae* Type b conjugate vaccines. *JAMA* **267**, 1489–1494.

33. Clements, M. L. (1995) Combination live respiratory virus vaccines. *Ann. NY Acad. Sci.* **754**, 351–355.

34. Olin, P. (1995) Defining surrogate serologic tests with respect to predicting protective vaccine efficacy: pertussis vaccination. *Ann. NY Acad. Sci.* **754**, 273–277.

35. Plotkin, S. A. and Fletcher, M. A. (1996) Combination vaccines and immunization visits. *Ped. Infect. Dis. J.* **15**, 103–105.

36. Paradiso, P. R., Hogerman, D. A., Madore, D. V., Keyserling, H., King, J., Reisinger, K. S., Blatter, M. M., Rothstein, E., Bernstein, H. H., Pennridge Pediatric Associates, and Hackell, J. (1993) Safety and immunogenicity of a combined diphtheria, tetanus, pertussis and *Haemophilus influenzae* type b vaccine in young infants. *Pediatrics* **92**, 827–832.

37. Clements, J. D., Ferreccio, C., Levine, M. M., Horowitz, I., Rao, M. R., Eng, M., Edwards, K. M., and Fritzell, B. (1992) Impact of *Haemophilus influenzae* type b polysaccharide-tetanus protein conjugate vaccine on responses to concurrently administered diphtheria-tetanus-pertussis vaccine. *JAMA* **267**, 673–678.

38. Sabin, A. B. (1959) Recent studies and field tests with a live attenuated poliovirus vaccine, in *Live Poliovirus Vaccines: Papers Presented and Discussions Held at the First International Conference on Live Poliovirus Vaccines.* Pan American Sanitary Bureau (Special Publication No. 44). Washington, DC, 14–38.

39. Lee, C. J. (1983) The quantitative immunochemical determination of pneumococcal and meningococcal capsular polysaccharides by light scattering rate nephelometry. *J. Biol. Stand.* **11**, 55–64.

40. Bevilacqua. J. M., Young, L., Chiu, S. W., Sparkes, J. D., and Kreeftenberg, J. G. (1996) Rat immunogenicity assay of inactivated poliovirus. *Dev. Biol. Stand.* **86**, 121–127.

41. Blackwelder, W. C. (1995) Similarity/equivalence trials for combination vaccines. *Ann. NY Acad. Sci.* **754**, 321–328.

42. Corkill, J. M. (1967). The stability of the components in DPT-poliomyelitis and DPT-poliomyelitis-measles vaccines. *Symposia Series in Immunobiological Standardization.* Vol. 7, Basel, Karger, pp. 165–178.
43. Usonis, V., Bakasenas, V., Taylor, D., and Vandepapeliere, P. (1996) Immunogenicity and reactogenicity of a combined DTPw-hepatitis B vaccine in Lithuanian infants. *Eur. J. Pediatr.* **155,** 189–193.
44. Gardner, R. A. and Pittman, M. (1965). Relative stability of pertussis vaccine preserved with merthiolate, benzethonium chloride, or the parabens. *Appl. Microbiol.* **13,** 564–569.
45. Davisson, E. O., Powell, H. M., MacFarlane, J. O., Hodgson, R., Stone, R. L., and Culbertson, C. G. (1956). The preservation of poliomyelitis vaccine with stabilized merthiolate. *J. Lab. Clin. Med.* **47,** 8–19.
46. Sawyer, L. A., McInnis, J., Patel, A., Horne, A. D., and Albrecht, P. (1994) Deleterious effect of thimerosal on the potency of inactivated poliovirus vaccine. *Vaccine* **12,** 851–856.
47. Eskola, J., Olander, R.-M., Litmanen, L., Saarinen, L., Bogaerts, H., and Kayhty, H. (1995) Hib antibody response after two doses of combined DTPa-Hib conjugate vaccine as compared to separate injections. Interscience Conference on Antimicrobial Agents and Chemotherapy, 160. Abstract No. G11.
48. Corbel, M. J. (1996) Reasons for instability of bacterial vaccines. *Dev. Biol. Stand.* **87,** 113–124.
49. Vogel, F. R. (1995) Immunologic adjuvants for modern vaccine formulations. *Ann. NY Acad. Sci.* **754,** 153–160.
50. Gupta, R. K. (1998) Aluminum compounds as vaccine adjuvants. *Adv. Drug Del. Rev.* **32,** 155–172.
51. Chang, M. F., White, J. L., Nail, S. L., and Hem, S. L. (1997) Role of the electrostatic attractive force in the adsorption of proteins by aluminum hydroxide adjuvant. *PDA J. Pharm. Sci. Technol.* **51(1),** 25–29.
52. Ellis, R. W. and Douglas, R. G., Jr. (1994) Combination vaccines. *Int. J. Technol. Assess. Health Care* **10,** 185–192.
53. Ellis, R. W. and Brown, K. R. (1997) Combination vaccines, in *Advances in Pharmacology*, August, J. T., Anders, M. W., Murad, F., and Coyle, J. T. (eds.), Academic, San Diego, CA, pp. 393–423.
54. Grabenstein, J. D. (1990) Drug interactions involving immunologic agents. Part I. Vaccine-vaccine, vaccine-immunoglobin, and vaccine-drug interactions, DICP *Ann. Pharmacother.* **24,** 67–81.
55. Gallili, G. E. (1990) Use of combined viral vaccines, in *Viral Vaccines* (Mizrahi, A., ed.), Wiley-Liss, New York, NY, pp. 147–157.
56. Andre, F. E. and Peetermans, J. (1986) Effect of simultaneous administration of live measles vaccine on the "take rate" of live mumps vaccine. *Dev. Biol. Stand.* **65,** 101–107.
57. Meyer, H. M., Jr., Hopps, H. E., Bernheim, B. C., and Douglas, R. D. (1967) Combined measles-smallpox and other vaccines, in *First International Conference on Vaccines Against Viral and Rickettsia Diseases in Man*, Pan American Health Organization (Scientific Publication No. 147). Washington, DC, pp. 336–342.
58. Insel, R. A. (1995) Potential alterations in immunogenicity by combining or simultaneously administering vaccine components. *Ann. NY Acad. Sci.* **754,** 35–47.
59. Germain, R. N. (1995) The biochemistry and cell biology of antigen presentation by MHC Class I and Class II molecules. Implications for development of combination vaccines. *Ann. NY Acad. Sci.* **754,** 114–125.
60. Melnick, J. L. and Wallis, C. (1963) The effect of pH on thermal stabilization of oral polio virus by magnesium chloride. *Proc. Soc. Exp. Biol. Med.* **112,** 894–897.

61. Volkin, D. B., Burke, C. J., Sanyal, G., and Middaugh, C. R. (1996) Analysis of vaccine stability. *Dev. Biol. Stand.* **87,** 135–142.
62. *Federal Register,* Tuesday, September 30, 1997, Department of Health and Human Services. Natural rubber-containing medical devices; user labeling, pp. 51,021–51,030.
63. Maleckar, J., Fosseco, S., and Katkocin, D. (1996) Factors affecting the ability of experimental vaccines to protect guinea pigs against lethal challenge with diphtheria toxin. Presented at WHO/IABS/NIBSC International Meeting on the Control and Standardization of Acellular Pertussis Vaccines. NIBSC, Potters Bar, Hertfordshire, UK, September 26–27.
64. Brown, K. R. (1995) Industry perspective on clinical trial issues for combination vaccines. *Ann. NY Acad. Sci.* **754,** 241–249.
65. Mercer Management Consulting Report on the United States Vaccine Industry to the U. S. Dept. of Health and Human Services, June 14, 1995.
66. Nail, S. L., White, J. L., and Hern, S. L. (1976) Structure of aluminium hydroxide gel I. Initial precipitate. *J. Pharm. Sci.* **65,** 1188–1191.
67. Ada, G. (1994) Combination vaccines: present practices and future possibilities. *Biologicals* **22,** 329–331.
68. Daum, R. S., Jain, A., and Goldstein, K. P. (1995) Combination vaccines: some practical considerations. *Ann. NY Acad. Sci.* **754,** 383–387.
69. Peetermans, J. (1996) Factors affecting the stability of viral vaccines. *Dev. Biol. Stand.* **87,** 97–101.
70. Peetermans, J., Colinet, G., Stephenne, J., and Bouillet, A. (1978) Stability of freeze-dried and reconstituted measles vaccine. *Dev. Biol. Stand.* **41,** 259–264.
71. Needleless Injections from PowderJect (1997) SCRIP No. 2232, P. J. B. Publications, Ltd. May 16, p. 13.
72. Fox, J. L. (1997) Education seen as key in bringing vaccines to adults. *ASM News* **63,** 29–33.
73. Walker, R. I. (1994) New strategies for using mucosal vaccination to achieve more effective immunization. *Vaccine* **12,** 387–397.
74. Eskola, J. (1994) Epidemiological views into possible components of paediatric combined vaccines in 2015. *Biologicals* **22,** 323–327.

4   Pediatric Combination Vaccines

Clinical Issues

Peter R. Paradiso and Robert Kohberger

Introduction

Combination vaccines present a unique clinical research challenge because, while on the one hand they are treated as new vaccine entities, they also face the challenge of replacing existing, proven vaccines. Therefore, they must fulfill all of the criteria for new vaccines in terms of safety and efficacy and in addition must be shown to be as good as the components given separately.

This latter consideration creates a challenge which increases with the number of components being combined. The history of combination products is in fact one of interference as much as compatibility. The components of live viral vaccines such as oral polio vaccine (OPV) and measles-mumps-rubella vaccine (MMR) had to be carefully titered to overcome the potential for interference among live components to ensure adequate replication of each virus (1,2). The literature is also ripe with examples of interference among components of non-live vaccines (3–6). Diphtheria-tetanus-pertussis (DTP), a long-standing combination on its own, has always created a challenge when used in combination with yet one more component. Additions of inactivated polio components have been successful but not without difficulty whether because of more trivial issues like preservative incompatibility or because of apparent immunological interference (4). Addition of *Haemophilus influenzae* type b (Hib) components have had only partial success. In the case of whole-cell pertussis vaccines, these components have been compatible and in some cases the responses are enhanced by combination with Hib conjugate vaccine (7). In other cases, similar but not identical components have shown interference (5,6). More recently, the acellular pertussis (aP)-containing DTaP vaccines have presented a surprising challenge. Unlike their whole cell counterparts, interference among the DTaP and Hib components have been more the rule rather than the exception (8,9).

From: *Combination Vaccines: Development, Clinical Research, and Approval*
Edited by: R. W. Ellis © Humana Press Inc., Totowa, NJ

The lack of assurance in combining vaccine components creates unique challenges and problems for a clinical program. Clearly, the most difficult aspect is the demonstration of equivalence in the efficacy of the combined product, not in absolute terms, but in comparative terms. The issue is made more complex when the intangible benefits of combination products, such as the potential for increased compliance, are weighed against the potential for small reductions in efficacy.

This chapter will focus on the clinical path to development of a combination vaccine with emphasis on the types of studies that are needed and some of the statistical and clinical considerations which are common to all vaccines along with those that are unique to combination products. The emphasis will be on DTP combination vaccines as an example of a multidisease combination vaccine as opposed to multivalent combination vaccines such as pneumococcal conjugates, although many of the same principles apply.

Clinical Programs

Licensure of a combination vaccine product requires clinical demonstration of the following characteristics:

1. Safety in absolute terms and in comparison to the separately-administered components based on currently accepted practice.
2. Efficacy equivalent to or greater than that seen in separately-administered components.
3. Consistency of the immune response.
4. Compatibility with other vaccines given at the same time.

This chapter will deal with each of these issues in turn.

Equivalence

The goal of equivalence studies is to demonstrate that components given together induce an equivalent response to the individual components when given separately. Ideally, researchers would like to be able to demonstrate efficacy. Unfortunately this is rarely possible because, in general, the vaccine components are universally used in the population of interest. This makes a placebo control impossible and overall disease incidence too low to realistically undertake a comparative efficacy trial. Instead surrogate markers must be relied on to assess the efficacy of the vaccine components. In a separate section below, surrogate markers will be discussed in greater detail.

Equivalence studies are generally designed with at least two cohorts: the first receiving the individual vaccines as currently used in practice and the second receiving the combined product. It generally has been found desirable to use the same lots of vaccine in the separate and combined products in order to reduce

Table 1. Antibody Response:
Comparison of Combined Versus Separate Vaccines[a]

| | Antibody titer (GMT) | | |
Component	Combined	Separate	P-Value
Hemophilus b, μg/mL *(n)*			
Pre	0.09 (181)	0.09 (183)	.762
Post 1	0.12 (170)	0.09 (172)	.002
Post 2	0.66 (168)	0.34 (166)	<.001
Post 3	6.67 (167)	4.42 (163)	.034
Diphtheria, IU/mL *(n)*			
Pre	0.04 (89)	0.05 (91)	.624
Post 3	0.71 (89)	0.40 (91)	.009
Tetanus, U/mL *(n)*			
Pre	0.45 (128)	0.50 (120)	.404
Post 3	8.20 (124)	4.51 (125)	<.001
Pertussis agglutinins, dilution^{-1} *(n)*			
Pre	6.53 (89)	4.69 (91)	.121
Post 3	51.93 (89)	23.34 (91)	.008

[a]GMT, geometric mean titer; *(n)*, number of sera. Reprinted with permission from *Pediatrics*, 1993; **92,** 827–832.

the number of variables which could contribute to differences in the measured response. Since it is important to demonstrate that the combined product is consistently equivalent to the separately administered vaccine, it is necessary to include two and often three different lots of each component in the clinical trials. In some cases, three lots of a combined product have been compared to one lot of separately-administered vaccine (that vaccine being derived from the same lots as used in one of the combined products). This three-to-one study design has the disadvantage that if the directly-compared combined vaccine is less immunogenic than the equivalent component, even if only marginally, it is not clear whether those differences will be seen consistently from lot to lot.

In a study of a combined product of DTP and Hib conjugate *(7)*, the limits of a four-cohort study were avoided by using six cohorts: three of the combined product (DTP-Hib) and three of the separately administered DTP and Hib components. In this case, each of the separate lots matched the lots in the combined product such that it would be possible to compare groups of children whose only difference was whether they had received the same lots separately or combined. *Tables 1* and *2* show the immune responses to the individual components of the vaccines. In this case the response to several of the components was actually higher after two or three doses in the combined product than when the vaccines were administered separately to infants.

Table 2. Immunogenicity of Three Lots of DTP-HbOC[a]

Component	Antibody titer (GMT)			P-Value[b]
	Lot 1	Lot 2	Lot 3	
Hemophilus b, µg/mL *(n)*				
Pre	0.10 (57)	0.08 (63)	0.08 (61)	.489
Post 1	0.15 (55)	0.11 (57)	0.10 (58)	.121
Post 2	0.73 (53)	0.71 (55)	0.55 (60)	.583
Post 3	5.72 (54)	8.84 (54)	5.94 (59)	.361
Diphtheria, IU/mL *(n)*				
Pre	0.04 (26)	0.05 (30)	0.04 (33)	.625
Post 3	0.61 (26)	0.67 (30)	0.84 (33)	.667
Tetanus, U/mL *(n)*				
Pre	0.42 (43)	0.50 (40)	0.45 (45)	.813
Post 3	8.69 (39)	7.52 (43)	8.50 (42)	.604
Pertussis agglutinins, dilution^{-1} *(n)*				
Pre	5.08 (26)	6.06 (30)	8.52 (33)	.490
Post 3	79.21 (26)	54.66 (30)	35.54 (33)	.251

[a]One of three diphtheria-tetanus-pertussis (DTP)-HbOC vaccine lots given at 2, 4, and 6 months of age. GMT, geometric mean titer; *(n)* number of sera tested.
[b]P-Values are based on a comparison of lots using one-way analyses of variance.
Reprinted with permission from *Pediatrics,* 1993; **92,** 827–832.

In general, the ability to combine the Hib conjugate vaccines with the DTaP vaccines has been much more difficult and inconsistent. Several studies have clearly shown interference in the response to the Hib component. A recent study by Pichichero et al. *(9)* used the 3:1 combined:separate design described above. In this study, three different manufactured lots of DTaP and Hib were combined and tested in a randomized fashion. The fourth arm of the study was separate administration of DTaP and Hib from one of the combined vaccines. In this case, there was a reduction in the immune response to the Hib component in the one lot that could be directly compared in the combined and separate vaccines. The question of whether this difference was clinically significant was hindered by the fact that the consistency of this reduction could not be addressed, since only one lot could be directly compared and the three combined lots did not produce a consistent response.

Safety

Generally, safety studies of combination products are not different from those for other vaccines, except that they are compared to the separately-administered components yielding not only absolute, but also comparative endpoints. Immediate adverse events are usually measured within 4–5 days postvaccination, with rarer events measured over a several month period after immunization. One of the difficulties with these comparisons is that blinding is often not possible because the separate products are given in two shots and the combined in one. Therefore, the cohort receiving the experimental vaccine is clear. This failure in blinding could lead to an unfair disadvantage for the combined product because of heightened awareness of its experimental nature. A solution is to use a placebo to be given with the combined product either in the form of another vaccine or as a true placebo such as saline or saline/aluminum. The latter is preferable from an adverse event standpoint because it eliminates the potential confounding effects of another vaccine antigen, but not ideal since administration of a true placebo obviously has no value to the subject.

Safety evaluations in combination vaccine studies generally compare local and systemic reactions to those seen in the separately-administered cohort. Systemic reaction comparisons are straightforward. Comparison of local reactions is more complex since there are two vaccine sites, and therefore two sets of adverse reaction data are generated in the separate cohort. To date, no attempt has been made to sum the local reaction data from two sites to compare to the combined product, but rather the later is compared to the most reactogenic component of the separately-administered vaccines. In the case of the DTP-Hib studies, local reactions of the combined product were compared to DTP injection site (7).

The last safety consideration is the generation of a large safety database which permits measurement of rarer adverse events in the period postvaccination. These studies can be designed in a number of ways, but because of the large numbers of subjects, generally 1–5000, they are not always placebo-controlled, double-blinded studies. Again, using the example of DTP-Hib combinations, Black et al. (10) studied a group prospectively randomized to receive either the combined or separately administered vaccine to look particularly at adverse events immediately after vaccination, but then vaccinated a larger cohort in a nonrandomized fashion to obtain sufficient subjects to look at rarer adverse events occurring up to 30 and 60 days postvaccination. This latter study used the database of the population receiving the separate vaccine as part of their routine well-child care as the control group.

Consistency of Manufacture

Licensure of all vaccines requires the demonstration of consistency. Consistency is generally defined in two ways. The first is consistency of manufacture in which it is demonstrated that the vaccine can be consistently produced to pass the specifications required to release it for use in people. The second definition is a clinical one and requires the demonstration of a consistent immune response to multiple vaccine lots. Three lots generally are considered sufficient for both parameters and in fact for practical reasons are often the same lots for both parameters. The clinical demonstration of equivalence from a consistency standpoint is not unlike the studies showing the equivalence of combined vs separate vaccines. In some cases these studies are done simultaneously (7), but this is not required.

One of the problems related to the current methods for demonstrating clinical consistency is that these trials are contrived from the standpoint of being totally unlike standard practice. Once a vaccine is licensed, it is very unlikely that infants will receive even two doses of vaccine from the same manufacturing run since, over a six-month period, providers are likely to have purchased new vaccine from a different lot. Therefore, studies where infants receive all three doses of the same lot of vaccine are well-controlled but perhaps not the only way to demonstrate consistency. Another example would be to measure consistency in the context of, for example, a large-scale efficacy trial. Most large-scale efficacy trials are done over a several year period using multiple lots of vaccine over that period. Vaccine lots are generally introduced sequentially over time and children are likely to receive different lots of vaccine. In such situations, random measures of antibody response at preset times within the population could be used to demonstrate that infants consistently respond to vaccine. Although possible only if enough different lots of vaccine are used over a sufficient period of time, this approach might measure more accurately the clinical consistency parameters that mimic vaccine use after licensure.

Compatibility With Other Routinely Administered Vaccines

Clinical studies which demonstrate that a new vaccine does not inhibit and is not inhibited by other routine vaccines given at the same time is routinely required for licensure (11). From an immunological standpoint, combination of two routinely used vaccines are not likely to create interference problems with other vaccines. However, at least for the purposes of use recommendations, such studies are still important.

These studies have become more complex with the introduction of new vaccines and the acceptance of alternative vaccine strategies. Recent examples are the introduction of DTaP vaccines (12), the increased use of inactivated poliomyelitis vaccine (IPV) in the polio vaccination schedule (13), and the availability of several different Hib conjugate vaccines. Studies initiated five years ago may have used vaccines which are no longer used in the same way. Similarly, compatibility with vaccines given in the second year of life are confounded by the fact that these vaccines are often not given simultaneously and there are many permutations of multiple vaccinations that must be considered when planning compatibility trials. Finally, there are often multiple products of a particu-

Table 3. Correlate of Immunity

Antigen	Protective correlate[a]
Diphtheria	>0.01 antitoxin U/mL
Tetanus	>.01 antitoxin U/mL
Polio	Seroconversion[b]
Hepatitis B	>10 U/mL

[a]Refs. *15–18*.
[b]By neutralization antibody assay.

lar type (e.g., hepatitis b [HB] vaccine from two manufacturers). In general, this latter point has not been an issue, but could become one in situations where vaccines for the same disease are significantly different in character.

Correlates of Immunity

Probably the most difficult issue associated with the clinical testing of combination vaccines is the satisfactory demonstration of equivalent efficacy. The demonstration of efficacy is dependent on correlating efficacy to some immune parameter, since true placebo controlled efficacy trials are not feasible. For many antigens, this does not present a significant problem since correlates are known and well accepted. Probably the best examples are the bacterial toxoids for immunity to diphtheria and tetanus. In this case, the ability of >90% of the population to achieve antibody titers in excess of the long-term protective levels is considered sufficient to demonstrate efficacy. Similar correlates have been accepted for polio and HB *(see Table 3) (14–17)*. The obvious advantage of such correlates is that if the geometric mean antibody response to these antigens is reduced in the combination vaccine, the clinical significance of those reductions can be assessed. Obviously these reductions are of lesser concern when responses are well above the protective titers in close to 100% of the population. However, as that percentage is reduced, the implications become more difficult to assess.

This is particularly true in the case of vaccines such as the aP and Hib conjugate vaccines for which correlates of immunity have not been established. Recently this issue has been in the literature because of interference encountered when combining the two vaccines in the form of DTaP-Hib. Studies with these components from various manufacturers have shown that in particular, the response to the Hib conjugate is reduced in the combined products after a primary series of vaccine is given to infants. This decrease in response, as measured by geometric mean titers (GMT), has ranged from 3- to 10-fold *(9,18)*. Because there is not a clear correlate of immunity for Hib vaccines, the clinical significance of reductions in immune response are difficult to assess.

For Hib, the generally accepted measures of immune status are the percentage of vaccinees who achieve titers of either 0.15 µg/mL or 1.0 µg/mL of anti-polysaccharide antibody which correspond to short term and long term protection respectively *(19,20)*. Using the 1.0 µg/mL level, the percentage of the population achieving this level can be measured and assessed with the assumption that the efficacy will be high (e.g., >90%) in the portion of the population with titers above this level. It follows therefore that if the majority of the population has titers that are well above the 1.0 µg/mL level, then at some point higher titers will have a marginal effect on efficacy.

However, the exact efficacy at any given titer is not known for these vaccines. This is especially true between titers of 0.15 and 1.0 µg/mL. It seems unlikely that "protection" has an all-or-none relationship with any titer but rather that there is a gradual decrease in efficacy with decreasing titer. Regardless of the exact relationship between titer and efficacy, a reduction in titer within a population will equate to a reduction in efficacy. The greater the percentage of the population that is below 1 µg/mL, the greater the potential for changes to effect efficacy. Assuming that titers have a log-normal distribution with a standard deviation of 1.5 (typically seen in studies), with a GMT = 4.0 µg/mL, approx 20% of the population will have a titer <1.0 µg/mL. A twofold reduction in GMT to 2.0 µg/mL would increase that percentage to 30%.

The clinical implications of such a reduction are unknown but are not zero. The difference in percentage "responders" increases as the differences in mean titers increase and as the absolute titers decrease. It then becomes an issue of what theoretical reduction in efficacy is acceptable. One could argue that no reduction is ethically acceptable since the separately administered vaccines are available and in use. However, it can also be argued that the increased convenience of combination products increases the utilization not only of the components in the questioned combination, but in the other vaccines given at the same time.

Statistical Methods

The last important issue in combination trial design is the issue of statistical methods for designing and analyzing trials for comparing combined administration with separate administration. These trials are not the same as trials where the desire is to demonstrate a difference between a treatment and a placebo. In the usual difference trials, the null hypothesis (i.e., the hypothesis that researchers wish to reject) is that there is no difference between treatments. Rejecting this null hypothesis means that there is a difference between treatments, but not rejecting the hypothesis does not mean that there is no difference. With difference testing, the inability to show a difference may be very dependent on the sample size. If the sample size is too small, the power to show differences will be small. In combination vaccine trials, it is desired to test whether the different administrations are equivalent. This requires a different approach to hypothesis testing than the more familiar difference testing.

In more formal statistical terms, the hypothesis may be formulated as:

$$H_o: \text{difference} \leq L \text{ or difference} \geq U$$

$$H_a: L < \text{difference} < U$$

The null hypothesis (H_o) that researchers hope to reject is that the difference between treatments does not lie within certain lower and upper limits (defined by L and U), and the alternate hypothesis (H_a) is that the difference lies within these limits, which is the goal in showing equivalence. The Type I error is the chance of rejecting H_o when the true difference is < L or > U, i.e., making a mistake. Typically, normal practice will set this = 0.05, or only a 5% chance of that occurring. The Type II error is the chance of not rejecting H_o when the true difference lies within L and U. In practical terms if H_o is rejected, it has been statistically demonstrated that the combined administration is equivalent to separate administration as defined by the limits L and U.

The statistical methods for testing this equivalence hypothesis can be shown to use two-sided 90% confidence limits (assuming a Type I error = 0.05) on the difference between treatments *(21)*. If the confidence limit lies entirely within the interval L to U, then the hypothesis may be rejected. It should be noted that it may be appropriate to use one-sided tests, since it may only be of interest whether the combined administration decreases immunogenicity, not whether it increases immunogenicity. In such a case the null hypothesis is a difference < L.

There are two major issues in these types of equivalency trials. The first is the definition of L and U, which is the numeric way of stating exactly what we mean by "equivalent" and the second is how to determine sample sizes in such trials. It is not possible to demonstrate that two treatments are exactly equal. Researchers must define how different the treatments could be and still be acceptable (e.g., L and U). For example, do GMTs need to be within a two-, four-, or higher-fold range, or do percent responders need to be within 10, 20, or 30%? This is a very difficult question which must rely on clinical judgment and historical experience.

Exact methods for sample size determination have not been thoroughly determined. Consider that in combination trials there are multiple antigens that must be tested and all null hypotheses must be rejected before the combination product can be declared equivalent to separate administration. There is a defined power *(p)* for comparing each antigen. If the responses to the individual antigens are independent, then the overall power in a combination containing n components is p^n. Consider a combination product such as DTaP–Hib, which could have seven antigens tested. If it is assumed that all are independent, for an overall power of 90%, each individual test needs a power of 98.51%. As a result, sample sizes must increase dramatically to achieve the desired power. Moreover, in combination trials not only are GMTs tested, but also the percentage responders for each antigen, so the number of comparisons can be doubled.

To demonstrate the sample size issues, consider a combination product with seven antigens that have log-normal distributions with a standard deviation = 1.2. This assumption is about what is seen in DTaP–Hib combination products. Furthermore, assume that the seven antigens are independent. Sample sizes will be developed just for the situation where GMT are to be tested. A two-sided test with an error = 0.05 also is assumed.

The sample size required to show equivalence when L and U are within 50% and 200% of the comparator (e.g., within twofold) or with 66% and 150% (1.5-fold difference) can be seen here.

Equivalence criteria L, U	Sample size individual test
50, 200%	102
66, 150%	290

The required sample size is very sensitive to the equivalence definition.

The difficulty with this example is that antigens are not independent and, perhaps more importantly, if percentage responders are included in the required equivalence definition, these also are correlated with GMT. The methods for sample size calculation in these correlated situations are still being examined.

Conclusions

With the recent introduction of new biological products and expectation of new products in the next several years, issues regarding the design of clinical trials will become critical. Currently, infants in the United States and in many parts of the world receive various combinations of DTaP (DTP), Hib conjugate, IPV, and HB. Work is being done by numerous groups to try to combine all or some of these components. The more components, the greater the complexity of the trials and the analyses.

New products in clinical trials will face many of the same issues outlined above. A particularly good example is the pneumococcal conjugate vaccine. This vaccine contains several conjugate vaccines in order to cover the most prevalent pneumococcal serotypes and is in itself a combination vaccine. While it will be necessary to show a consistent response to each serotype, since it is a new vaccine, comparison to individual components will not be necessary. However, work is already underway to combine this vaccine with other glyco-conjugates such as for *Neisseria meningitidis* groups A and C along with the Hib conjugate. Such a combination could contain as many as 14 components. Combining this formulation with the standard infant DTP or DTaP would provide a global product which comprehensively covers the most important vaccine preventable infant. The headaches from a clinical plan perspective are as daunting as the prospect for the vaccine is exciting!

References

1. Sabin, A. B. and Boulger, L. R. (1973) History of Sabin attenuated poliovirus oral live vaccine strains. *Biol. Stand* **1**, 115–125.
2. Stokes J., Weibel, R. E., Villarejos, V. M., Arguedes, G., Bunyak, E. B., and Hilleman, M. R. (1971) Trivalent combined measles-mumps-rubella vaccine. Findings in clinical laboratory studies. *JAMA* **218**, 57–61.
3. Dagan, R., Botujancky, C., Watemberg, N., Arbelli, Y., Belmaker, I., Ethevenaux, C., and Fritzell, B. (1994) Safety and immunogenicity in young infants of Haemophilus b-tetanus protein conjugate vaccine, mixed in the same syringe with diphtheria-tetanus-pertussis-enhanced inactivated polio vaccine. *Ped. Infant Dis. J.* **13**, 356–361.
4. Halperin, S. A., Langley, J. M., and Eastwood, B. J. (1996) Effect of inactivated poliovirus vaccine on the antibody response to *Bordatella pertussis* antigens when combined with diphtheria-pertussis-tetanus vaccine. *Clin. Infct. Dis.* **22**, 59–62.
5. Ferreccio, C., Clemens, J., Arendano, A. Horwitz, I., Flores, C., Avila, L., Cayazzo, M., Fritzell, B., Cadoz, M., and Levine, M. (1991) The clinical and immunology response of Chilean infants to *Haemophilus influenzae* type b polysaccharide-tetanus conjugate vaccine coadministered in the same syringe with diphtheria-tetanus toxoids-pertussis vaccine at two, four, and six months of age. *Ped. Infant Dis. J.* **10**, 764–771.
6. Clemens, J. D., Ferrecio, C., Levine, M. M. Horwitz, I., Rao, M. R., Edwards, K. M., and Fritzell, B (1992) Impact of *Haemophilus influenzae* type b polysaccharide-tetanus protein conjugate vaccine on responses to concurrently administered diphtheria-tetanus-pertussis vaccine. *JAMA* **267**, 673–678.
7. Paradiso, P. R, Hogerman, D. A., Madore, D. V., Keyserling, H., King, J., Reisinger, K. S., Blatter, M. M., Rotherstien, E., Bernstein, H. H., Pennridge Pediatric Associates, and Hackell, J. (1993) Safety and Immunogenicity of a Combined Diphtheria-tetanus, pertussis and *Haemophilus influenzae* type b vaccine in young infants. *Pediatrics* **92**, 827–832.
8. Eskola, J., Olander, R-M., Hovi, T., Litmanen, L., Peltola, S., and Kayhty, H. (1996) Randomised trial of the effect of co-administration with acellular pertusis DTP vaccine on immunogenicity of *Haemophilus influenzae* type b conjugate vaccine. *Lancet* **348**, 1688–1692.
9. Pichichero, M. E., Latiolais, T., Bernstein, D. I., Hosbach, P., Christian, E., Vidor, E., Meschievitz, C., and Dacum, R. S. (1997) Vaccine antigen interactions after a combination diphtheria-tetanus toxoid-acellular pertussis/purified capsular polysaccharide of *Haemophilus influenzae* type b-tetanus toxoid vaccine in two, four, and six month old infants. *PIDJ* **16**, 863–870.
10. Black, S. B., Shinefield, H. R., Ray, P., Lewis, E. M., Fireman, B., Hiatt, R., Madore, D. V., and Johnson, C. L. (1993) Safety of combined oligosaccharide conjugate *Haemophilus influenzae* type b (HbOC) and whole cell diphtheria-tetanus toxoids-pertussis vaccine in infancy. *Pediatr. Infect. Dis. J.* **12(12)**, 981–985.
11. Halsey, N. A., Blatter, M., Bader, G., Thoms, M. L., Willingham, F. F., O'Donovan, J. C., Pakula, L., Berut, F., Reisinger, K. S., and Meschievitz, C. (1997) Inactivated poliovirus vaccine alone or sequential inactivated and oral poliovirus vaccine in two, four, and six month old infants with combination *Haemophilus influenzae* type b hepatitis b vaccine. *Pediatr. Infect. Dis. J.* **16(7)**, 675–679.

12. Pertussis vaccination: use of acellular pertussis vaccines among infants and young children (1997) *MMWR* **46(RR-7),** 1–25.
13. Poliomyelitis prevention in the United States: introduction of a sequential vaccination schedule of inactivated polio vaccine followed by oral polio vaccine. (1997) *MMWR* **46(RR-3),** 1–25.
14. Recommendations of the Immunization Practices Advisory Committee (ACIP). Poliomyelitis prevention (1982) *MMWR* **31(3),** 22–34.
15. *Federal Register Notice*, Friday, December 13, 1985, vol. 50, no. 240.
16. Pappenheimer, A. M. (1984) Diptheria, *Bacterial Vaccines*. Academic, New York, pp. 1–36.
17. Hollinger, F. B. (1996) Hepatitis b virus, *Fields Virology*, 3rd ed. (Fields, B. N., ed.), Lippincott-Raven, Philadelphia, PA, pp. 2739–2807.
18. Edwards, K. M. and M. D. Decker (1997) Combination vaccines consisting of acellular pertusis vaccines. *Pediatr. Infect. Dis. J.* **16(4),** S97–S102.
19. Anderson, P. (1984) The protective level of serum antibodies to the capsular polysaccharide of *Haemophilus influenzae* type b (letter). *J. Infect. Dis.* **149(6),** 1034,1035.
20. Kayhty, H., Peltola, H., Karanko, V., and Makela, P. H. (1983) The protective level of serum antibodies to the capsular polysaccharide of *Haemophilus influenzae* type b. *J. Infect. Dis.* **147(6),** 1100.
21. Blackwelder, W. C. (1982) Proving the Null Hypothesis in clinical trials. *Cont. Clin. Trials* **3,** 345–353.

5   Immunological Correlates for Efficacy of Combination Vaccines

Ronald W. Ellis

Introduction

Vaccines are licensed on the basis of their efficacy in preventing or treating a disease or infection. Such efficacy typically is demonstrated in a Phase 3 clinical trial with disease as an endpoint. The group receiving the vaccine is compared to a control group (e.g., receiving placebo, historical control, case control) in order to calculate the level of efficacy.

Once efficacy has been demonstrated at a high enough level for a vaccine to be licensed initially, the vaccine may undergo changes as part of the evolution of the product. Such changes may include manufacturing with a different process or at a different scale, changing the dosage level or formulation, or creating combination vaccines by mixing with other vaccine(s). Combination vaccines are attractive as products, since they can reduce the number of immunizations and can lead to increased use for the many available vaccines *(1,2)*. Is it necessary for the developer to demonstrate clinical efficacy yet again in case of any such change in the product, especially for creating a new combination vaccine? There may be significant or impenetrable hurdles to running another efficacy trial, including a vaccine-mediated reduction in the incidence of disease that is significant enough to make the trial impractical, or the ethical dilemma of repeating the trial with a control group once a known efficacious product has become available. Because vaccines function through immunological means, there may be an immune response to a particular vaccine that correlates well with its protective efficacy. Ideally, such an immune response is qualitatively or quantitatively low or absent in individuals who are shown to be susceptible to disease or infection and is present or at higher levels through naturally acquired immunity or in those who are protected following prior immunization. The

From: *Combination Vaccines: Development, Clinical Research, and Approval*
Edited by: R. W. Ellis © Humana Press Inc., Totowa, NJ

laboratory parameter that is used to measure such an immune response associated with protection is called an "immunological correlate of efficacy." Such correlates may be used effectively in the evaluation and licensure of combination vaccines. The best correlate of efficacy is one where there is a clearly identified assay, known as a "surrogate assay." A defined quantitative level of antibodies (or measurement of another type of immune response) associated with protection is known as the "seroprotective level" of antibodies (although it should be noted that a seroprotective level typically is relative, not absolute). For some infectious diseases, especially those with relatively long incubation periods, induction of seroconversion by vaccines is paralleled by the induction of immunological memory, the latter providing a mechanism for long-term protection even if antibody titers wane.

Relevance of Correlates of Efficacy to Different Types of Combination Vaccines

The basic principle is that if there is a demonstrated immunological correlate of efficacy for a particular vaccine, then the combination of that vaccine with other vaccines can be qualified for regulatory purposes by a clinical trial that measures the correlate by serological endpoints, thereby obviating a new efficacy trial. Before clinical trials of a vaccine are undertaken, correlates may be inferred by serological studies in animal models of infection, by studying serology in a large human population which is susceptible to infection, or by evaluating the level of protection afforded by immune globulin (IG) specific for a given infection.

MULTIDISEASE

Multidisease combinations vaccines are for diseases caused by different microorganisms, e.g., DTP (diphtheria-tetanus-pertussis); MMR (measles-mumps-rubella). These usually are combinations of licensed components. Thus, it would not be expected that efficacy would need to be shown again for components with demonstrated efficacy, assuming comparable immunogenicity. Correlates of efficacy are useful for demonstrating that a given vaccine is as effective in combination as it is *per se*. One challenge arises when a vaccine being developed into a combination does not have a validated correlate of efficacy, e.g., acellular pertussis and varicella. In such cases, the combination may be qualified on the basis of serologically comparable immunogenicity. While one might argue that using serological comparability is an unsound basis for qualifying such a combination, the only alternatives would be to mandate another efficacy trial (with its possible attendant ethical or other practical concerns) or to skip developing the combination vaccine entirely. Given the benefits of having combination vaccines, using serological comparability at least provides some degree of rigor in qualifying the combination. Postmarketing surveillance could confirm the continued effectiveness of each component in the combination vaccine.

MULTIVALENT

A multivalent combination is for a disease caused by one microorganism with multiple antigenic types (serotypes) or groups (serogroups), e.g., *Streptococcus pneumoniae* (pneumococcal) or poliovirus (polio). In order to have a significant impact on a disease, a multivalent combination usually is licensed initially as a combination rather than as individual serotypes. It is assumed that each serotype of the same microorganism causes disease by the same or similar mechanism and that a vaccine against each serotype functions through similar immunological mechanisms. Thus, once a correlate has been established for one serotype of vaccine, it is expected that the correlate could be used to qualify other serotypes for the same vaccine. One complication is that although the correlate would measure the same qualitative type of immune response for all serotypes, the seroprotective level may vary among serotypes or serogroups.

It should be noted that a vaccine also can be multicomponent, i.e., consists of several different vaccine antigens. Prominent examples are the multicomponent acellular pertussis (aP) vaccines, described later. Such a vaccine is not considered a combination *per se*, but may be combined with other vaccines (diphtheria, tetanus) into a combination vaccine.

Assays for Measuring Immune Responses

The overwhelming majority of protective immune responses that have been identified for available vaccines are measured by antibody assays. Such assays usually are performed on serum samples from subjects in clinical studies, although for studies involving mucosal immunization such as rotavirus and cholera, assays also are performed on mucosal fluids such as saliva and feces. Techniques commonly used to measure antibodies include enzyme-linked immunosorbent assay (ELISA), radioimmunoassay (RIA), neutralization (Nt), passive hemagglutination (PHA), hemagglutination inhibition (HI), complement fixation (CF), and immunofluorescence (IF) *(3)*. It is most practical if the assay which measures the correlate is easy to perform with large numbers of clinical samples, with common reagents, and with routinely trained (not necessarily highly specialized) personnel. Although all of the above assays are amenable to accurate quantification, ELISA and RIA generally are preferred for reasons of objectivity, throughput, relatively low variability, and interlaboratory comparisons. With the movement in many groups to eliminate the unnecessary use of radioactive isotopes, it is expected that ELISAs will continue to become the most commonly used assays for evaluating immune responses in clinical trials. Nevertheless, there are cases in which cellular immune responses may be correlates of immunity, especially for some experimental vaccines. Thus, techniques such as T-cell proliferation and ELISPOT (ELISA on individual antibody-secreting B-cells) *(4)* may become used increasingly, notwithstanding their technical challenges in widespread use, reproducibility, and validation.

In all serological assays that measure antibodies, the concentration of specific antibodies in each clinical sample can be calculated in terms of units or ng or µg/mL. This calculation is made relative to a serum standard with a precalculated level of the specific antibodies being measured. The titer is measured against a predetermined endpoint in a serological assay. Once the titer has been determined for each sample, the geometric mean titer (GMT) is calculated for the entire clinical cohort. Conclusions regarding the immunogenicity of a component vaccine by itself relative to the component in combination are made based upon the comparison of GMTs of cohorts receiving each vaccine. In these assays, seroconversion is defined as the appearance of any detectable antibody (according to the assay parameters) in a previously seronegative subject, and the seroconversion rate can be calculated for each cohort. Similarly, the seroprotection rate above a predetermined cutoff is defined as the percent of a cohort achieving seroprotective levels of antibody following immunization (where the correlate is known). In addition to measuring the actual level of antibodies, other properties of the induced antibodies may be measured, including affinity, avidity, epitope recognition, and functionality in tests like Nt and opsonization.

Protective Immune Responses for Different Vaccines

The following sections review the status of knowledge of correlates of efficacy for most widely-used vaccines and a summary of the general properties of the vaccine and its target population. These form the framework for evaluating and interpreting correlates of efficacy for combinations of these vaccines (as well as for other vaccines not listed here) in the context of how the vaccine is used in the field. Surrogate antibody assays for evaluating correlates of efficacy are summarized in *Table 1*. It should be noted that all of the following vaccines are administered parenterally, except for rotavirus and oral polio. All of the following vaccines have a single component which elicits group-common immunity, except for four (polio, pneumococcal, influenza, and rotavirus) that are multivalent.

Diphtheria

The diptheria (D) vaccine antigen is a toxin secreted from *Corynebacterium diphtheriae*. The D toxin is purified and inactivated with formalin, which was shown to eliminate toxicity without destroying immunogenicity *(5)*. The potency of the vaccine is quantified by flocculation with standard antiserum and is

Table 1. Surrogate Antibody Assays for Individual Vaccines in Combination

Vaccine	Type of assay	Specificity of assay	Surrogate
Diphtheria	RIA, ELISA, Nt	Toxoid	+
Tetanus	RIA, ELISA, Nt	Toxoid	+
Pertussis (whole cell)	Nt, ELISA, agglutination	Various antigens	−
Pertussis (acellular)	Nt, ELISA, agglutination	Various antigens	?
Measles	HI, ELISA, Nt	Whole virion	+
Mumps	HI, ELISA, Nt	Whole virion	+
Rubella	HI, ELISA, Nt	Whole virion	+
Varicella	ELISA, Nt	Whole virion, glycoproteins	?
Influenza	HI, Nt	Whole virion	+
Polio	Nt	Whole virion	+
Hepatitis B	RIA, ELISA	Surface protein	+
Hepatitis A	RIA, ELISA	Whole virion	+
Rotavirus	Nt, ELISA	Whole virion	−
Hib conjugate	RIA, ELISA	Capsular polysaccharide	+
Pneumococcal	RIA, ELISA	Capsular polysaccharide	+
Pneumococcal conjugate	ELISA	Capsular polysaccharide	?

measured in units called limits of flocculation (Lf). For enhancing immunogenicity, the D toxin is adsorbed to aluminum salts (6), whether monovalent or combined with other vaccines. The D toxin has been combined for over 50 years with T toxoid and pertussis vaccine into DTP vaccine, which has been the world's first and most widely used multidisease combination vaccine. Lower levels of D toxoid have been combined with T toxoid, and this Td vaccine has been used to immunize adults. In countries in which immunization has been widely used, diphtheria has disappeared almost completely. The degree of protection against clinical disease has been shown to be correlated with the level of serum antibody against the toxin and standardized to international units (IU) IU/mL relative to an international serum reference standard (7). The level of 0.01 IU anti-D/mL is accepted as the protective level of antibodies, although a titer >0.05 IU anti-D/mL is considered to indicate optimal protection (8). The vaccine typically is given (as part of DTP vaccine) three times in the first year of life, with boosters at ages 2 and 5–6. Anti-D titers wane into adulthood to below protective levels in many individuals. This has been of concern in developed countries, even though the incidence of C. diphtheriae infection is very low. Therefore, as a conservative measure many authorities recommend booster immunization with Td vaccine every 10 years during adulthood (9).

Tetanus

The tetanus (T) vaccine antigen is a toxin secreted from *Clostridium tetani*. In the production process, the T toxin is purified. Based on success with D toxin in achieving inactivation and retaining immunogenicity, T toxin is inactivated with formalin *(10)*. The potency of the vaccine is quantified by flocculation and measured as Lf units. The adsorption of T toxoid onto aluminum hydroxide or phosphate as adjuvant also has been shown to enhance immunogenicity *(11)*; adsorbed toxoid is mixed with D and P into DTP vaccine or with D into Td vaccine. Where it is widely used, immunization with T toxoid has resulted in the virtual disappearance of tetanus in children and adults. However, in many areas of the world without adequate levels of hygiene, infants in their first month of life can contract infection by *C. tetani*; this neonatal form of tetanus can occur in infants whose mothers did not possess adequate neutralizing levels of anti-toxin antibodies *(12)*. Serum antibodies to T toxoid have been quantified historically by Nt and PHA *(13)*. More recently, RIA and ELISA have been employed as assays that are more reproducible and amenable to automation *(14)*. Protection against clinical disease has been considered to be correlated with a serum anti-T titer >0.01 IU/mL, as standardized to an international reference serum *(7)*. The vaccine typically is given (as part of DTP vaccine) three times in the first year of life, with boosters at ages 2 and 5–6. Given that booster immunizations should maintain long-term immunity *(15)*, it has been recommended that routine boosters using Td vaccine be given to adults every 10 years *(9)*.

Pertussis

The historically widely used whole-cell pertussis (P) vaccine (wP) consists of intact bacterial cells of *Bordetella pertussis* that are collected and inactivated by treatment with one of a variety of agents, which include formalin, glutaral-dehyde, and heat *(16)*. The wP vaccine is adsorbed to aluminum salts, which increase immunogenicity and reduce reactogenicity (especially to lipopolysac-charide in the vaccine). As a whole-cell vaccine with many antigens, establishing a potency test needed to have a different focus from those of other vaccines that used purified antigens or live viruses or bacteria. The wP vaccine is quantified for use on the basis of opacity units, which is a measure of the number of *B. pertussis* organisms in a dose. However, the potency is measured in a mouse protection test in which immunized mice are challenged intracerebrally with live *B. pertussis* organisms *(17)*; data from this test have been shown historically to correlate with protection in humans *(18)*. Nevertheless, even data from this test are not necessarily predictive of efficacy, since vaccine lots which had passed this test were shown to confer low rates of protective efficacy when used as controls in efficacy trials of aP vaccines *(19)*. The wP vaccine is administered as part of DTP vaccine. The immunogenicity of wP vaccines has been measured by RIA or ELISA using specific *B. pertussis* protein antigens, e.g., pertussis toxoid (PT), filamentous hemagglutinin (FHA), agglutinogens (Agg), and pertactin (Pert) *(20)*. However, data from these serological assays have not been shown to correlate with protection against clinical infection, so that there has been no reliable accepted correlate of efficacy for the wP vaccine.

Because of the relatively poor tolerability of the wP vaccine, second-generation P vaccines have been developed (aP vaccines) that use 1–5 purified *B. pertussis* proteins as vaccine antigens. These vaccines all include PT as antigen; all but one also include FHA, and some include Pert and Agg *(19)*. The vaccine antigens are purified from cultures of native *B. pertussis*, and the PT is inactivated chemically. However, one of the aP vaccines utilizes a purified genetically-inactivated PT as well as other proteins purified from the same recombinant *B. pertussis* strain *(21)*. The aP antigens are adsorbed to aluminum adjuvant and mixed with D and T to constitute DTaP vaccines. Most of the DTaP vaccines have shown rates of protective efficacy >70% in controlled efficacy trials and have been shown to be well-tolerated *(19)*. Immune responses in clinical trials have been measured with ELISAs specific to each vaccine antigen used in the trials. However, there has been no clear indication from these trials as to which type of immune response might be a useful correlate of efficacy *(19)*. It should be noted that virtually all trials of aP vaccines have been as DTaP vaccine. Therefore, the DTwP and DTaP vaccines each have been treated as a licensed component to be mixed with other components such as Hib conjugate, hepatitis B (HB), and polio vaccines in pediatric multidisease combination vaccines.

Polio

There are two types of polio vaccine which have been in widespread use. One type, oral polio vaccine (OPV), is a trivalent mixture of live attenuated viruses which are grown in culture *(22)*. The idea behind the use of a live vaccine was to reproduce the natural infection and thereby stimulate longer-lasting protection against reinfection, since the natural infection confers lifelong immunity. Attenuation was made possible by the passage of polioviruses in non-nervous system tissues. This resulted in a loss of their ability to replicate in the nervous system, thereby losing virulence *(23)*. Potency of each component of the vaccine is quantified by infectious units in cell culture *(24)*. Owing to differences in their relative infectivities, 6-fold as much type 3 and 10-fold as much type 1 poliovirus is included relative to the amount of infectious type 2 poliovirus *(25)*. These viruses interfere with one another in vivo, hence the full regimen of three doses is required for full immunization. Having been used worldwide for decades, OPV is on its way to potentially eradicating polio worldwide by the middle of the next decade, an achievement matched to date only by smallpox vaccine.

Immunization at 2–4–6 months of age with OPV elicits serum neutralizing antibodies in close to 100% of infants and children following three doses *(26)*. Immunization also elicits immunity in the gut, based on secretory IgA, which may exist even when levels of serum antibody are low *(27)*. There is priming for persistent antibody levels and for immunological memory *(28)*. Given the relative ease of measuring serum antibodies as opposed to antibodies in gut secretions, the presence of detectable serum neutralizing antibodies is accepted as the serological correlate of protection, as commonly measured by a micro-Nt assay *(29)*.

The second type of vaccine, inactivated polio vaccine (IPV), is made by growing and collecting poliovirus, which then is purified and inactivated with formalin *(30)*. Like OPV, this vaccine is trivalent. Changes to the original production process resulted in an enhanced IPV (eIPV) which is in widespread use *(31)*. Potency of IPV is quantified in vitro in terms of D-antigen units and also can be tested in animals relative to an international vaccine reference *(31)*. One advantage to the use of IPV in developed countries is that its use does not result in vaccine-associated polio paralysis, which is a rare complication of the use of OPV. The current recommendation for polio vaccination in the United States is the use of IPV at 2 and 4 months and OPV at 6 and 15 months of age *(32)*. Immunization at 2–4–6 months of age with IPV elicits neutralizing antibodies after the first dose in close to 100% of infants and children and secretory IgA following the second and third doses *(33)*. There also is long-term persistence of neutralizing antibodies and priming for long-term memory *(34)*. As for OPV, the micro-Nt assay is used as a surrogate assays for the detection of serum neutralization antibodies, the correlate of efficacy *(29)*.

Measles

This vaccine consists of live attenuated measles virus grown in cells in culture, usually chicken embryo fibroblasts *(35,36)*. The virus is collected in culture medium and diluted in stabilizer to its final use level, (may be mixed with other vaccines [mumps, rubella]), then lyophilized. The potency of the vaccine is quantified on the basis of its in vitro infectivity in appropriate indicator cells, in assays which measure plaque forming units (pfu) or tissue-culture-infectious-dose ($TCID_{50}$). The vaccine is indicated for immunization at 12–18 months of age. Some countries with a high incidence of disease in early childhood immunize children as early as 9 months of age, with some experimental vaccines having been tested as early as 6 months of age *(37)*. In developed countries, the vaccine is administered together with mumps and rubella as MMR and is given in a two-dose series, with the booster dose being given on entry to primary or secondary school *(32,38)*. The accepted immunological correlate of efficacy is titer of antivirion antibodies, with neutralizing antibodies being most directly related to clinical protection *(39)*. Surrogate assays are either Nt assays or are based on the detection of such antibodies and comparison with neutralizing antibody titrations *(36)* utilizing a range of serological techniques including HI, CF, and ELISA, with seroprotective levels defined according to the assay *(39)*.

Mumps

The vaccine consists of live attenuated mumps virus grown in cells in culture, usually chicken embryo fibroblasts *(40)*. The virus is produced and its potency quantified as for measles vaccine. Primary immunization is indicated at 12–18 months of life. In developed countries, the vaccine is administered together with mumps and rubella as MMR and is given in a two-dose series, with the booster dose upon entry to primary school or secondary school *(32,38)*. As for measles vaccine, the immunological correlate of efficacy against mumps has been accepted to be antibodies directed against the virion, especially virus-neutralizing antibodies. Surrogate assays are either Nt assays or based upon the detection of such antibodies and demonstration of correlation with neutralizing antibody titrations *(41)*, utilizing serological techniques including HI and ELISA with seroprotective levels defined accordingly.

Rubella

The vaccine consists of live attenuated rubella virus grown in cells in culture, usually human diploid fibroblasts *(42)*. The virus is produced and its potency quantified as for measles vaccine. The vaccine is indicated for immunization at 12–18 months of life. In developed countries, the vaccine is administered together with mumps and rubella as MMR and is given in a two-dose series, with the booster dose upon entry to primary school or secondary school *(32,38)*. Some countries have focused their immunization practice upon teenage girls, with the goal of establishing a high level of rubella-specific antibodies during the child-bearing period which can be transmitted transplacentally to the fetus in order to minimize the likelihood of *in utero* infection with rubella virus and its teratogenic consequences *(43)*. However, this strategy has proven suboptimal for control. As for measles and mumps vaccines, the immunological correlate of efficacy has been accepted to be antibodies directed against the virion, especially virus-neutralizing antibodies. Surrogate assays are either Nt assays or are based upon the detection of such antibodies *(44)* utilizing serological techniques including HI, CF, and ELISA, with seroprotective levels defined according to each assay.

Varicella

Varicella (chickenpox) vaccine consists of live attenuated varicella-zoster virus (VZV) grown in human diploid fibroblasts *(45)*. Very little infectious virus is secreted into culture medium. Thus, the infected cells are lysed in buffer and sonicated, diluted in stabilizer to its final use level, and lyophilized. The potency of the varicella vaccine (VV) is quantified by pfu following infection of human diploid fibroblasts in vitro. For combination with other live attenuated vaccines (measles, mumps, rubella) as an experimental vaccine, the VZV-infected cell lysate is diluted appropriately, mixed with diluted culture media containing the other viruses, and lyophilized. The VV is administered once in children over 15 months of age, although it would not be unexpected that the vaccine be indicated in the future for a second dose later in childhood at a time similar to that for MMR vaccine. The immune response to VV in most United States clinical trials has been measured by an ELISA using VZV-infected cell glyco-protein (gp) as solid-phase antigen. Because the neutralizing antibody response against VZV is directed at VZV envelope glycoproteins *(46)*, serum titers mea-sured by this gpELISA have shown good correlation with neutralizing antibody titers. The definition of an immunological correlate of efficacy for VV is more complicated than for the other live viral vaccines, where protection against clinical disease after immunization is complete. For VV, 1–3% per year of immunized children develop a mild breakthrough infection, known as modified varicella-like syndrome (MVLS), following significant exposure to wild-type VZV *(47)*. MVLS is characterized by a reduced number of lesions (usually <50) and little fever >38°C compared with hundreds of lesions and a high rate of fever following natural varicella. The initial anti-VZV IgG response following VV immunization shows a rough overall correlation with protection against infec-tion during the next 2 years *(48)*. There are general inverse relationships both between gpELISA titer and breakthrough rate to the development of MVLS as well as between gpELISA and the median number of lesions in breakthrough cases. Thus, gpELISA or another assay qualified in a similar fashion would appear to be a useful general immunological correlate of efficacy for VV. However, this is only a trend rather than a solid correlation as for other vaccines such as HB and other live virus vaccines. Long-term persistence of immunity also can be followed by a number of assays, including those based on cell-mediated immunity *(49)*.

Hepatitis B

The HB virus (HBV) has a major envelope protein, the surface (S) protein or antigen, which also presents in virions as surface polypeptides containing pre-S antigens cotranslationally linked to the S protein. During HBV infection, excess S protein is secreted from infected cells as 20-nm noninfectious particles known as HB surface antigen (HBsAg) particles. These HBsAg particles were the basis for the first-generation plasma-derived HB vaccine. The S gene sub-sequently was expressed as recombinant proteins in eukaryotic cells, in particu-lar bakers' yeast *(Saccharomyces cerevisiae)*, in the form of 20-nm particles which are the basis for the second-generation recombinant-derived HB vaccine *(50)*. The HBsAg vaccine antigen is quantified for potency on the basis of its protein content, with dosage levels in the range of 5–20 μg. The vaccines are typically given to all age groups in three doses at a schedule such as 0–1–6 months, where the third dose serves to establish long-term immunological memory following the two priming doses. Both types of HBsAg particles contain a major conformational epitope (*a* epitope) that elicits anti-HBsAg antibodies that do not recognize individual S polypeptides. Anti-HBsAg antibodies (anti-HBs) were shown to be associated with protection against HBV infection, and efficacy studies with the plasma-derived HB vaccine demonstrated that following immunization the presence of at least 10 milli-International units (mIU) anti-HBs/mL of serum (quantified by RIA and subsequently by ELISA as surrogate assays, relative to an international reference standard) confers protection against clinical infection *(51,52)*. Subsequent studies demonstrated that immunization with recombinant-derived HB vaccine elicits a similar level of protective immunity as the plasma-derived vaccine *(53)* as well as biologically-equivalent antibodies *(54)*. Thus, the induction of ≥10 mIU anti-HBs/mL has become accepted as the correlate of efficacy for HB. Immunological memory more than 5 years after primary vaccination has been demonstrated by ELISPOT and by the ability of a booster dose of vaccine to elicit a rapid anti-HBs response *(55)*. Despite waning levels of anti-HBs (<10 mIU/mL down to undetectable levels) at 5–12 years after immunization, there have been very few reports of clinical HB disease among vaccinees who achieved the seroprotective level of ≥10 mIU anti-HBs/mL after primary immunization *(56)*. Thus, the correlate of efficacy (≥10 mIU/mL) appears to be valid for long-term protection from HBV disease, although whether this extends to a period of time longer than 5–12 years will be established only by further studies.

Hepatitis A

Like poliovirus, the Hepatitis A (HA) virus (HAV) is a picornavirus which can be used as an inactivated whole-virus vaccine. However, HAV is not efficiently released by cells in culture and therefore is purified from infected mammalian cells grown in vitro. The virus is inactivated by treatment with a chemical such as formalin *(57)*. The vaccine antigen is quantified for potency on the basis of protein content or units of reactivity in a specific ELISA. The vaccine is administered as a two-dose series, where the first priming dose is followed 6 months later by a dose that should establish long-term immunological memory. The major epitopes on HAV are conformational and are not present on individual capsid polypeptides. Anti-HAV antibodies (anti-HA) specific to such epitopes have been quantified by RIA. It first was demonstrated that passive protection against HAV infection was conferred by IG, since minute levels of anti-HA IG confer protection (levels below the limits of detectability of current assays). There is only a partially quantified correlation with the presence of detectable anti-HA *(58)*; however, any individual with a postvaccinal detectable titer (>10 mIU anti-HA/mL) is protected. Immunization with inactivated HA vaccine then was shown to elicit protective efficacy against HAV disease, which also was shown to correlate with the appearance of RIA-detectable anti-HA *(59)* and parallel induction of immunological memory *(60)*. As has been shown for HB vaccine, despite waning levels of anti-HA postvaccination, immunological memory can be shown by ELISPOT and T-cell proliferation assays *(61)* and by the rapid anti-HA response following booster vaccination *(62)*. The extent to which long-term memory is established by primary immunization with HA vaccine will be established following long-term studies of vaccinees, given that HA vaccines have been available for only a few years. Thus, RIA for the detection of anti-HA is a surrogate assay for the correlate of efficacy. However, it should be noted that since anti-HA in IG is qualitatively distinguishable in other serological assays from anti-HA in vaccinee sera during the (postimmunization) prebooster period *(63)*. Therefore, an international reference standard of vaccine-induced anti-HA needs to be established for serological endpoint analyses of correlates of efficacy in clinical studies HA vaccine during the first 6 months after the priming dose of vaccine.

Haemophilus influenzae *type* b

The first-generation *Haemophilus influenzae* type *b* (Hib) vaccine was the Hib capsular polysaccharide (Ps) Polyribosyl Ribitol Phosphate (PRP), which is shed from Hib organisms grown in culture. This vaccine antigen was shown to be immunogenic and to elicit protective immunity in >18- to 24-month-old children *(64)*, but not in younger children who suffer the highest incidence of invasive Hib diseases. To improve immunogenicity in infants, who have the highest rates of Hib diseases, PRP is conjugated to a carrier protein. There are four Hib conjugate vaccines currently available, each with a different carrier protein and conjugation chemistry *(65)*. The potency of each vaccine is quantified on the basis of Ps content and is in the range of 5–20 µg. The vaccines are administered as two or three doses (depending on the vaccine) in the first year of life followed by a booster dose at age 2, in a schedule which conforms to that of DTP vaccine. Immunization with Hib conjugate vaccines has been shown to elicit antibodies to PRP (anti-PRP) and to confer high rates of protective efficacy in infants as young as 2 months of age *(66)*. While anti-PRP antibodies have been shown to be the immunological correlate of efficacy, the seroprotective level of anti-PRP has been the subject of many retrospective studies and is not yet completely agreed upon *(67)*. Most determinations of anti-

PRP have been by RIA as the surrogate assay *(68)*. The interlaboratory variability of ELISA has been noted *(69)*, even though ELISA generally is considered a technique quite amenable to standardization. Early estimations of protective levels of anti-PRP in serum were based on the rarity of invasive Hib disease in adults, presumably due to the presence of protective antibodies; adults were found to have 0.04–0.10 or >0.15 µg anti-PRP/mL *(68,70)*. Passive immunization with IG enriched in anti-PRP antibodies resulted in protection of high-risk infants from invasive Hib diseases; measuring anti-PRP levels in vaccinees together with calculating the $t_{1/2}$ of antibodies gave an estimate of 0.05–0.15 µg anti-PRP/mL as protective *(71)*. Because infants passively acquire anti-PRP from their mothers and do not begin to suffer invasive Hib diseases for a few months, protective levels of anti-PRP may be inferred. Based on levels in newborns of 0.3 µg anti-PRP/mL, with disease not observed in Finland until 4–6 months of age, a protective level of 0.03 µg anti-PRP/mL was inferred; with disease observed among Alaskan natives starting at 2 months of age (at a frequency much higher than that observed in the era before Hib conjugate vaccines), a protective level of 0.1 µg anti-PRP/mL was inferred *(67)*. Thus, values in the range of 0.03–0.15 µg anti-PRP/mL appear to be naturally protective. Following immunization of young children with the PRP vaccine and based on correlating protection with anti-PRP levels, it appeared that >1 µg anti-PRP/mL of vaccine-induced antibody would protect against Hib diseases for 1 year *(72)*. Immunization with Hib conjugate vaccines is associated with the development of immunological memory, as shown by the rapid and high-level of anti-PRP response following a booster dose with either conjugate vaccine or PRP vaccine *(73)*. A calculation of the protective level of anti-PRP following immunization with conjugate vaccines has not been straightforward, since the presence of memory in an immunologically primed child may mean that a lower level of anti-PRP need be present upon challenge with Hib organisms *(67)*. Nevertheless, numbers in the range of >0.15–0.50 µg anti-PRP/mL have been used as reference values for protection following immunization with Hib conjugate vaccines. Once Hib conjugate vaccines had been approved for the immunization of infants, it became very difficult ethically to conduct further efficacy studies for licensure. Therefore, the Food and Drug Administration (FDA) made use of a range of immunological surrogates to license additional Hib conjugate vaccines: comparative immunogenicity trials relative to licensed vaccines with respect to class and subclass of anti-PRP, measurements of anti-PRP persistence before the booster dose, priming for a booster response, and demonstration of in vitro functional activity (opsonization) of anti-PRP *(74)*. These criteria, adapted to combination vaccines containing a Hib conjugate, also serve as a useful framework for licensure.

Pneumococcal

The Pneumococcal (Pn) vaccine for use in adults consists of a mixture of 23 Ps, each specific to a different Pn serotype *(75)*. Each Pn organism type is grown in culture, into which each Ps type is shed. The Pn Ps are mixed and lyophilized. The potency of the vaccine is quantified on the basis of the content of each Ps as determined in an immunological assay. The multivalent vaccine is given as a single dose to individuals >65 years of age. RIA has been used as the surrogate assay to measure anti-Pn Ps, the immunological correlate of efficacy.

The Ps are immunogenic in older children and adults, but not in young infants. As was done for Hib conjugate vaccines, each Pn Ps type is conjugated to a carrier protein. The same four carrier proteins as used for Hib conjugate vaccines have been used for Pn conjugate vaccines. The potency of each vaccine antigen is quantified on the basis of content of Ps in each conjugate. The resultant conjugates have been shown to be immunogenic in infants as young as 2 months of age *(76)*, where they are given in a regimen of immunization like that of Hib conjugate vaccines. Mixtures of 7–11 conjugates of different Pn Ps serotypes are in Phases 2–3 clinical trials for the prevention of invasive Pn diseases in infants. It is expected that ELISA will be used as the surrogate assay for Pn conjugate vaccines and that anti-Pn Ps will be the immunological correlate of efficacy.

Influenza

The most commonly used influenza vaccines are inactivated whole-virus vaccines. These are prepared following the growth of influenza virus (usually in chick eggs), collection of fluids, inactivation with formalin, and dilution. Vaccines in worldwide use are trivalent; the composition of vaccine is selected each year to contain three influenza virus serotypes (two type A and one type B) based on the prevalent serotypes of the virion surface glycoprotein hemagglutinin (HA) in sentinel areas worldwide *(77)*. The potency of the vaccine is quantified on the basis of the amount of each of the three viral HA proteins *(77)*. Since vaccines do not elicit group-common immunity and since virus serotypes can vary each year, annual immunization is indicated. Antibodies to HA are quantified by the HI assay using red blood cells and the same antigens as in the vaccine being evaluated *(78)*. The titer is defined as the final serum dilution inhibiting a set number of HA units of virus. Serological analyses also have employed a virus Nt assay *(79)*. The HI and Nt assays have been used as surrogate assays for measuring anti-HA or anti-virion antibodies as the correlate of efficacy. The protective level of HI antibodies has been estimated at 1:32 on an calibrated scale in some studies *(80,81)*. However, the determination of efficacy and protective level of antibodies in placebo-controlled efficacy studies has been complicated by the presence of specific antibodies in sera of preimmunization subjects, for which adjustment should be made in calculating the rate of efficacy *(82)*.

Rotavirus

This oral vaccine consists of live attenuated rotavirus grown in subhuman primate cells in culture. The virus, which has a segmented genome, is collected from culture media, diluted in stabilizer, and lyophilized. The potency of the vaccine is quantified on the basis of infectious units of each virus type in a primate cell line such as Vero *(83,84)*. Clinical trials typically have employed a schedule of three doses in the first year of life with a booster dose in the second year, all given at the same time as other childhood vaccines such as DTP, polio, and Hib conjugate vaccine. Early vaccines, which consisted of Rhesus *(83)* or bovine *(84)* rotaviruses, showed variable levels of efficacy in clinical trials. There are two types of vaccines currently licensed or in Phase 2–3 clinical trials. Multivalent reassortant rotaviruses consist of Rhesus or bovine rotaviruses which, through and genetic reassortment following coinfection with human rotavirus, contain one (sometimes two) human rotavirus segment encoding VP7 or VP4, the virion surface proteins. Given that there are four VP7 types and one VP4 type that cause >90% of infections in infants, such vaccines are multivalent mixtures of 4–5 reassortant rotavirus types *(85,86)*. The second type of vaccine in development is a live attenuated human rotavirus (or mixture of human rotaviruses) grown in primate cells in culture *(87)*. In the 10 years in which rotavirus clinical trials have been conducted, no clear correlate of efficacy has been found. In an analysis of a United States multicenter Phase 3 trial with monovalent reassortant and tetravalent reassortant rotavirus vaccines (in which there was 50% efficacy against all rotavirus disease and 80% efficacy against severe disease *[85]*), there was no consistent relationship observed between protection and serum neutralizing antibody titers *(88)*. In an analysis of a larger United States multicenter Phase 3 trial with higher dosage levels of the same vaccines, serum antibody responses following immunization show some general relationship with protection; however, such relationships were weak and inconsistent and do not indicate a reliable correlate of efficacy *(89)*. Because rotavirus infection is mucosal, intestinal or other mucosal antibody may provide a more reliable measure of protection although not necessarily as a correlate of protection.

Applying Immunological Correlates
to the Evaluation of Combination Vaccines

The goal of the serological evaluations for any combination vaccine is to establish its immunogenicity profile, hence indirectly the efficacy profile of its component vaccines. Each component may be comparably immunogenic in combination as by itself. However, immunological interactions have been observed among components in both multidisease and multivalent combinations. "Interference" is the reduction in the immunogenicity of one or more components when placed in combination. Conversely, "enhancement" is an increase in such immunogenicity. Both phenomena have been observed in the combination of DTwP vaccines with other component vaccines, e.g., IPV and Hib conjugate vaccines *(20,90)*. Although there are several hypotheses to explain interference and enhancement, these observations remain mostly empirical.

Multidisease Combinations

There generally are four different scenarios for the application of serological assays to the analysis of each component in a combination vaccine.

1. There is a correlate of protection which is well-established qualitatively and quantitatively, meaning that there is a well-defined surrogate assay and seroprotective level of antibodies.
2. The correlate is established qualitatively (well-defined surrogate assay) but not quantitatively.
3. The correlate is not well-established or may bear only a rough correlation with efficacy.
4. There is no known correlate.

Each of these scenarios now is considered with respect to the immunological evaluation of multidisease combinations. The basic question which is asked in such evaluations is whether a component of the combination vaccine is as immunogenic (and indirectly as efficacious) as part of the combination as it is when administered by itself and, if there is reduced immunogenicity, whether the reduction is clinically significant. This question typically is studied in a comparative controlled trial of subjects who are randomized to receive either the component vaccines separately or the new combination vaccine containing that component *(91)*. In the trial, there needs to be a sufficient number of subjects to be able to draw statistically valid conclusions regarding comparative immunogenicity. The larger the number of subjects in the study, the greater the statistical power around precalculated 95% confidence intervals to be able to draw conclusions from the study about the comparative immunogenicity of vaccines in different study groups. However, the actual sizes of the study groups depend upon the criteria of statistics as well as scientific and clinical judgment with respect to the objectives of the study and the hypothesis which is being addressed by the study *(92)*.

There are some vaccines for which the correlate is accepted both qualitatively and quantitatively, such that there is a level of antibodies which is accepted as protective. Such vaccines include D, T, Pol, MMR, and HB. In such cases, there are four levels at which the comparison can be done for those immunized with the component vaccine alone relative to those immunized with the component in combination. At one level, the GMTs elicited by the component in each of the groups are compared; if the GMTs are statistically equivalent, then it may be concluded that the component is as immunogenic in combination as alone. At the second level, the seroprotection rates in each cohort can be calculated. If these are statistically equivalent, then the vaccines can be considered comparably protective. There may be cases in which there is a statistically significant difference in the GMTs of the two groups, but the seroprotection rates are equivalent, such that the difference in GMTs is not considered clinically significant. Such a component in a combination vaccine may be acceptable as equivalently efficacious to the component alone. The third level is to compare seroconversion rates for each cohort as another measure of comparative immunogenicity; however, this parameter is generally less informative than GMTs or seroprotection rates. The fourth level is to statistically compare reverse cumulative distribution curves for antibody levels *(93)*. A complication to all such analyses is the issue of persistence of antibody levels, which usually are assayed within a few weeks or months after the completion of the immunization regimen. It is expected that antibody levels following immunization decay at the same rate in different cohorts, i.e., parallel line decay. If seroprotection rates are comparable, but the GMT is lower in the combination group a few months after immunization, then after a longer period of time (such as a few years) the seroprotection rate of the combination group may become lower than that of the component-only group. In this situation, it is important to demonstrate that there is satisfactory immunological memory, as demonstrated by the attainment of antibody levels following a further booster dose at least as high as has been achieved following the primary immunization. Such studies have been performed extensively with HB vaccine *(56)*.

The surrogate assay may be well-established for some vaccines, but the protective level is not completely agreed upon. Such vaccines include the Hib conjugate and influenza. For comparing combination vaccine vs component vaccine alone, the GMTs for each cohort are compared for statistical equivalence. In addition, given the lack of agreement on a seroprotective level of antibodies, two different putative seroprotection levels of antibody, e.g., 0.15 and 1.0 µg anti-PRP/mL for the Hib conjugate vaccine, may be selected as the basis for comparison. The seroprotection rates based on each level are compared for the two cohorts which, if equivalent, may validate the combination vaccine containing the Hib conjugate as comparably immunogenic to the conjugate vaccine alone; seroconversion rates also can be compared. The persistence of antibody needs to be addressed for certain vaccines as discussed later, especially for the time-period during which the individuals remain susceptible to infection.

There are vaccines, such as varicella, for which various serological assays have been performed but for which the data from one or more of these assays show only a rough overall relationship with protection. In such cases, several serological assays for the given vaccine may be performed and the GMTs for the component vaccine alone vs the combination vaccine then compared. For assays where there is some indication of a correlation with protection or clinical outcome (e.g., gpELISA for varicella vaccine), the seroprotection rates for the two groups can be compared over a range of different numerical values for seroprotection, given that the seroprotective level of antibodies has not been established firmly. This provides additional comfort, although not formal proof, that the component is equally efficacious alone vs in combination and represents almost the only type of analysis that can be performed within the constraints of available assays.

Some vaccines have no known immunological correlate of efficacy. The wP vaccine has been used for decades, with a demonstrated high level of efficacy. The recently completed efficacy studies of seven different P_a vaccines were accompanied by arguably the most extensively conducted serological evaluations of any vaccine in terms of different assays and vaccines. Nevertheless, no immunological correlate of efficacy has been found for any of these two types of vaccines *(19)*. This complicates the issue of accurately comparing the immunogenicity of a combination of wP or aP vaccines with the vaccine alone. There are a large number of antigens of *B. pertussis* that have been defined as vaccine antigens, including PT, FHA, Agg, and Pert. For the wP vaccine, serological assays can be performed with specificity for each of these antigens. If all these assays are used to evaluate the GMTs and seroconversion rates of the wP vaccine vs its combination with other vaccines, there is additional comfort (as opposed to "proof," given that there is no correlate of efficacy) that the two vaccines are equally immunogenic. Similarly for the aP vaccines, serological assays corresponding to each of the *B. pertussis* antigens in the vaccine can be performed in order to provide the best evidence that the vaccine in combination is comparably immunogenic to the vaccine alone by all measurable assays.

Multivalent Combinations

The main challenge to the demonstration of efficacy of such combinations, whose individual serotypes usually are unlicensed, is that the incidence of disease attributable to each serotype may be very low. As a consequence, it ordinarily would not be possible with diseases of relatively low incidence (pneumococcal) to establish the efficacy of each individual serotype in the vaccine without running an extremely and impracticably large efficacy study. In such cases, efficacy can be evaluated for all serotypes of disease in aggregate and for the most abundant serotype of disease. The serological evaluations of individual serotypes in the combination may be handled differently depending on whether or not there is a known immunological correlate of efficacy.

Once efficacy has been established for all serotypes in aggregate and for at least one individual serotype in the case of a low-incidence disease (e.g., pediatric invasive pneumococcal disease), a correlate of efficacy and seroprotective level of antibodies may be established for that serotype and may be inferred for all serotypes in general. The correlate would be expected to be relevant to all serotypes in the vaccine, given that all serotypes of virus or bacteria are expected to be structurally similar. However, it is not possible to conclude that all serotypes would be associated with the same seroprotective level of antibodies, since the types may have different levels of virulence. This represents a major challenge, because all serotypes other than the one for which efficacy is proven may be dosed based on "blind faith" comparison to the lead serotype or adjusted correspondingly following the results of an efficacy trial. In the case of a high-incidence disease (e.g., influenza), it may be possible to establish a correlate of efficacy for all serotypes.

There are combination vaccines with no correlate of efficacy. If the disease is of high incidence, as in the case of rotavirus, it may be possible to establish efficacy for each vaccine serotype. If the disease is of low incidence and efficacy is established for all serotypes collectively and for one individually, then serological comparisons by different assays, especially functional antibody assays (Nt, opsonization) and comparability of the potency of each component may be used as the basis for defining the vaccine *(94)*. As long as the addition of minor serotypes does not compromise the safety of the multivalent product and does not interfere significantly with the immunogenicity of the type shown to be efficacious, then it may be justified to add additional serotypes.

Conclusions

There is an increased momentum toward the development and licensure of combination vaccines, both multidisease and multivalent. For multidisease combinations, where the licensure of individual components typically has been established by efficacy trials, serological endpoint evaluations offer the opportunity to evaluate that a component is as immunogenic or clinically effective in combination as by itself. For multivalent combinations, where efficacy cannot always be established for every serotype in the vaccine, serological endpoint evaluations enable minor serotypes to be evaluated relative to major serotypes for inclusion in the final product. All serological evaluations are most informative where there is a known immunological correlate of efficacy, preferably with both a well-established surrogate assay and a seroprotective level. Therefore, there is increased attention toward the identification of correlates of efficacy and toward the design of assays with specificity appropriate to be a surrogate assay. While most such assays to date have made use of whole immunogens (e.g., viruses, bacteria, or individual proteins), assays which probe specific epitopes on proteins or whole pathogens represent a promising direction in the identification if new surrogate assays. In cases where no correlate of efficacy has been identified for a particular component vaccine, more extensive comparative serological evaluations may need to be conducted in order to establish that the immunogenicity profile of the component in combination is satisfactory for licensure.

References

1. Goldenthal, K. L., Burns, D. L., McVittie, L. D., Lewis, B. P., and Williams, J. C. (1995) Overview—Combination vaccines and simultaneous administration. Past, present and future, in *Combined Vaccines and Simultaneous Administration: Current Issues and Perspectives* (Williams, J. C., Goldenthal, K. L., Burns, D. L., and Lewis, B. P., eds.), *Ann. NY Acad. Sci.* **754,** xi–xv.
2. Ellis, R. W. and Brown, K. R. (1997) Combination Vaccines, in *Advances in Pharmacology* (August, J. T., Anders, M. W., Murad, F., and Coyle, J. T., eds.). Academic, San Diego, CA, pp. 393–423.
3. Prescott, L. M., Harley, J. P., and Klein, D. A., eds. (1990) *Microbiology.* W. C. Brown, Dubuque, IA, pp. 636–656.
4. Czerkinsky, C. C., Nilsson, L. A., Nygren, H., Ouchterlony, O., and Tarkowski, A. (1983) A solid-phase enzyme-lined immunospot (ELISA) assay for enumeration of specific antibody-secreting cells. *J. Immunol. Meth.* **65,** 109–116.
5. Ramon, G. (1923) Sur le pouvoir floculant et sur les proprietes immunisantes d'une toxin diphtherique rendue anatoxique (anatoxine). *Compt. Rend. Aca. Sci.* **177,** 1228–1240.
6. Glenny, A. T., Pope, C. G., Waddington, H., and Wallace, U. (1926) Immunological notes. XIII. The antigenic value of toxoid precipitated by potassium alum. *J. Path. Bacteriol.* **29,** 38,39.
7. Fayet, M. T., Vincent-Falquet, J. C., Tayot, J. L., and Trian, J. (1978) Interest in the evaluation of tetanus antibodies by RIA. Presented at the Fifth International Conference on Pertussis, Ronely, Sweden, June 18–23, 1978.
8. Volk, V. K., Gottchall, R. Y., Anderson, H. D., et al. (1962) Antigenic responses to booster dose of diphtheria and tetanus toxoids: Seven to thirteen years after primary inoculation of noninstitutionalized children. *Public Health Rep.* **77,** 185–194.
9. Centers for Disease Control (1991) Update on adult immunization. Recommendations of the Immune Practices Advisory Committee (ACIP). *MMWR* **40(RR12),** 1–94.
10. Weinstein, L. (1973) Tetanus. *N. Engl. J. Med.* **289,** 1293–1296.
11. Jones, F. G. and Moss, J. M. (1936) Studies on tetanus toxoid. I. The antitoxic titer of human subjects following immunization with tetanus toxoid and tetanus alum precipitated toxoid. *J. Immunol.* **30,** 115–125.
12. Stanfield, J. P and Galazka, A. (1984) Neonatal tetanus in the world today. *Bull. WHO* **62,** 647–669.
13. Hardegree, M. C., Barile, M. F., Pittman, M., et al. (1970) Immunization against neonatal tetanus in New Guinea. 4. Comparison of tetanus antitoxin titers obtained by haemagglutination and toxin neutralization in mice. *Bull. WHO* **43,** 461–468.
14. Simonsen, O., Schou, C., and Heron, I. (1987) Modification of the ELISA for the estimation of tetanus antitoxin in human sera. *J. Biol. Stand.* **15,** 143–157.

15. McCarroll, J. R., Abrahams, I., and Skudder, P. A. (1962) Antibody response to tetanus toxoid 15 years after initial immunization. *Am. J. Public Health* **52,** 1669–1675.
16. Manclark, C. R. and Cowell, J. L. (1984) Pertussis, in *Bacterial Vaccines* (Germanier, R., ed.) Academic, New York, NY, pp. 69–106.
17. Kendrick, P. L., Eldering, G., Dixon, M. K., et al. (1947) Mouse protection tests in the study of pertussis vaccine: a comparative series using intracerebral route for challenge. *Am. J. Public. Health* **37,** 803–810.
18. Medical Research Council (1956) Vaccination against whooping cough: relation between protection in children and results of laboratory tests. *Br. Med. J.* **2,** 454–462.
19. Plotkin, S. A. and Cadoz, M. (1997) The acellular pertussis vaccine trials: an interpretation. *Pediatr. Inf. Dis. J.* **16,** 508–517.
20. Paradiso, P. R., Hogerman, D. A., Madore, D. V., Keyserling, H., King, J., Reisinger, K. S., Blattner, M. M., Rothstein, E., Bernstein, H. H., Pennridge Pediatric Associates, and Hackell, J. (1993) Safety and immunogenicity of a combined diphtheria, tetanus, pertussis and *Haemophilus influenzae* type *b* vaccine in young infants. *Pediatrics* **92,** 827–832.
21. Rappuoli, R., Podda, A., Pizza, M., Covacci, A., Bartolini, A., de Magistris, M. T., and Nencioni, L. (1992) Progress toward the development of new vaccines against whooping cough. *Vaccine* **10,** 1027–1032.
22. Sabin, A. B. (1957) Properties and behavior of orally administered attenuated poliovirus vaccine. *JAMA* **164,** 1216–1223.
23. Enders, J. F., Robbins, F. C., and Weller, T. H. (1955) The cultivation of the poliomyelitis viruses in tissue culture. *Les Prix Nobel*, Stockholm, Sweden, 1954.
24. Melnick, J. L., Benyesh-Melnick, M., and Brennan, J. C. (1959) Studies on live poliovirus vaccine. Its neurotropic activity in monkeys and its increased neurovirulence after multiplication in vaccinated children. *JAMA* **171,** 1165–1172.
25. Katz, S. L. (1995) Combination live enteric virus vaccines, in *Combined Vaccines and Simultaneous Administration: Current Issues and Perspectives.* (Williams, J. C., Goldenthal, K. L., Burns, D. L., and Lewis, B. P., eds.), *Ann. NY Acad. Sci.* **754,** 347–355.
26. World Health Organization Consultative Group (1969) Evidence on the safety and efficacy of live poliovirus vaccines currently in use, with special reference to type 3 poliovirus. *Bull. WHO* **40,** 925–945.
27. Sabin, A. B., Michaels, R. H., Ziring, P., et al. (1963) Effect of oral poliovirus vaccine in newborn children. II. Intestinal resistance and antibody response at 6 months in children fed type 1 vaccine at birth. *Pediatrics* **31,** 641–650.
28. Sabin, A. B. (1985) Oral poliovirus vaccine: history of its development and use and current challenge to eliminate poliovirus from the world. *J. Infect. Dis.* **151,** 420–436.
29. Grenier, B., Hamza, B., Biron, G., Xuref, C., Viame, F., and Roumiantzeff, M. (1984) Seroimmunity following vaccination in infants by an inactivated poliovirus preparation on Vero cells. *Rev. Infect. Dis.* **6(2),** 545–547.
30. Salk, J. and Gori, G. B. (1960) A review of theoretical, experimental, and practical considerations in the use of formaldehyde for the inactivation of poliovirus. *Ann. NY Acad. Sci.* **83,** 609–637.
31. Montagnon, B., Fanget, B., and Vincent-Falquet, J. C. (1984) Industrial-scale production of inactivated poliovirus vaccine prepared by culture of Vero cells and microcarrier. *Rev. Infect. Dis.* **6,** S341–S344.
32. Centers for Disease Control (1998) Recommended Childhood Immunization Schedule—United States, 1998. *MMWR* **47,** 8–12.
33. Carlsson, B., Zaman, S., Mellander, L., et al. (1985) Secretory and serum immunoglobulin class-specific antibodies to poliovirus after immunization. *J. Infect. Dis.* **152,** 1238–1244.
34. Salk, J. (1960) Persistence of immunity after administration of formalin-treated poliovirus vaccine. *Lancet* **2,** 715–723.

35. Schwartz, A. J. F. and Anderson, J. T. (1965) Immunization with a further attenuated live measles vaccine. *Arch. Virusforsch.* **16,** 273–278.
36. Hilleman, M. R., Buynak, E. B., Weibel, R. E., Stokes, J. Jr., Whitman, J. E. Jr., and Leagus, M. B. (1968) Development and evaluation of the Moraten measles virus vaccine. *JAMA* **206,** 587–590.
37. Expanded Programme on Immunization. Safety of high-titre measles vaccines. *Wkly. Epidemiol. Rec.* **67,** 357–361.
38. Paunio, M., Virtanen, M., Peltola, H., et al. (1991) Increase of vaccination coverage by mass media and individual approach: intensified measles, mumps and rubella prevention program in Finland. *Am. J. Epidemiol.* **133,** 1152–1160.
39. Black, F. L. (1989) Measles, in *Viral Infections of Humans. Epidemiology and Control,* 3rd ed. (Evans, A. S., ed.), Plenum, New York, pp. 451–465.
40. Buynak, E. B. and Hilleman, M. R. (1966) Live attenuated mumps virus vaccine. 1. Vaccine development. *Proc. Soc. Exp. Biol. Med.* **123,** 768–775.
41. Shehab, Z. M., Brunell, P. A., and Cobb, E. (1984) Epidemiological standardization of a test for the susceptibility to mumps. *J. Infect. Dis.* **149,** 810–812.
42. Plotkin, S. A. and Buser, F. (1985) History of RA27/3 rubella vaccine. *Rev. Infect. Dis.* **7,** S77,S78.
43. Dudgeon, J. A. (1980) Selective immunization: protection of the individual. *Rev. Infect. Dis.* **7,** S185–S190.
44. Weibel, R. E., Villarejos, V. M., Klein, E. B., et al. (1980) Clinical and laboratory studies of live attenuated RA27/3 and HPV-77DE rubella virus vaccines. *Proc. Soc. Exp. Biol. Med.* **165,** 44–49.
45. Takahashi, M. (1996) Vaccine development, in *Varicella Vaccine* (Ellis, R. W. and White, C. J., eds.) Saunders, Philadelphia, PA, pp. 469–488.
46. Provost, P. J., Krah, D. L., Kuter, B. J., Morton, D. H., Schofield, T. L., Wasmuth, E. H., White, C. J., Miller, W. J., and Ellis, R. W. (1991) Antibody assays suitable for assessing responses to live varicella vaccine. *Vaccine* **9,** 111–116.
47. Bernstein, H. H., Rothstein, E. P., Watson, B. M., et al. (1993) Clinical survey of natural varicella compared with breakthrough varicella after immunization with live attenuated Oka/Merck varicella vaccine. *Pediatrics* **92,** 833–837.
48. White, C. J., Kuter, B. J., Ngai, A., Hildebrand, C. S., Isganitis, K. L., Patterson, C. M., Capra, A., Miller, W. J., Krah, D. L., Provost, P. J., Ellis, R. W., and Calandra, G. B. (1992) Modified cases of chickenpox after varicella vaccination: correlation of protection with antibody response. *Pediatr. Infect. Dis. J.* **11,** 19–23.
49. Arvin, A. (1996) Immune responses to varicella-zoster virus, in *Varicella Vaccine* (Ellis, R. W. and White, C. J., eds.) Saunders, Philadelphia, PA, pp. 529–570.
50. Krugman, S. and Stevens, C. E. (1992) Hepatitis B vaccine, in *Vaccines,* 2nd ed. (Plotkin, S. A. and Mortimer, E. A., eds.) W. B. Saunders, Philadelphia, PA, pp. 419–438.
51. Szmuness, W., Steven, C. E., Zang, E. A., Harley, E. J., and Kellner, A. (1981) A controlled clinical trial of the efficacy of the hepatitis B vaccine (Heptavax B): a final report. *Hepatology* **1,** 377–385.
52. Francis, D. P., Hadler, S. C., Thompson, S. E., et al. (1982) The prevention of hepatitis B with vaccine: report of the Centers for Disease Control multi-center efficacy trail among homosexual men. *Ann. Int. Med.* **97,** 362–366.
53. West, D. J. (1989) Clinical experience with hepatitis B vaccines. *Am. J. Infect Control.* **17,** 172–180.
54. Emini, E. A., Ellis, R. W., Miller, W. J., McAleer, W. J., Scolnick, E. M., and Gerety, R. J. (1986) Production and immunological analysis of recombinant hepatitis B vaccine. *J. Infect.* **13A,** 3–9.

55. Van Hattum, J., Maikoe, T., Poel, J., and deGast, G. C. (1991) *In vitro* anti-HBs production by individual B cells of responders to hepatitis B vaccine who subsequently lost antibody, in *Viral Hepatitis and Liver Disease* (Hollinger, F. B., Lemon, S. M., and Margolis, H. S., eds.), Williams and Wilkins, Baltimore, MD, pp. 774–776.

56. West, D. A. and Calandra, G. B. (1996) Vaccine-induced immunologic memory for hepatitis B surface antigen: implications for policy on booster vaccination. *Vaccine* **14,** 1019–1027.

57. Provost, P. J., Hughes, J. V., Miller, W. J., Giesa, P. A., Banker, F. S., and Emini, E. A. (1986) An inactivated hepatitis A vaccine of cell culture origin. *J. Med. Virol.* **19,** 23–31.

58. Conrad, M. E. and Lemon, S. M. (1987) Prevention of icteric viral hepatitis by administration of immune serum gamma globulin. *J. Infect. Dis.* **156,** 56–63.

59. Werzberger, A., Mensch, B., Kuter, B., Brown, L., Lewis, J., Sitrin, R., Miller, W., Shouval, D., Wiens, B., Calandra, G., Ryan, J., Provost, P., and Nalin, D. (1992) A controlled trial of a formalin-inactivated hepatitis A vaccine in healthy children. *N. Engl. J. Med.* **327,** 453–457.

60. Werzberger, A., Kuter, B., and Nalin, D. (1998) Six years follow-up after hepatitis A vaccination. *N. Engl. J. Med.* **338,** 1160.

61. Chen, X. Q., Boland, G. J., de Gast, G. C., and van Hattum, J. (1997) Immune memory after hepatitis A vaccination. *Proc. Am. Gastroenterol. Assoc. Am. Assoc. Study Liver Dis.* **A76**.

62. Nalin, D. R. (1995) Hepatitis A vaccine, purified inactivated. *Drugs Future* **20,** 24–29.

63. Lemon, S. M., Murphy, P. C., Provost, P. J., Chalikonda, I., Davide, J. P., Schofield, T. L., Nalin, D. A., and Lewis, J. A. (1997) Immunoprecipitation and virus neutralization assays demonstrate qualitative differences between protective antibody responses to inactivated hepatitis A vaccine and passive immunization with immune globulin. *J. Infect. Dis.* **176,** 9–19.

64. Peltola, H., Kayhty, H., Sivonen, A., and Makela, P. H. (1977) *Haemophilus influenzae* type *b* capsular polysaccharide vaccine in children: a double-blind field study of 100,000 vaccinees 3 months to 5 years of age in Finland. *Pediatrics* **60,** 730–737.

65. Kniskern, P. J., Marburg, S., and Ellis, R. W. (1995) *Haemophilus influenzae* type *b* Conjugate Vaccines, in *Vaccine Design: The Subunit Approach* (Powell, M. and Newman, M., eds.) Plenum, New York, NY, pp. 673–694.

66. Wenger, J. D., Booy, R., Heath, P. T., and Moxon, R. (1997) Epidemiologic impact of conjugate vaccines on invasive disease caused by *Haemophilus influenzae* type *b*, in *New Generation Vaccines*, 2nd ed. (Levine, M. L., Woodrow, G. C., Kaper, J. B., and Cobon, G. S., eds.), Marcel Dekker, New York, NY, pp. 489–502.

67. Kayhty, H. (1994) Difficulties in establishing a serological correlate of protection after immunization with *Haemophilus influenzae* conjugate vaccines. *Biologicals* **22,** 397–402.

68. Robbins, J. B., Parke, J. C., Schneerson, R., and Whisnant, J. K. (1973) Quantitative measurement of "natural" and immunization-induced *Haemophilus influenzae* type *b* capsular polysaccharide antibodies. *Pediatrics* **7,** 103–110.

69. Madore, D. V., Anderson, P., Baxter, B. D., Carlone, G. M., Edwards, K. M., Hamilton, R. G., Holder, P., Kayhty, H., Phipps, D. C., Schneerson, R., Siber, G. R., Ward, G. I., and Frasch, C. E. (1996) Interlaboratory study evaluating quantitation of antibodies to *Haemophilus influenzae* type *b* polysaccharide by enzyme-linked immunosorbent assay. *Clin. Diag. Lab. Immunol.* **3,** 84–88.

70. Makela, P. H., Peltola, H., Kayhty, H., et al. (1977) Polysaccharide vaccines of group A *Neiserria meningitidis* and *Haemophilus influenzae* type *b*. *J. Infect. Dis.* **136,** S43–S50.

71. Santosham, M., Reid, R., Ambrosino, D., et al. (1987) Prevention of *Haemophilus influenzae* type *b* infections in high-risk infants treated with bacterial polysaccharide immune globulin. *N. Engl. J. Med.* **317,** 923–929.

72. Kayhty, H., Peltola, H., Karanko, V., and Makela, P. H. (1983). The protective level of serum antibodies to the capsular polysaccharide of *Haemophilus influenzae* type *b*. *J. Infect. Dis.* **147,** 1100.

73. Kayhty, H., Eskola, J., Peltola, H., et al. (1992) High antibody responses to booster doses of either *Haemophilus influenzae* capsular polysaccharide or conjugate vaccine after primary immunization with conjugate vaccines. *J. Infect. Dis.* **165,** 165–175.

74. Frasch, C. E. (1995) Regulatory perspectives in vaccine licensure, in *Development and Clinical Uses of Haemophilus influenzae type b Conjugate Vaccines* (Ellis, R. W. and Granoff, D. M., eds.). Marcel-Dekker, New York, NY, pp. 435–453.

75. Austrian, R. (1989) Pneumococcal polysaccharide vaccines. *Rev. Infect. Dis.* **11,** S598–S602.

76. Ahman, H., Kayhty, H., Tamminen, P., Vuorela, A., Malinoski, F., and Eskola, J. (1996) Pentavalent pneumococcal oligosaccharide conjugate vaccine PnCRM is well tolerated and able to induce an antibody response in infants. *Pediatr. Infect. Dis. J.* **15,** 134–139.

77. Kilbourne, E. D. (1994) Inactivated influenza vaccines, in *Vaccines*, 2nd ed. (Plotkin, S. A. and Mortimer E. A., eds.) W. B. Saunders, Philadelphia, PA, pp. 565–581.

78. Dowdle, W. N., Kendall, A. P., and Nobel, G. R. (1979) Influenza viruses, in *Diagnostic Procedures for Viral, Rickettsial and Chlamydial Infections,* 5th ed. (Lennart, E. H. and Schmidt, N. J., eds.) American Public Health Association. Washington, DC, pp. 603–605.

79. Frank, A. L., Puck, J., Hughes, B. J., and Cate, T. R. (1980) Microneutralization test for influenza A and B and parainfluenza 1 and 2 viruses that uses continuous cell lines and fresh serum enhancement. *J. Clin. Microbiol.* **12,** 426–432.

80. Quinnan, G. V., Schooley, R., Doli, R., Ennis, F. A., Gross, P., and Gwaltney, J. M. (1983) Serologic responses and systemic reactions in adults after vaccination with monovalent A/USSR/77 and trivalent A/USSR/77, A/Texas/77 and B/HongKong/72 influenza vaccines. *Rev. Infect. Dis.* **5,** 748–757.

81. Belshe, R. B., van Voris, L. P., Bartram, J., and Crookshank, F. K. (1984) Live attenuated influenza A virus vaccines in children: results of a field trial. *J. Infect. Dis.* **150,** 834–840.

82. Hirota, Y., Kaji, M., Ide, S., Kajiwara, S., Goto, S., and Oka, T. (1997) Antibody efficacy as a keen index to evaluate influenza vaccine effectiveness. *Vaccine* **15,** 962–967.

83. Gothefors, L., Wadell, G., Juto, P., et al. (1989) Prolonged efficacy of rhesus rotavirus vaccine in Swedish children. *J. Infect. Dis.* **159,** 753–757.

84. Clark, H. F., Borian, F. E., Bell, L. M., et al. (1988) Protective effect of WC3 vaccine against rotavirus diarrhea in infants during a predominantly serotype 1 rotavirus season. *J. Infect. Dis.* **158,** 570–587.

85. Bernstein, D. I., Glass, R. I., Rodgers, G., Davidson, B. L., Sack, D. A., and United States Rotavirus Vaccine Efficacy Group (1995) Evaluation of rhesus rotavirus monovalent and tetravalent reassortant vaccines in United States children. *JAMA* **273,** 1191–1196.

86. Clark, H. F., Offit, P. A., Ellis, R. W., Krah, D., Shaw, A. R., Eiden, J., Pichichero, M., and Treanor, J. J. (1996) WC3 reassortant vaccines in children. Brief review. *Arch. Virol.* **12,** 187–198.

87. Bernstein, D. I., Smith, V. E., Sherwood, J. R., et al. (1998) Safety and immunogenicity of live, attenuated human rotavirus vaccine 89-12. *Vaccine* **16,** 381–387.

88. Ward, R. L., Bernstein, D. I., and United States Rotavirus Efficacy Group (1995) Lack of correlation between serum rotavirus antibody titers and protection following vaccination with reassortant RRV vaccines. *Vaccine* **13,** 1226–1232.

89. Ward, R. L., Knowlton, D. R., Zito, E. T., Davidson, B. L., Rappaport, R., Mack, M. E., and United States Rotavirus Vaccine Efficacy Group (1997) Serological correlates of immunity in a tetravalent reassortant rotavirus vaccine trial. *J. Infect. Dis.* **176,** 570–577.

90. Pichichero, M. E., Latiolais, T., Bernstein, D. I., Hosbach, P., Christian, E., Vidor, E., Meschievitz, C., and Daum, R. S. (1997) Vaccine antigen interactions after a combination diphtheria-tetanus toxoid-acellular pertussis/purified capsular polysaccharide of *Haemophilus influenzae* type *b*-tetanus toxoid vaccine in two-, four- and six-month-old infants. *Pediatr. Infect. Dis. J.* **16,** 863–870.

91. Decker, M. D. and Edwards, K. M. (1995) Issues in design of clinical trials of combination vaccines, in *Combined Vaccines and Simultaneous Administration Current Issues and Perspectives* (Williams, J. C., Goldenthal, K. L., Burns, D. L. and Lewis, B. P., eds.), *Ann. NY Acad. Sci.* **754,** 234–240.

92. Center For Biologics Evaluation and Research, United States Food and Drug Administration (1997) *Guidance for Industry for the Evaluation of Combination Vaccines for Preventable Diseases: Production, Testing and Clinical Studies.*

93. Reed, G. F., Meade, B. D. and Steinhoff, M. C. (1995) The reverse cumulative distribution plot: a graphic method for exploratory analysis of antibody data. *Pediatrics* **96(Suppl),** 600–603.

94. Paradiso, P. R. and Lindberg, A. A. (1996) Glycoconjugate vaccines: future combinations. *Dev. Biol. Stand.* **87,** 269–275.

6   Influenza Vaccines

Bert E. Johansson

Introduction

Disease caused by influenza virus infection is not a trivial matter. In the United States influenza can kill 10,000 people in a nonpandemic year and 30,000 people after an acute epidemic *(1)*. Additionally, in terms of physician and hospital expenses and time away from work, the dollar cost to the United States economy is immense. The Surgeon General of the United States Public Health Service estimated that at least 43 million Americans are at risk of death from influenza by virtue of their underlying medical illness and should be immunized *(2)*. Persons over 60 years of age and children less than one year of age have increased case-fatality rates for influenza, probably resulting from decreased immune response with age and complicating cardiopulmonary disease. As the proportion of elderly and children surviving with congenital heart and lung disease increases, so will the need for control of influenza. Additionally, pregnant women, asthmatics, diabetics, and patients receiving immuno-suppressive drugs for organ transplants or neoplastic diseases are at high risk for severe influenza.

This chapter will discuss basic influenza virology and immunology, with emphasis on the inherent problems of vaccination against influenza. Discussion will focus on the problem of antigenic competition among the components of this multivalent combination vaccine, a situation that is not unique to influenza immunology.

Influenza and Influenza Viruses

Influenza is an acute respiratory tract infection that can result in a mild inapparent infection or a severe incapacitating illness. Influenza viruses, the causative agents of influenza, are members of the *Orthomyxoviridae*; they are further divided into types A, B, and C, a classification based on genetic differences and antigenic differences among surface proteins and the major internal proteins M and NP. Influenza A viruses are described by a nomenclature which includes the

From: *Combination Vaccines: Development, Clinical Research, and Approval*
Edited by: R. W. Ellis © Humana Press Inc., Totowa, NJ

host of origin, geographic origin, strain number, and year of isolation. The antigenic classification of the two major surface glycoproteins, hemagglutinin (HA) and neuraminidase (NA) are given in parenthesis (e.g., A/Turkey/ Massachusetts/360/75 [H6N2]). There are 13 antigenic subtypes of HA (H1–H14) and nine subtypes of NA (N1–N9). All subtypes are found in birds, but thankfully only a few in humans (H1, H2, H3; N1, N2), swine, and horses. Influenza virus has a genome composed of eight negative sense RNA segments that encode ten viral proteins *(3)*. Two of these genes encode for the surface glycoproteins, HA and NA. The HA mediates the initial attachment of the virion to cells via sialic acid residues *(4)* and possesses a fusion capability that enables the virus envelope to integrate with a lysoendosomal membrane, thereby allowing the internal viral components access to the host cell cytoplasm *(5)*. The HA molecule is present in the virus as a trimer. Each monomer exist as two chains, HA_1 and HA_2, linked by a disulfide bond. Antibodies to HA neutralize viral infectivity; antigenic variation in this molecule is mainly responsible for frequent outbreaks of influenza and for the poor control of infection by immunization. The NA is a tetrameric enzyme which cleaves terminal sialic acid residues from any oligosaccharide chain possessing that terminal sugar *(6)*, including terminal keto-groups on the HA and NA molecules *(7)*. This reaction permits transport of the virion through mucin and destroys the HA receptor on the host cell, thereby allowing release of progeny virus from infected cells *(6)*. Furthermore, the removal of sialic acid from oligosaccharide chains on newly synthesized HA and NA probably prevents self-aggregation of viral particles *(7)*. Immunization of mice *(8,9)* or humans *(10)* induces a specific response to NA which, although infection-permissive across a broad range of NA-antibody levels, results in the reduction of pulmonary virus titers below a pathogenic threshold *(8,11)*. As a result of the greater selective pressure of HA antibodies that force the more rapid emergence of escape mutants, NA antigenically evolves more slowly *(12)*. Intact virions also contain a third major envelope-associated protein called matrix (M_1) protein, which is the major virus protein and is associated with the inside of the membrane *(13)*. There is another surface protein found in variable amounts in the viral membrane, the M_2 protein, which functions as an ion-channel *(14,15)*. Inside the viral envelope are the eight RNA segments, the polymerase proteins (PA, PB_1, PB_2) which supply the enzymatic machinery for viral RNA synthesis, and nucleoprotein (NP) that associates with RNA segments to form ribonucleoprotein (RNP) *(16,17)*.

Serological Methods

Increases in serum antibody responses during influenza are usually demonstrable no earlier than the end of the first week of illness. Therefore, specific responses diagnostic of infection can be documented by comparative measurements of antibody in sera obtained during the acute phase and in convalescent phase sera obtained

10 days or more following the onset of illness. A single serum specimen is inadequate for diagnosis because the mere presence of antibody permits no valid inference about when antibody to these ubiquitous viruses may have been acquired.

Hemagglutination Inhibition

In the presence of virus, cells containing neuraminic acid receptors are agglutinated in the hemagglutination reaction. This reaction can serve as an in vitro measure for the quantification of serially-diluted viruses; its inhibition can be used to measure specific antibody in serum. Serum may contain nonspecific inhibitors to which the virus may bind; prior treatment of serum with receptor-destroying enzyme (RDE) is necessary before use in hemagglutination inhibition (HI) assay. The HI test is a simple and commonly used technique for the measurement of antibody reactive to the HA of influenza virus and, because the HI test detects principally anti-HA antibody which mediates viral attachment, usually is concordant with the neutralization test. However, the HI test can be influenced by the binding avidity of the virus and species of RBC used *(71)*. Additionally, antibody to the viral NA can sterically block access of the HA to RBC receptors and thereby falsely inhibit hemagglutination *(71)*. Therefore, antigenically hybrid reassortant viruses containing an NA alien to the immunizing experience of the test animal are required for valid and reliable measurement of HI antibody. Finally, as with any twofold dilution series, titer increases of fourfold or greater are considered significant.

Neuraminidase Inhibition

Detection of antibody to the viral NA has relied upon the neuraminidase inhibition (NI) assay, which requires that anti-NA antibodies sterically block access of NA to substrate *(21)*. This test does not measure antibodies that may aggregate virus particles; enzyme-linked immunoassay (ELISA) is more sensitive *(8,21)*. The NI test is costly and imprecise and consequently does not play a major role in diagnostic virology. Its importance lies in epidemiological and clinical research. Just as with the HI assay, as with any twofold dilution series, titer increases of fourfold or greater are considered significant.

There are other assays of the immune response to influenza virus such as neutralization assay, complement fixation, single radial hemolysis, and ELISA, which are well described in many basic immunology texts.

Antigenic Properties of Viral Proteins

B-Cell Recognition

Locations of major antigenic sites on the HA molecule have been described using two complementary techniques: generation of a panel of monoclonal anti-

HA antibodies for selecting viral mutants expressing antigenically-changed HA molecules and an analysis of the three-dimensional structure of HA molecules and a comparison of the amino acid sequences of the HA from related epidemic and mutant strains. There is consensus that these approaches show four principal antigenic determinants which have been designated for the H3 molecule as: A, B, C, and D *(18)* and for the H1 molecules as: Sa, Sb, Ca, and Cb *(19,20)*. The antigenic sites of PR8 H1-HA correlate with the structure of the Hong Kong H3-HA, indicating that the HA molecules of these two subtypes must share many related structural features, although there is less than 25% sequence similarity between H1 and H3. However, Caton et al. *(20)* suggest that the presence of carbohydrate moieties at certain sites could result in some of the differences in antigenicity observed between H3 and H1.

HA as the major antigen of influenza viruses possesses both specific and cross-reacting determinants *(21,22)*. With conventional serological methods significant cross-reactivity is limited to strains within a subtype although minor cross-reactions can be found *(21)*. Rabbits immunized with either intact or purified HA produced antibodies reactive with either HA_1 or HA_2, and some antibodies to the HA_2 showed a limited amount of cross-reactivity *(22)*. Using purified HA_1 or HA_2 in radioimmunoassay (RIA), it was observed that serum raised against H1N1 virus contained two populations of antibody binding to HA_1 or HA_2 *(23)*. The HA_2-specific antibodies to H1-HA had some homotypic cross-reactivity (i.e., to H3-HA). This possibly can be explained by the sequence similarity of HA genes; HA_2 subunits are highly conserved among influenza A viruses *(24)*.

Approaches similar to those used to study the antigenic properties of HA are being used to examine NA *(25,26)*. Variation in amino acid sequence has been observed to occur in regions that form a nearly continuous surface at the top of the subunit *(25,26)*. The catalytic site, which is a large pocket of the distal surface, appears to be surrounded by variable regions *(26)*. Studies with monoclonal antibodies have shown that these variable areas are also antigenic *(27)*. Despite immunogenic equivalence to HA *(8)*, the immune response to the NA is dominated by the anti-HA response *(21,28)*. Furthermore, NA evolves at a slower rate than HA as a result of the greater selective pressure of HA antibodies *(12)*.

During the past decade much effort has been made to explore the immune response to the internal proteins of Influenza A virus, especially M_1 and NP. Both of these proteins are highly conserved *(29–32)*. These studies focused primarily on the cross-reactive cytotoxic T-cell (CTL) and T-helper response. Antibodies to M_1 and NP can be found in the sera of animals immunized with whole virus vaccines, purified protein preparations, and after infection *(33–35)*. But recent studies have failed to demonstrate a significant role for these antibodies in the amelioration of disease *(33,36)*, and their presence in conventional vaccine preparations *(37)* does not result in a diminution or enhancement of the immune response to the surface glycoproteins *(33)*.

T-Cell Recognition

The requirement of T-helper (T_H) cells for the induction of specific immunity to influenza virus proteins has been extensively well documented *(38–40)*. An intact T_H cell function is needed for the production of neutralizing antibodies during both primary *(38,39)* and secondary *(40)* immune responses. Immunization with whole influenza virus gives rise to populations of MHC-restricted T_H cells in both humans and mice directed toward the major glycoproteins, HA and NA, and internal proteins, M and NP *(33,41,42)*. Two major groups of T_H cells have been described, one that recognizes antigenic determinants common to all influenza A viruses and the other that is reactive only to determinants within a given subtype *(43)*. Analysis of a panel of human T_H cell clones induced with intact influenza virus revealed that approx 50% were subtype cross-reactive; the majority of these clones were reactive with M or NP *(43)*. Similar results have been obtained in mice, where at the clonal level 58% of the T_H hybridomas were reactive to M or NP and were subtype-crossreactive, whereas the HA- and NA-specific hybridomas were subtype-specific *(44)*. It has been shown that both subtype-specific and cross-reactive T_H cells can be stimulated by both HA_1 and HA_2 polypeptide chains of the HA molecule.

Interestingly, both human and murine T_H cells specific for internal components of the virion are able to collaborate with B cells in the production of HA- and NA-specific antibody *(33,45–47)*. Studies have shown that T_H cells specific for the internal proteins M and NP, are as effective in vivo as an HA-specific T_H clone in providing help for HA-specific B cells during a primary immune response. This study also showed evidence that the observed help followed the rules of a "cognate interaction" (i.e., direct T–B cell interaction), and therefore supports the concept of intermolecular/intrastructural T–B interaction in the anti-influenza response. The proposed mechanism for this phenomenon is that B cells specific for the surface glycoproteins, HA and NA, capture intact whole influenza virus particles via their surface Ig, but after internalization and processing present the various processed protein components (e.g., M, NP) of the virus *(33,47,48)*.

Cytotoxic T cells kill virus-infected cells when their T-cell receptors recognize viral proteins on the surface of infected cells. Shortly after demonstration that CTLs could be generated against influenza virus *(49)*, several groups showed that CTLs raised to one A strain of virus could lyse target cells infected with any A strain, but not with a B strain *(50–52)*. Early studies indicated that CTLs generated during the course of infection in mice show two types of specificity, one specific to the stimulating virus and another broadly reactive with other influenza subtypes *(52,53)*. It had been thought that CTLs would predominantly recognize surface glycoproteins and in particular HA. There is little doubt that in both murine and human studies HA is recognized by CTLs, but the evidence suggest that only 10–15% of CTL precursor cells recognize HA *(54,55)* and that approx 90% of CTLs recognize internal proteins. A significant number of cross-reactive CTLs recognize M_1 and NP *(55–57)*. Indeed, both of these proteins are highly conserved *(29–31)* and induce a cross-reactive CTL response *(56–59)*. Many studies using a variety of immunization schemes, including purified proteins *(60)*, isolated peptides *(61)*, vaccinia recombinants expressing influenza viral proteins *(62)*, and injection of DNA encoding viral protein *(63,64)*, have shown an induction of immune response to heterotypic influenza A viruses. However, other studies have failed to demonstrate protection from infection despite the presence of M_1- and NP-specific CTLs *(36,49)*. Furthermore, despite evidence that live and inactivated influenza vaccines induce cross-reactive T-cells in humans *(65,66)* and mice *(67,68)*, reinfection with homologous or heterotypic virus does occur *(33)*.

Vaccination Against Influenza

Influenza remains a pervasive public health problem in spite of the wide availability of a specific whole-virus vaccine that is 60–80% effective under optimal conditions *(69,70)*. Currently licensed trivalent influenza vaccines are derived from high-yield reassortant viruses comprised of formalin-inactivated strains that possess the HA and NA of recently prevalent influenza A viruses predicted to cause widespread infection (i.e., H3N2 and H1N1), the internal proteins from the A/PR/8/34 high-yield donor parent, and similar antigens from the prevalent B influenza strain *(33,37,71)*. Antibody to both major glycoproteins can be found in the serum of individuals immunized with these vaccines *(33,72,73)*. When these vaccines are effective illness is prevented usually by preventing infection *(8,71,73)*. These conventional vaccines are effective only if the HA of the vaccine strain is closely matched in antigenic structure to the expected wild-type strain HA. Furthermore, immunity produced in this way is of short duration *(74)*; consequently, annual vaccination may be necessary to perpetuate immunity. Also, in part, inadequacy of disease control reflects less than optimal utilization of the vaccine even in those at high risk for serious illness and restricted use of the vaccine because of its reactogenicity in very young children, a group at high risk for serious illness.

Inactivated Virus Vaccines

Inactivated influenza virus vaccines are prepared from the allantoic fluid of virus-infected eggs. Virus is purified and concentrated by zonal centrifugation or chromatography. Purified virus can be inactivated by a number of procedures, including treatment with formalin, β-propionolactone or ultraviolet irradiation. Whole-virus vaccines contain intact inactivated virus. Split-product vaccines are prepared from purified formalin-treated virus disrupted with organic solvents or detergents to solubilize the surface glycoproteins. The principle value of split-product vaccines is their relatively low toxicity. Virtually all contemporary inactivated influenza vaccines are derived from reassortant viruses and are standardized according to the antigenic content of HA only *(71)*.

Questions have been raised concerning the immunogenicity and efficacy of inactivated virus vaccines. Additionally, concerns about inactivated virus vaccines include potential toxicity, possible escape from inactivation, brevity of immunity, and the presentation of influenza viral antigens by an abnormal route (i.e., parenteral injection). Parenteral administration of inactivated virus vaccine will induce antibody formation in man *(75)* and mice *(8,76)*. In primed individuals (e.g., people with serologic evidence of exposure to H3N2 influenza virus), parenteral vaccination with either an H3N2 whole virus vaccine or split-product vaccine induced "protective" levels of antibody against HA, which prevented infection in 89% of recipients shortly after vaccination. In contrast, in unprimed recipients of whole-virus vaccine, only 65% developed protective levels of serum anti-HA antibodies *(72,77)*. Similar findings were reported on the serological responses to H1N1 virus (A/NJ/70). Wise et al. *(78)* observed that levels of anti-HA antibody were generally low after a single dose of vaccine, but increased significantly in response to a second dose. Differences in response to whole vaccine prepared by different manufacturers have been noted; these different serologic responses correlated to the HA content of the vaccines. Additionally, split-virus vaccines were less immunogenic than whole-virus vaccines, especially in younger vaccinees *(78)*. Other studies showed no difference between these two types of vaccines *(79)*. Results from several studies demonstrate that the serologic response to influenza virus vaccine varied with the age of the recipient and previous exposure to influenza virus *(78–81)*. Results of studies in mice are concordant with those found in humans, i.e., split-virus and whole-virus vaccines were less immunogenic in unprimed subjects. However, the immunogenicity of both types of vaccine were enhanced in subjects primed by previous influenza immunization or infection *(80)*.

Vaccination with conventional, inactivated influenza virus vaccines, containing both HA and NA, stimulates immunity against both antigens *(74,77, 82,83)*, although the immunological response to NA is severely suppressed in primed subjects as a result of HA dominant antigenic competition *(8,28,33, 48,84)*. Studies have shown that only 20% of children vaccinated with conventional trivalent influenza vaccine had detectable antibody to the viral NAs after vaccination *(82)*. In immunologically primed adults, the NA antibody responses to a single dose of H1N1 or H3N2 vaccine were 38% and 54%, respectively.

Similarly studies with conventional trivalent inactivated vaccine showed a 20–68% response to one or more of the NAs contained in the vaccine. Interestingly, there are no reports of a diminution of the anti-HA response in the trivalent vaccine despite the presence of two other HAs *(33,77,83)*.

It has been shown that T_H cells are stimulated in response to influenza virus vaccine *(84,85)*. However, several groups have shown that inactivated virus vaccines are not as effective as infectious virus in induction of CTLs *(53,60)*. Differences in the immunogenicity of inactivated virus vaccines with respect to ability to stimulate the host for a CTL response have been related to different methods of inactivation *(86)*. In studies with mice, virus inactivated by UV irradiation or formalin induced a poor primary CTL response and was relatively ineffective in priming for a secondary CTL response *(60,86)*. Virus inactivated by gamma-irradiation stimulated a cross-reactive primary CTL response *(87)* and a secondary CTL response *(88)* in mice. In primed humans, inactivated virus stimulated a cross-reactive CTL response *(66)*. The ability of inactivated vaccine to stimulate a CTL response in unprimed humans has not been determined.

The protective efficacy of inactivated vaccine against influenza virus infection has been 70–90% in studies of vaccinated military personnel, but protection of persons in high-risk categories (e.g., the elderly) has been variable (0–80%) *(89–92)*. In view of antigenic drift, how effective is inactivated vaccine in induction of protection against challenge with a heterotypic virus? This question was addressed experimentally in a study by Hoskins et al. *(93)*, who showed that the first vaccination of young schoolboys with prevailing influenza virus strain provided protection against that strain, but that the next annual vaccination with a subsequent variant did not induce protection against the second strain. The cumulative influenza attack rate was the same for unvaccinated as for vaccinated boys; however, disease in vaccinated boys was shifted toward later epidemics *(93)*. Vaccine studies in mice have shown that the likelihood of infection from a challenge virus is correlated to the antigenic relatedness of the HA from the challenge strain to the immunizing strain. Furthermore, the severity of infection (i.e., manifestation of disease) is also mediated by the antigenic relatedness of the NAs involved *(9,33,94)*. These data suggest that optimal protection against epidemic influenza illness is probably afforded by a combination of antibodies against both HA and NA of the circulating strain *(77,94)*.

Live Attenuated Virus Vaccines

Live attenuated virus vaccines have been studied in several countries. However, the World Health Organization (WHO) has not formulated recommendations on their routine use. Live attenuated vaccines have a theoretical advantage over inactivated vaccines in that they mimic natural infection and therefore could produce a longer lasting immunity.

A live vaccine virus must be attenuated and not produce clinical illness in vaccinees or their contacts. The virus should also be infectious and induce a protective immunity; furthermore, the vaccine virus should be genetically stable. There are four main approaches to the production of live attenuated influenza vaccines:

1. Generation of virus "deadapted" to humans by passage of the virus in a nonhuman host (e.g., chick embryo);
2. Selection of viruses with specific genetic markers for viral attenuation (e.g., cold-adapted [ca] or temperature sensitive [ts] mutants);
3. Recombine naturally occurring avian influenza viruses attenuated for replication in nonhumans with human influenza viruses; and
4. Use of genetic engineering techniques to create attenuated mutants containing lesions or deletions in one or more genes.

Clinical studies in man suggest that live influenza A vaccines can afford protection from disease. However, the type and amount of protection afforded varies with the sort of live virus agent used (90,95–97). Recent studies in children (96) and adults (90,97) comparing serum antibody production and protective efficacy of ca mutants with inactivated influenza vaccine have shown that ca mutants can induce an immunity equivalent to that induced by conventional inactivated vaccine. This includes the lack of interference of the immune response to a specific HA by other HAs present in the vaccine while retaining the relative suppression of the immune response to NA (90,97). However in other studies ca mutants were 100-fold less efficient than the inactivated counterpart in the induction of influenza virus-specific antibody (95). Clements et al. (98) evaluated an avian–human reassortant influenza virus in adults. The avian–human reassortant virus, like its avian influenza virus parent (A/Pintail/119/79) was restricted 100-fold in replication relative to wild-type human influenza virus (A/Washington/897/80). Despite this restriction of replication, infection of human volunteers with the reassortant virus induced resistance to an antigenically homologous wild-type human influenza A virus. However, difficulty in confirming attenuation and genetic instability have restricted this approach. There are no studies using combinations of avian-reassortants containing the HAs of currently circulating A subtype influenza viruses or any studies of B subtype reassortants.

The ts mutant strains have not been directly used as vaccines but have contributed genes bearing ts defects to reassortant viruses (72,99). A new approach to the generation of live attenuated influenza A virus vaccine candidates was made possible by the development of techniques to introduce influenza A virus RNA genes, produced in vitro from cDNA, into infectious virus (99–102). Using this methodology, a large number of attenuating mutations have been introduced into the HA *(103)*, NA *(104)*, polymerase gene products *(99,105)*, M_1, and NP *(105)*. However, attenuating mutations on the HA and NA genes are not useful as the transferable attenuating genes of an influenza A donor virus, since the HA and NA genes must be derived from a newly emerged epidemic or pandemic strain. As with other live attenuated viral vaccines, there can be rapid loss of temperature sensitivity in the host *(99,106)*. Multivalent vaccines containing live attenuated influenza A strains have been associated with variable frequencies of virus shedding and serologic response to both HA and NA for each H1N1 and H3N2 subtype contained in the vaccine preparation *(107–111)*. The evidence from these studies indicates that the response to the viral HA is dependent on the amount of viral replication, as reflected in viral shedding. Furthermore, once strain differences in viral replication are controlled, there is no evidence of interference of the immune response to any of the HAs contained in the vaccine preparations *(90,97,108)*. The immune response to the NAs contained in these vaccines was significantly less than the response to HA, when measured by frequency of seroconversion and comparison of NA antibody titers, again an apparent manifestation of HA-dominant antigenic competition.

Despite restriction of replication and promises of better immunization, use of live ca and ts mutant viruses has been limited by their genetic instability, leading to reversion to virulence *(99,107,108)*.

New Approaches to Influenza Virus Vaccination

New approaches to influenza virus vaccine development include:

1. Synthesis of the appropriate oligopeptides *(42,112)*;
2. Synthesis of influenza virus proteins in transformed prokaryotes *(113)*, mammalian *(114)*, or insect *(115,116)* cells;
3. Production of anti-idiotype antibodies *(117,118)*;
4. Use of infectious organisms as vectors of influenza viral genes, such as vaccinia *(119)*, herpes *(120)*, and adenovirus *(121)*; and
5. The use of naked DNA vaccines *(63,64)*.

None of these vaccines has enjoyed wide experimental usage in animals or humans therefore, further discussion of them is beyond the ambit of this paper. However, each of these novel approaches to immunization against influenza holds promise of reduced reactogenicity and avoidance of HA-NA antigenic competition.

There is another alternative approach to immunization against influenza that is the product of studies investigating antigenic competition and therefore has relevance here; it is infection permissive immunization induced by vaccination with influenza viral NA. The usual object of immunization against influenza virus is complete inhibition or restriction of infection. Another strategy is infection-permissive immunization. The basic premise of this approach involves immunization with viral proteins, such as the NA, that do not elicit neutralizing antibody but do restrict viral replication below a pathogenic threshold, thereby allowing infection but not disease *(33,74,122,123)*. Influenza virus NA, whether administered as a purified protein without adjuvant *(8,9,37)* or administered in viral antigenic hybrids containing an HA novel to human experience (e.g., H7N2) *(11,74,122)*, has been shown to engender protective immunity both in a murine model *(9)* and in humans *(37,74,122)*. Immunization of mice with either N1 or N2 alone or combined together induces a specific immune response to NA which, although infection-permissive across a broad range of NA-antibody levels *(8,9,124)*, is free of intra-NA antigenic competition (i.e., no reduction of the anti-N2 NA response in the presence of the N1 NA and vv) and results in the significant reduction of viral titers as measured by plaque-forming units in tissue culture *(8,9,11,124)* and lessens the severity of viral infection as measured by the reduction of weight loss *(125)*. Recent studies have shown that purified NA vaccine *(10,37)*, purified HA preparations and conventional commercial whole virus vaccine contain significant amounts of matrix (M_1) and nucleoprotein (NP) as measured by immunoblotting and assay of polyclonal sera made against "purified" HA preparations. The presence of these "bystander" proteins neither enhanced or reduced the immune response to the surface glycoproteins *(33)*, consistent with earlier work with purified HA and NA demonstrating that an immune response to the surface glycoproteins affords the same protection as whole virus immunization *(8,33,124)*.

Antigenic Competition Between HA and NA

Although there has been relatively limited information regarding immunological interactions among different HAs in trivalent combination influenza vaccine, there have been many studies of antigenic competition between HA and NA in this combination. Both HA and NA are immunogenic and are the antigens primarily involved in the induction of specific immunity to influenza. HA is generally the superior immunogen, inducing antibody that directly neutralizes virus infectivity. Antibody to the NA, although not neutralizing, limits viral replication in multicycle infections. "NA-specific" immunization can be carried out with antigenically hybrid viruses that contain the HA of an animal strain irrelevant to human experience. Comparative studies of such "NA-specific" and conventional vaccines in populations primed to prevalent influenza virus subtypes have shown that the H7N2 and H7N1 reassortant vaccines (NA-specific) evoke greater NA antibody response than H3N2 and H1N1 equivalent in NA immunogenicity *(21,85,122)*. Diminished NA antibody response in HA primed populations has also been remarked by Kendal et al. *(82)*.

The first observation of this phenomenon was in groups of college students with serologic evidence of experience with H3N2 viruses, who then received either a conventional H3N2 vaccine (A/England/42/72), an antigenic hybrid H7N2 virus vaccine (A/Equine/Prague/56 × A/England/42/72) or a placebo injection *(21)*. All subjects had antibody to N2-NA before immunization, and the mean initial HI and NI were comparable in both vaccine groups. Yet, the mean antibody response to N2 was twofold greater in those vaccinated with H7N2 reassortant virus vaccine. In a similar study, school-age children were immunized with an H3N2 (A/Port Chalmers/73) vaccine, a NA-specific H7N2 reassortant virus vaccine (A/Equine/Prague/56 × A/Port Chalmers/73), or a placebo *(122)*. Before vaccination, all of the children were seronegative for H7, 80% were seronegative for H3-Port Chalmers, and 90% were negative for N2-Port Chalmers. Vaccination induced seroconversion for the Port Chalmers HA- and NA-specific antibody in children receiving the conventional vaccine, while the NA-specific vaccine induced only N2-Port Chalmers-specific antibody. Two natural outbreaks of H3N2 influenza A virus infection occurred during the study period: one caused by the Port Chalmers strain in the winter of 1974–75; the other by the Victoria strain in the winter of 1975–76. Analysis of antibody titers after infection with the Victoria strain indicated that uninfected children had relatively high titers of anti-H3 and anti-N2 Port Chalmers-specific antibody regardless of the vaccine they had received. It was observed that the antigenically hybrid H7N2 virus vaccine induced a greater frequency and magnitude of response to the NA antigen. Children who were asymptomatically infected with the Victoria strain had mean N2-Port Chalmer specific NA antibody titers three to fivefold greater than those symptomatically infected. In fact, children vaccinated with H7N2 virus demonstrated significantly higher N2 Port Chalmers antibody titers than children who received H3N2 vaccine, both before and after exposure to the Victoria strain. All groups demonstrated equivalent anti-H3 Victoria antibody titers. Furthermore, cell-mediated immunity measured by lymphocyte transformation assay showed that blood lymphocyte cultures from children immunized with H7N2 virus vaccine proliferated threefold greater than cells from H3N2 vaccinees in response to in vitro stimulation with N2 antigen *(85)*. The children were initially seronegative or manifested low titers of H3-Port Chalmers or N2-Port Chalmers antibody activity before immunization. The H7N2 vaccine induced no increase in H3 antibody, but all subjects demonstrated an increase in N2-Port Chalmers antibody titers after immunization. Vaccination with the conventional (H3N2) vaccine resulted in seroconversion for H3-Port Chalmers and N2-Port Chalmers in all subjects, but the NA antibody titers in the H3N2 vaccine group were four to tenfold less than those in the H7N2 vaccine group despite the twofold higher NA activity of the H3N2 vaccine *(85)*.

The immunological response to influenza virus NA has been examined in initially primed and unprimed vaccinees in whom vaccination with a conventional H1N1 vaccine or H7N1 antigenic reassortant vaccine was followed by natural infection with an H1N1 influenza virus *(126)*. Both vaccines were only marginally immunogenic for NA in initially seronegative subjects, yet in vaccinees initially seropositive for H1 significant NA antibody titer increases occurred with H7N1 vaccine. Furthermore, subsequent infection with an H1N1 influenza virus boosted NA antibody less effectively in the initially infection-primed vaccinees than in the initially seronegative subjects primed by vaccination. Kilbourne et al. *(126)* concluded that prior experience with influenza virus HA has a suppressive influence on immune response to NA. This is consistent with an earlier proposal that the superiority of the NA-specific vaccine (H7N2 or H7N1) as an immunogen for antibody to NA might reflect different processing of NA when it is associated with a HA to which the study population had not been primed, presumably because subjects were primed to the HA (H1 or H3) and the anti-HA anamnestic response depresses the concomitant NA response apparently by antigenic competition *(21)*.

Mechanism of HA–NA Antigenic Competition

In BALB/c mice primed to H3–HA and N2–NA by infection, the presentation of N2 in association with a heterotypic HA (H6N2) resulted, as expected, in production of a greater amount of N2 antibody than was found with homologous (H3N2) reimmunization *(28)*. Titration of primed T_H activity by adoptive transfer of purified T cells to athymic mice given H6N2 vaccine demonstrated a lesser number of N2-specific T_H cells in mice subjected to homologous (H3N2-H3N2) reimmunization *(48,84)*. These observations demonstrated the participation of T_H cells in the mediation of intermolecular intravirionic antigenic competition between influenza HA and NA. In further exploration of the mechanism, the in vitro reaction of purified splenic B and T lymphocytes from mice immunized by various immunization schedules was investigated. Assay of the proliferation response of T cells in B/T cell mixtures stimulated by HA- and NA-specific reassortant viruses in vitro enabled differentiation of cellular responses to HA and NA antigens. It was shown that intravirionic HA is dominant over NA in both T- and B-cell priming and memory B-cells functioned as antigen-presenting cells and interacted with memory T_H cells in the mediation of intravirionic HA/NA antigenic competition in favor of HA. Thus, the damping of the response to the NA in favor of HA prohibited a balanced response to the two virion antigens under ordinary conditions of immunization, whether by whole virus vaccine or by infection *(48,84)*. Finally, BALB/c mice immunized with graded doses of chromatographically purified HA and NA antigens derived from A/Hong

Kong/1/68 (H3N2) influenza virus demonstrated equivalent responses when HA- and NA-specific serum antibodies were measured by ELISA. Antibody responses measured by HI or NI titrations showed similar kinetic patterns, except for more rapid decline in HI antibody *(8,124,126)*.

The model proposed for intravirionic antigenic competition assumes that antigen presentation by macrophages probably precedes or coincides with antigen presentation by B cells. This assumption is based on work indicating that B cells present antigen efficiently only in secondary immune responses or late in the primary response *(127)*. It can be postulated that, in the initial recognition of influenza virus antigens by the immune system, the antigens are probably engulfed by macrophages or dendritic cells, processed and presented to T cells. Because HA is found in greater molar amounts on the virion surface than NA, despite immunogenic equivalence as purified antigens, the immune response is skewed toward HA. However, when infection or vaccination occurs with a virus containing a previously encountered NA and an HA to which the host is immunologically naive, NA-specific memory B cells expanded by previous exposure more efficiently capture viral particles and present antigen to memory T_H cells, resulting in B- and T-cell activation. Resting B cells recognizing the novel HA are probably competitively blocked by the more efficient activated NA-specific B cell. Additionally in support of this model, recent work has shown that for intravirionic antigenic competition to occur the competing antigens must be on the same viral particle *(9)*.

Summary

Combining several antigens into single vaccine preparations is not novel or unique to influenza vaccines and is often driven by administrative and financial considerations. However, presenting multiple antigens in a given vaccine with the goal of attaining immunization and subsequent protection equivalent to that seen with the individual components can be problematic. Barr and Llewellyn-Jones *(128–130)* observed "immunologic interference" among components of the diphtheria-pertussis-tetanus (DTP) vaccine in humans. Taussig *(131)* described this form of antigenic competition (i.e., a relative decrease in immune response to an antigen when presented within a mixture) as intermolecular antigenic competition. The solution to avoid competition when mixed antigens were injected was to adjust the relative ratios of antigens to "balance" the immune response. In contrast, intravirionic antigenic competition *(84)* is dependent not only on the concomitant administration of antigens but on the fact that these antigens are physically linked (i.e., as antigens on the same viral particle) and therefore are taken up and processed together *(28,48,84)*. Studies of NA-specific antigenic hybrid vaccines and purified NA and HA have shown that the diminished antibody response to NA occurs only when both NA and HA are presented on the same viral particle despite evidence that the surface glycoproteins are equivalent antigens *(8,9,21,33)*. HA immunogenicity is dominant over NA in both B- and T-cell priming as a result of intravirionic antigenic competition. Further studies found no indication of intramolecular or of intravirionic antigenic competition within mixed but physically dissociated N1 and N2 NAs *(9)*, or any evidence of antigenic competition from the internal proteins, M and NP *(11)*.

The impact of antigenic competition on current commercial inactivated vaccines is limited to the potential diminution of the immune response to NA. However, recently proposed DTP-HA *(132)*, DTP-NA (B. Johansson, unpublished data) and other noninfluenza vaccines *(133)* highlight the need for vaccine designers to be aware of potential changes in the immunogenicity of vaccine components as a result of the presence of other antigens in the injection mixture.

References

1. Frank, J., Henderson, M., and McMurray, L. (1985) Influenza vaccination in the elderly. I. Determinants of acceptance. *Can. Med. Assoc. J.* **132,** 371.
2. Mostow, S. (1985) Influenza: a preventable disease not being prevented. *Am. Rev. Respir. Dis.* **134,** 1.
3. Mahy, B. (1983) Mutants of influenza virus, in *Genetics of Influenza Viruses* (Palese, P. and Kingsbury, D. W., eds.), Spring-Verlag, New York, pp. 192–254.
4. Choppin, P. and Tamm, I. (1960) Studies of two kinds of virus particles which comprise influenza A2 virus strains. II. Reactivity with virus inhibitors in normal sera. *J. Exp. Med.* **112,** 921.
5. Yoshimura, A. and Ohnishi, S. (1984) Uncoating of influenza virus in endosomes. *J. Virol.* **51,** 497–504.
6. Gottschalk, A. (1957) Neuraminidase: The specific enzyme of influenza virus and *Vibro cholerae. Biochem. Biophys. Acta.* **23,** 645.
7. Palese, P., Tobita, K., Ueda, M., and Compans, R. W. (1974) Characterization of temperature sensitive influenza virus mutants defective in neuraminidase. *Virology* **61,** 397.
8. Johansson, B., Bucher, D., and Kilbourne, E. (1989) Purified influenza virus hemagglutinin and neuraminidase are equivalent in stimulation of antibody response but induce contrasting types of immunity to infection. *J. Virol.* **63,** 1239.
9. Johansson, B. and Kilbourne, E. (1994) Immunization with purified N1 and N2 influenza virus neuraminidases demonstrates cross-reactivity without antigenic competition. *Proc. Natl. Acad. Sci. USA* **91,** 2358.
10. Kilbourne, E., Couch, R., Kasel, J., Keitel, J., Cate, T., Quarles, J., Grajower, B., Pokorny, B., and Johansson, B. (1995) Purified influenza A virus N2 neuraminidase vaccine is immunogenic and non-toxic in humans. *Vaccine* **13,** 1799.
11. Johansson, B. and Kilbourne, E. (1991) Comparative long term effects in a mouse model system of influenza whole virus vaccine and purified neuraminidase vaccine followed by sequential infections. *J. Infect. Dis.* **162,** 800–809.
12. Kilbourne, E., Grajower, B, and Johansson, B. (1990) Independent and disparate evolution in nature of influenza A virus hemagglutinin and neuraminidase. *Proc. Natl. Acad. Sci. USA* **87,** 786.
13. Compans, R., Klenk, H-D., Caliguiri, L., and Choppin, P. (1970) Influenza virus proteins. I. Analysis of polypeptides of the virion and identification of spike glycoproteins. *Virology* **42,** 880.

14. Lamb, R. and Choppin, P. (1983) Gene structure and replication of influenza virus. *Virology* **81**, 382.

15. Zebedee, S., Richardson, C., and Lamb, R. (1985) Characterization of the influenza virus M2 integral membrane protein and expression at the infected-cell surfacefrom cloned cDNA. *J. Virol.* **56**, 502.

16. Krug, R. (1971) Cytoplasmic and nucleoplasmic viral RNPs newly synthesized during the latent period of viral growth in MDCK cells. *Virology* **44**, 125.

17. Krug, R. (1972) Cytoplasmic and nucleoplasmic viral RNPs in influenza viral infected MDCK cells. *Virology* **50**, 103.

18. Wiley, D., Wilson, I., and Skehel, J. (1981) Structural identification of the antibody-binding sites of Hong Kong influenza hemagglutinin and their involvment in antigenic variation. *Nature* **289**, 373.

19. Gerhard, W., Yewdell, J., Frankel, M., and Webster, R. (1981) Antigenic structure of influenza virus hemagglutinin defined by hybridoma antibodies. *Nature* **290**, 713.

20. Caton, A., Brownlee, G., Yewdell, J., and Gerhard, W. (1982) The antigenic structure of the influenza virus A/PR/8/34 hemagglutinin (H1 subtype). *Cell* **31**, 417.

21. Kilbourne, E. (1976) Comparative efficacy of neuraminidase-specific and conventional influenza virus vaccines in the induction of anti-neuraminidase antibody in man. *J. Infect. Dis.* **134**, 384.

22. Noble, G., Kaye, H., Kendal, A., and Dowdle, W. (1977) Age rrelated heterologous antibody responses to influenza virus vaccination. *J. Infect Dis.* **136**, 5686.

23. Graves, P., Schulman, J., Young, J., and Palese, P. (1983) Preparation of influenza virus subviral particles lacking the HA1 subunit of hemagglutinin: Umasking of cross-reactive HA2 determinants. *Virology* **126**, 106.

24. Krystal, M., Elliot, R., Bergz, E., Young, J., and Palese, P. (1982) Evolution of influenza A and B viruses: conservation of structural features in the hemagglutinin genes. *Proc. Natl. Acad. Sci. USA* **79**, 4800.

25. Air, G., Els, M., Brown, L. et al. (1985) Location of antigenic sites on the three-dimensional structure of the influenza N2 virus neuraminidase. *Virology* **145**, 237.

26. Coleman, P, Varghese, J., and Laver, W. (1983) Structure of the catalytic and antigenic sites in influenza virus neuraminidase. *Nature* **303**, 41.

27. Biddison, W. E., Doherty, P. C., and Webster, R. (1977) Antibody to influenza virus matrix protein detects a common antigen on the surface of cells infected with type A influenza viruses. *J. Exp. Med.* **146**, 690.

28. Johansson, B., Moran, T., Bona, C., Popple, S., and Kilbourne, E. (1987) Immunologic response to influenza virus neuraminidase is influenced by prior experience with the associated viral hemagglutinin. II. Sequential infection of mice simulates human experience. *J. Immunol.* **139**, 2010.

29. Class, E. C., Kawaoka, Y., DeJong, J. C., Masurel, N., and Webster, R. (1994) Infection of children with avian-human reassortant influenza virus from pigs in Europe. *Virology* **204**, 453.

30. Huddelston, J. and Brownlee, G. (1982) The sequence of the nucleoprotein gene of human influenza virus strain A/NT/60/68. *Nucleic Acids Res.* **10**, 1029.

31. Kida, H., Ito, T., Yasuda, J., Shimizu, Y., Itakura, C., Shortridge, K., Kawaoka, Y., and Webster, R. (1994) Potential for transmission of avian viruses to pigs. *J. Gen. Virol.* **75**, 2183.

32. Mandler, J. and Scholtissek, C. (1989) Localization of the temperature sensitive defect in the nucleoprotein of an influenza A/FPV/Rostock/34. *J. Virol.* **12(2)**, 113.

33. Johansson, B. and Kilbourne, E. (1996) Immunization with dissociated neuraminidase, matrix, and nucleoproteins from influenza A virus eliminates cognate help and antigenic competition. *Virology* **225**, 136.

34. Van Wyke, K., Hinshaw, V., Lu, C., and Allen, P. (1980) Antigen presentation: Comments on its regulation and mechanism. *J. Virol.* **35,** 24.
35. Van Wyke, K., Yewdell, J., Peck, L., and Murphy, B. (1984) Antigenic characterization of influenza virus matrix protein with monoclonal antibodies. *J. Virol.* **49,** 248.
36. Lawson, C., Bennink, J., Restifo, N., Yewdell, J., and Murphy, B. R. (1994) Primary pulmonary cytotoxic T lymphocytes induced by immunization with a vaccinia virus recombinant expressing influenza A virus nucleoprotein peptide do not protect mice against challenge. *J. Virol.* **68,** 3505.
37. Hocart, M., Grajower, B., Donabedian, A., Pokorny, B., Whitaker, C., and Kilbourne, E. (1995) Preparation and characterization of a purified influenza virus neuraminidase vaccine. *Vaccine* **13,** 1793.
38. Virelizier, J., Postlewaite, R., Schild, G., and Allison, A. (1974) Antibody response to antigenic determinants of influenza virus hemagglutinin. Thymus dependence and antibody formation and thymus independence of immunmological memory. *J. Exp Med.* **140,** 1559.
39. Burns, W., and Billups, L., and Notkins, A. (1975) Thymus dependence of viral antigens. *Nature* **256,** 654.
40. Anders, E., Peppard, P., Burns, W., and White, D. (1979) *In vitro* antibody response to influenza virus. I. T cell dependence of secondary immune response to hemagglutinin. *J. Immunol.* **127,** 669.
41. Hurwitz, J., Heber-Katz, E., Hackett, C., and Gerhard, W. (1984) Characterization of the murine T helper response to influenza virus hemagglutinin: Evidence for three major specificities. *J. Immunol.* **133,** 3371.
42. Hackett, C., Hurwitz, J., Dietzschold, B., and Gerhard, W. (1985) A synthetic decapeptide of influenza virus hemagglutinin elicits T helper cells with the same fine recognition specifies as occur in response to whole virus. *J. Immunol.* **135,** 1391.
43. Lamb, R., Eckels, D., Lake, P., Woody, J., and Green, N. (1982) Human T cell clones recognize chemically synthesized peptides of influenza hemagglutinin. *Nature* **300,** 66.
44. Hurwitz, J., Hackett, C., McAndrew, E., and Gerhard, W. (1985) Murine helper response to influenza virus: Recognition of hemagglutinin, neuraminidase, matrix and nucleoprotein. *J. Immunol.* **134,** 1994.
45. Russell, S. and Liew, F. (1979) T cells primed by influenza viron internal components can cooperate in the antibody response to hemagglutinin. *Nature* **280,** 147.
46. Russell, S. and Liew, F. (1980) Cell cooperation in antibody responses to influenza virus. I. Priming of helper T cells by internal components. *Eur. J. Immunol.* **10,** 791.
47. Scherle, P. A. and Gerhard, W. A. (1986) Functional analysis of influenza-specific helper T-cell clones *in vivo*. *J. Exp. Med.* **164,** 1114.
48. Johansson, B., Moran, T., and Kilbourne, E. (1987) Antigen-presenting B cells and helper T cells cooperatively mediate intravirionic antigenic competition between influenza A virus surface glycoproteins. *Proc. Natl. Acad. Sci. USA* **84,** 6869.
49. Yap, K. L. and Ada, G. L. (1977) Cytotoxic T cells specific for influenza virus-infected target cells. *Immunology* **32,** 151.
50. Doherty, P., Biddison, W., Bennick, J., and Knowles, B. (1978) Cytotoxic T cell responses in mice infected with influenza and vaccinia viruses vary in magnitude with H2 genotype. *J. Exp. Med.* **148,** 534.
51. Zweerink, H., Askonas, B., Millican, D., Courtneidge, S., and Skehel, J. (1977) Cytotoxic T cells to type A influenza virus: Viral hemagglutinin induces A strain specificity while infected cells confer cross-reactive cytotoxicity. *Eur. J. Immunol.* **7,** 30.
52. Braciale, T. J. (1977) Immunologic recognition of influenza virus infected cells. *Cell Immunol.* **33,** 423.
53. Braciale, T. J. and Yap, K. L. (1978) Role of viral infectivity oin the induction of influenza virus-specific cytotoxic T cells. *J. Exp. Med.* **147,** 1236.

54. Owen, J., Allouche, M., and Doherty, P. (1982) Limiting dilution analysis of the specificity of influenza immune cytotoxic T cells. *Cell Immunol.* **67,** 49.
55. Andrew, M. E., Coupar, B. E., Ada, G. L., and Boyle, D. B. (1986) Cell-mediated immune responses to influenza virus antigens expressed by vaccinia virus recombinants. *Microb. Pathol.* **1,** 443.
56. Yewdell, J. W., Bennink, J. R., Smith, G. L., and Moss, B. (1985) Influenza A virus nucleoprotein is a major target antigen for cross-reactive anti-influenza A virus cytotoxic T lymphocytes. *Proc. Natl. Acad. Sci. USA* **83,** 1785.
57. Fleischer, B., Becht, H., and Rott. R. (1985) Recognition of viral antigens by human influenza A virus-specific T lymphocyte clones. *J. Immunol.* **135,** 2800.
58. McMicheal, A., Michie, C., Grotch, F., Smith, G., and Moss, B. (1986) Recognition of influenza A virus nucleoprotein by human cytotoxic T lymphocytes. *J. Gen. Virol.* **164,** 1367.
59. Reiss, C. and Schulman, J. (1980) Influenza type A virus M protein expression on infected cells is responsible for cross reactive recognition by cytotoxic thymus-derived lymphocytes. *Infect. Immunol.* **29,** 719.
60. Webster, R. G. and Askonas, B. A. (1980) Cross-protection and cross-reactive cytotoxic T cells induced by influenza virus vaccines in mice. *Eur. J. Immunol.* **10,** 396.
61. Townsend, A. R. M., McMicheal, A. J., Carter, N. P., Huddelston, J. A., and Brownlee, G. G. (1984) Cytotoxic T cell recognition of the influenza nucleoprotein and hemagglutinin expressed in transfected mouse L cells. *Cell* **39,** 13.
62. Andrew, M. E., Coupar, B. E., Boyle, D. B., and Ada, G. L (1987) The roles of influenza virus hemagglutinin and nucleoprotein in protection: analysis using vaccinia virus recombinants. *Scand. J. Immunol.* **25,** 21.
63. Ulmer, J. B., Donnelly, J. J., Parker, S. E., et al. (1993) Heterologous protection against influenza by injection of DNA encoding a viral protein. *Science* **259,** 1745.
64. Donnelly, J. J., Friedman, A., Ulmer, J. B., and Liu, M. A. (1997) Further protection against antigenic drift of influenza virus in a ferret model by DNA vaccination. *Vaccine* **15,** 865.
65. McMicheal, A., Grotch, F., Cullen, P., Askonas, B., and Webster, R. (1981) The human cytotoxic T cell response to influenza vaccination. *Clin. Exp. Immunol.* **43,** 276.
66. McMicheal, A., Grotch, F., Noble, G., and Beare, P. (1983) Cytotoxic T-cell immunity to influenza. *N. Engl. J. Med.* **309,** 13.
67. Ennis, F. A., Rock, A. H., Qi, K. L., Schild, G. C., Riley, D., Pratt, R., and Potter, C. W. (1981) HLA-restricted virus-specific cytotoxic T-lyphocyte responses to live and inactivated influenza vaccines. *Lancet* **2,** 887.
68. Wraith, D. C. (1986) Induction of influenza A virus cross reactive cytotoxic lymphocytes by purified viral proteins, in *Options for the Control of Influenza* (Kendal, A. P. and Patriarca, P. A., eds.), A. R. Liss, New York, pp. 461–469.
69. Gross, P., Quinnan, G., Rodstein, M., et al. (1988) Association of influenza immunization with reduction in mortality in an elderly population: a prospective study. *Arch. Intern. Med.* **148,** 562.
70. Barker, W. and Mullooly, J. (1982) Pneumonia and influenza deaths during epidemics. Implications for prevention. *Arch. Intern. Med.* **142,** 85.
71. Kilbourne, E. (1980) Influenza: viral determinants of the pathogenicity and epidemicity of an invariant disease of variable occurrence. *Phil. Trans. R. Soc. L.* **288,** 291.
72. Murphy, B. and Chanock, R. (1985) Immunization against viruses, in *Virology* (Fields, B., ed.), Raven, New York, pp. 349–370.
73. Couch, R., Douglas, R., Fedson, D., and Kasel, J. (1971) Correlated studies of a recombinant influenza virus vaccine. III. Protection against experimental influenza in man. *J. Infect. Dis.* **124,** 473.

74. Couch, R., Kasel, J., Gerin, J., Schulman, J., and Kilbourne, E. (1974) Induction of partial immunity to influenza by a neuraminidase-specific influenza A virus vaccine in humans. *J. Infect. Dis.* **129**, 411.

75. Chenoweth, A., Waltz, A., Stokes, J., Jr., et al. (1936) Active immunization with the viruses of human and swine influenza. *Am. J. Dis. Child* **52**, 757.

76. Balkovic, E. and Six, R. (1986) Pulmonary and serum isotypic antibody responses of mice to live and inactivated influenza virus. *Am. Rev. Respir. Dis.* **134**, 6.

77. Powers, D., Kilbourne, E., and Johansson, B. (1996) Neuraminidase-specific antibody responses to inactivated influenza vaccine in young and elderly adults. *Clin. Diagn. Lab. Immunol.* **3**, 511.

78. Wise, T., Polin, R., Mazur, M., and Ennis, F. (1977) Serologic responses after two sequential doses of influenza A/New Jersey/76 virus vaccine in normal young adults. *J. Infect. Dis.* **136**, 5496.

79. Meiklejohn, G., Eichoff, T., and Graves, P. (1977) Antibody response of young adults to experimental influenza A/New Jersy/76 virus vaccine. *J. Infect. Dis.* **136**, 5456.

80. McLaren, C., Verbonitz, T., Daniel, S., Guggs, G., and Ennis, F. (1977) Effect of priming infection on serologic response to whole and subunit influenza virus vaccines in animals. *J. Immunol.* **125**, 2679.

81. Gonchoroff, N., Kendal, A., Phillips, D., and Reiner, C. (1982) Immunoglobulin M and G antibody response to type and sub-type specific antigens after primary and secondary exposures of mice to influenza A viruses. *Infect. Immunol.* **35**, 310.

82. Kendal, A., Noble, G., and Dowdle, W. (1977) Neuraminidase content of influenza vaccines and neuraminidase antibody responses after vaccination of immunologically primed and unprimed populations. *J. Infect. Dis.* **136**, S145.

83. Kilbourne, E., Palese, P., and Schulman, J. (1975) Inhibition of viral neuraminidase as a new approach to the prevention of influenza, in *Perspectives in Virology*, vol. 9 (Pollard, M., ed.), Academic, New York, pp. 99–113.

84. Johansson, B., Moran, T., Bona, C., and Kilbourne, E. (1987) Immunologic response to influenza virus neuraminidase is influenced by prior experience with the associated viral hemagglutinin. III. Reduced generation of neuraminidase-specific helper T cells in hemagglutinin-primed mice. *J. Immunol.* **139**, 2015.

85. Chow, T., Beutner, K., and Ogra, P. (1979) Cell-mediated immune response to the hemagglutinin and neuraminidase antigens of influenza virus after immunization in humans. *Infect. Immunol.* **25**, 103.

86. Ada, G., Laver, W., and Webster, R. (1987) An analysis of effector T cells infected with influenza viruses. *Immunochemistry* **14**, 643.

87. Wraith, D. and Askonas, B. (1985) Induction of influenza A virus specific cross-reactive T cells by a nucleoprotein/hemagglutinin preparation. *J. Gen. Virol.* **66**, 1327.

88. Owen, J., Dudzik, K., Klein, L., and Dorer, D. (1988) The kinetics of generation of influenza-specific cytotoxic T-lymphocyte precursor cells. *Cell Immunol.* **111**, 247.

89. Barker, W. and Mullooly, J. (1980) Influenza vaccination of elderly persons. *JAMA* **244**, 2547.

90. Keitel, W., Couch, R., Quarles, J., Cate, T., Baxter, B., and Maasab, H. (1993) Trivalent attenuated cold-adapted influenza virus vaccine; reduced viral shedding and serum antibody responses in susceptible adults. *J. Infect. Dis.* **167**, 305.

91. Gross, P., Ennis, F., Gaerlan, L., Denson, L., Denning, C., and Schiffman, D. (1977) A controlled double-blind comparison of the reactogenicity, immunogenicity, and protective efficacy of whole-virus and split-product influenza vaccines in children. *J. Infect. Dis.* **136**, 623.

92. Hobson, D., Curry, A., Beare, A., and Ward-Gardner, A. (1973) Hemagglutination inhibition antibody titers as a measure of protection against influenza in man. *Dev. Biol. Stand.* **20**, 164.

93. Hoskins, T., Davies, J., Smith, A., et al. (1979) Assessment of inactivated influenza A vaccine after three outbreaks of influenza at Christ's Hospital. *Lancet* **1,** 33.

94. Johansson, B., Matthews, J., and Kilbourne, E. Supplementation of conventional influenza A vaccine with purified viral neuraminidase results in a balanced and broadened immune response. *Vaccine* **16,** 1009.

95. Jones, P. and Ada, G. (1987) Influenza virus-specific antibody-secreting cell and B cell memory in the murine lung after immunization with wild-type, cold-adapted and inactivated influenza viruses. *Vaccine* **5,** 244.

96. King, J., Gross, P., Denning, P., et al. (1987) Comparison of live and inactivated influenza vaccine in high risk children. *Vaccine* **5,** 234.

97. Atmar, R., Keitel, W., Cate, T., Quarles, J., and Couch, R. (1995) Comparison of trivalent cold-adapted recombinant (CR) influenza virus vaccine with monovalent CR vaccines in healthy unselected adults. *J. Infect. Dis.* **172,** 253.

98. Clements, M., Snyder, M., Buckler-White, A. Tierney, E., London, W., and Murphy, B. (1986) Evaluation of avian-human reassortant influenza A/Washington/119/79 virus in monkeys and adult volunteers. *J. Clin. Microbiol.* **24,** 47.

99. Murphy, B., Park, E., Gottlieb, P., and Subbarao, K. (1997) An influenza A live attenuated reassortant virus possessing three temperature-sensitive mutations in the PB2 polymerase gene rapidly loses temperature sensitivity following replication in hamsters. *Vaccine* **15,** 1372.

100. Luytjes, W., Krystal, M., Enami, M., Parvin, J., and Palese, P. (1989) Amplification, expression and packaging of a foreign gene by influenza virus. *Cell* **59,** 1107.

101. Enami, M., Luytjes, W., Krystal, M., and Palese, P. (1990) Introduction of site specific mutations into the genome of influenza virus. *Proc. Natl. Acad. Sci. USA* **87,** 3802.

102. Enami, M. and Palese, P. (1991) High-frequency formation of influenza virus transfectants. *J. Virol.* **65,** 2711.

103. Horimoto, T. and Kawaoka, Y. (1994) Reverse genetics provides direct evidence for a correlation of hemagglutinin cleavability and virulence of an avian influenza virus. *J. Virol.* **68,** 3120.

104. Gastrucci, M. R., Bilsel, P., and Kawaoka, Y. (1992) Attenuation of influenza A virus by insertion of a foreign epitope into the neuraminidase. *J. Virol.* **66,** 4647.

105. Snyder, M., Buckler-White, A., London, W., Tierney, E., and Murphy, B. (1987) The avian influenza virus nucleoprotein gene and a specific constellation of avian and human virus polymerase genes each specify attenuation of avian-human influenza A/Pintail/79 reassortant viruses for monkeys. *J. Virol.* **61,** 123.

106. Snyder, M., Betts, R. F., DeBorde, D., et al. Four viral genes independently contribute to attenuation of live influenza A/Ann Arbor/6/60 (H2N2) cold-adapted reassortant virus vaccine. *J. Virol.* **62,** 488.

107. Gruber, W. C., Darden, P. M., Still, J. G., Lohr, J., Reed, G., and Wright, P. (1997) Evaluation of bivalent live attenuated influenza A vaccines in children 2 months to 3 years of age: safety, immunogenicity and dose-response. *Vaccine* **15,** 1379.

108. Gruber, W. C., Kirschner, K., Tollefson, S., et al. (1993) Comparison of monovalent and trivalent live attenuated influenza vaccines in young children. *J. Infect. Dis.* **168,** 53.

109. Piedra, P. A., Glezen, W. P., and Mbawuike, I., et al. (1993) Studies on reactogenicity and immunogenicity of attenuated bivalent cold recombinant influenza type A (CRA) and inactivated trivalent influenza (TI) vaccines in infants and young children. *Vaccine* **11,** 718.

110. Belshe, R., Swierkosz, E., Anderson, E., Newman, F., Nugent, S., and Maassab, H. (1992) Immunization of infants and young children with live attenuated trivalent cold-adapted recombinant influenza A H1N1, H3N2, and B vaccine. *J. Infect. Dis.* **165,** 727.

111. Swierkosz, E. M., Dupont, W. D., Westrich, M. K., et al. (1994) Multi-dose, live attenuated, cold-recombinant, trivalent influenza vaccine in infants and young children. *J. Infect. Dis.* **169,** 1121.

112. Green, N., Alexander, H., Olson, A., et al. (1982) Immunogenic structure of the influenza virus hemagglutinin. *Cell* **28,** 477.
113. Palese, P. and Kingsbury, D. (eds.) (1983) *The Genetics of Influenza Viruses*. Spring-Verlag, Vienna, New York, pp. 19–125.
114. Gething, M. and Sambrook, J. (1982) Construction of influenza hemagglutinin genes that code for intracellular and secreted forms of the protein. *Nature* **300,** 598.
115. Price, P., Reichelderfer, C., Johansson, B., Kilbourne, E., and Acs, G. (1989) Complementation of recombinant baculovirus by coinfection with wild-type virus facilitates production in insect larvae of antigenic proteins of hepatitis B virus and influenza virus. *Proc. Natl. Acad. Sci. USA* **86,** 1453.
116. Johansson, B., Price, P., and Kilbourne, E. (1995) Immunogenicity of influenza A virus N2 neuraminidase produced in insect larvae by baculovirus recombinants. *Vaccine* **9,** 841.
117. Dressman, G. and Kennedy, R. (1985) Anti-idiotypic antibodies: Implications of internal image based vaccines for infectious diseases. *J. Infect. Dis.* **151,** 761.
118. Bona, C. and Moran, T. (1985) Idiotype vaccines. Ann L'Instit Pasteur/Immunologie. **136,** 21.
119. Panicali, D. and Paoletti, E. (1982) Construction of poxviruses as cloning vectors: Insertion of the thymidine kinase gene from herpes simplex virus into the DNA of infectious vaccina virus. *Proc. Natl. Acad. Sci. USA* **79,** 4927.
120. Roizman, B. and Jenkins, F. (1985) Genetic engineering of novel genomes of large DNA viruses. *Science* **229,** 1208.
121. Davis, A., Kostek, B., Meeson, B., et al. (1985) Expression of hepatitis B surface antigen with a recombination adenovirus, in *Modern Approaches to Vaccines* (Chanock, P. and Lerner, R., eds.). Cold Spring Harbor Laboratory Press, Cold Spring Harbor, NY, p. 85.
122. Beutner, K., Chow, T., Rubi, E., Strussenberg, J., Clement, J., and Ogra, P. (1979) Evaluation of a neuraminidase-specific influenza vaccine in children: antibody responses and effects of the successive outbreak of natural infection. J. Virol. **140,** 844.
123. Kilbourne, E., Laver, W., Schulman, J., and Webster, R. (1968) Antiviral activity of antiserum specific for an influenza virus neuraminidase. I. *in vitro* effects. *J. Virol.* **2,** 281.
124. Johansson, B. and Kilbourne, E. (1993) Dissociation of influenza virus hemagglutinin and neuraminidase eliminates their intravirionic antigenic competition. *J. Virol.* **67,** 5721.
125. Johansson, B. E., Grajower, B., and Kilbourne, E. D. (1993) Infection permissive immunization with influenza virus neuraminidase prevents weight loss of infected mice. *Vaccine* **10,** 1037.
126. Kilbourne, E. D., Cerini, C. P., Khan, M. W., Mitchell, J. W., Jr., and Ogra, P. O. (1987) Immunologic response to the influenza virus neuraminidase is influenced by prior experience with the associated viral hemagglutinin. I. Studies in human vaccinees. *J. Immunol.* **138,** 3010.
127. Lanzavecchia, A. (1985) Antigen-specific interaction between T and B cells. *Nature* **314,** 537.
128. Barr, M. and Llewellyn-Jones, M. (1953) Some factors influencing the response of animals to immunization with combined prophylactics. *Br. J. Exp. Pathol.* **34,** 12.
129. Barr, M. and Llewellyn-Jones, M. (1953) Interferences with antitoxic responses in immunization with combined prophylactics. *Br. J. Exp. Pathol.* **34,** 233.
130. Barr, M. and Llewellyn-Jones, M. (1955) Some factors influencing the response to immunization with single 9' combined prophylactics. *Br. J. Exp. Pathol.* **36,** 147.
131. Taussig, M. (1977). Antigenic competition, in *The Antigens*, vol. IV (Sela, M., ed.), Academic, New York, pp. 333–368.
132. Gravenstein, S., Drinka, P., Duthie, E. H., Miller, B. A., Brown, C. S., Hensley, M., Circo, R., Langer, E., and Ershler, W. B. (1994) Efficacy of an influenza hemagglutinin-diphtheria toxoid conjugate vaccine in elderly nursing home subjects during an influenza outbreak. *J. Am. Geriatr. Soc.* **42(3),** 245.
133. Jahiel, R. and Kilbourne, E. (1966) Reduction in plaque number as differing indices of influenza virus-antibody reactions. *J. Bacteriol.* **92,** 1521.

7

Vaccines Against
Streptococcus pneumoniae

Kenneth R. Brown and Francis M. Ricci

Introduction

Streptococcus pneumoniae is an important bacterial pathogen, especially for the very young and the very old *(1)*. *S. pneumoniae*, also referred to as the pneumococcus, was formerly known as *Diplococcus pneumoniae.*

In the United States each year, there are approx 7 million cases of otitis media, 500,000 cases of pneumonia, 50,000 cases of bacteremia, and 3000 cases of meningitis caused by *S. pneumoniae (2)*. Invasive infections, i.e., meningitis, bacteremia, and infection of other normally sterile sites, may be life threatening, whereas otitis media, more common than all other pneumococcal diseases combined, exerts a huge financial burden on parents and threatens hearing but usually not life; sinusitis is also a common but usually non-life-threatening form of pneumococcal infection. In developing countries, pneumonia may cause up to 30% of the deaths in children under the age of 5 years and the pneumococcus is the most important bacterial cause *(3)*.

A discussion of pneumococcal vaccines serves as an opportunity to study the problems inherent in the development of combination vaccines, i.e., vaccines that have several or many specific components; the currently licensed vaccines are really many vaccines combined into a single dose. As a prelude to the discussion of pneumococcal vaccines, this chapter will first summarize information about the pneumococcus itself, its epidemiology, the pathogenesis of disease caused by these organisms, the host response, and the relationship of these factors to vaccine development. While the similarities in the nature of the capsular polysaccharides (CPS) making up the pneumococcal vaccines would suggest relative simplicity in making a polyvalent or combination pneumococcal vaccine, the contemporary development of multivalent products has become extremely complicated. In this chapter the authors attempt to point out the reasons for this and discuss methods which may help to rationalize the overall

From: *Combination Vaccines: Development, Clinical Research, and Approval*
Edited by: R. W. Ellis © Humana Press Inc., Totowa, NJ

Table 1. Common Pneumococcal Capsular Polysaccharide [CPS] Serotypes as Isolated from Various Populations and Areas, from Invasive or Noninvasive Disease, and as Represented in Early, Current, and Proposed Vaccines

A	B	C	D	E	F	G	H	J	K
			1[9]		1[5]	1			
2	2								
3	3	3[5]		3[6]			3		
4	4	4[2]	4[8]				4	4	4
5	5				5[4]	5			
6B	6A	6B[6]	6[2]	6[3]	6B[1]	6B	6B	6B	6B
7F	7F	7F[8]	7[7]			7F			
	8	8[11]			8[3]				
9N	9N		9[5]		9[7]		9		
9V		9V[4]				9V		9V	9V
10A									
11A									
12F	12F	12F[10]							
14	14	14[1]	14[1]	14[4]	14[2]		14	14	14
15B					15[10]				
17F									
18C	18C		18[4]	18[5]	18[9]	18C	18	18C	18C
19A	19F	19A[12]	19[3]	19[1]	19[6]		19		
19F		19F[9]				19F		19F	19F
	20								
22F		22F[7]							
23F	23F	23F[3]	23[6]	23[2]	23[8]	23F	23F	23F	23F
33F									

Arabic numbers not in parentheses represent serogroups, or data from studies which did not mention specific serotypes. Capital letters beside arabic numbers indicate specific serotypes. Numbers in parentheses in columns C, D, E, and F indicate the decreasing frequency of isolation of the serotypes, with 1 representing the most common CPS

A = Pneumococcal capsular polysaccharides [CPS] represented in currently licensed 23 valent pneumococcal vaccines[4,21]

B = CPS represented in 14 valent vaccines licensed in 1977[4,21]

C = CPS serotypes most commonly isolated from adults with lower respiratory or invasive diseases [US][7]

D = CPS serotypes most commonly from infections other than otitis media in children in developed countries[7]

E = CPS serotypes most commonly isolated from children with otitis media [US][45]

F = CPS most commonly isolated from children with infections other than otitis media in developing countries[7]

G = Proposed CPS serotypes which should be represented in an ideal vaccine for global use[7]

H = CPS serotypes included in the vaccine using tetanus toxoid/diptheria toxoid as protein carriers[30]

J = CPS serotypes included in the vaccine using CRM-197 as protein carrier; a formulation for developing countries will include types 1 and 5 also[30]

K = CPS serotypes included in the vaccine using OMPC as protein carrier[30]

development process. *Table 1* has been designed to illustrate the make up of the older and newer vaccines, and some of the correlations between the needs for specific serotypes by geographic or age considerations and vaccines in development. It will therefore, reflect material discussed in several sections of this chapter.

Streptococcus pneumoniae—The Organism

S. pneumoniae is a Gram-positive organism, usually occurring in pairs (hence its previous name *Diplococcus pneumoniae*) or in chains in broth culture. In the microbiology laboratory it is distinguished from other streptococci by its inhibition by optochin and its solubility in deoxycholate. Virulent pneumococci have a polysaccharide capsule which constitutes a chief factor in virulence *(4)*. Serotypes are defined by the chemical nature of their polysaccharide capsules; at present, there are more than 90 serotypes known *(5)* and they are widely distributed throughout the world. More recently a number or strains of pneumococci with intermediate resistance to penicillin have been recovered from clinical sites, and routine high-level susceptibility of pneumococci to penicillin can no longer be assumed *(6)*.

Epidemiology

Numbered serogroups of pneumococci are defined by reactivity with specific antisera to the capsular polysaccharides; these groups may have two or more closely related members which are serotypes, noted by a group number plus a capital letter, i.e., group 6 with types 6A and 6B. There are two systems of notation for *S. pneumoniae*, the Danish system, used here, and the American system.

The epidemiology of disease-causing serotypes is well-studied *(7)*, although the reasons for the geographical distribution are poorly understood. While 90 serotypes have been identified, most serious disease is caused by fewer than 25 *(4)*. The most important serotypes causing disease in children are not necessarily the most important serotypes causing disease in adults *(Table 1)*. Similarly, the serotypes are distributed differently in the US and Europe and the developing world.

Diseases Caused by the Pneumococcus

Lower respiratory infections and otitis media are the most common pneumococcal infections. Although we do not ordinarily think of the pneumococcus as a highly invasive organism such as streptococci and some staphylococci, *S. pneumoniae* is an important cause of some invasive diseases including bacteremia and meningitis, which are both serious and life-threatening; other less frequent infections include septicemia without a known primary site, endocarditis, osteomyelitis, pericarditis, and bone and joint infection. Since the development and widespread use of effective vaccines against *Haemophilus influenzae* type b *(8)*, and subsequent decline in *H. influenzae* meningitis in the US, pneumococcus has become the most common cause of bacterial meningitis in young children *(9)*.

Pathogenesis of Pneumococcal Disease

The pneumococcus is so-named because of its propensity to cause disease of the lung, including bronchitis as well as pneumonia and its complications. Such disease occurs when organisms colonizing in the nasal pharynx are inhaled in respiratory droplets through the upper airways evading the hairs in the nose, the mucus in the upper airways, and the attempted trapping of respiratory droplets containing the organisms by the mucus continuously propelled upward by the ciliated epithelium of the bronchi and the bronchioles. When trapped in the mucus, the organisms are coughed up in patients with a normal cough reflex, or they may come to rest in the alveolus where, if not phagocytosed, they multiply and cause disease.

In contrast to many other Gram-positive bacteria which exert their pathogenic effects by virtue of either exotoxins, lytic, or other enzymes, and in contrast to Gram-negative bacteria that usually release endotoxin, a component of the cell wall that exerts a broad range of adverse biologic effects, the pneumococci multiply and exert their pathogenic effects by their ability to resist phagocytosis and death. This defense is attributed to the polysaccharide capsule *(10)*.

Host Defenses and Immune Responses to *S. pneumoniae*

As previously noted, in order for pneumococci to become functionally pathogenic, they must evade a series of protective mechanisms, mostly physical barriers. However, pneumococci in the resident nasopharyngeal flora *(11)* and those that cause disease both stimulate the formation of antibodies directed against the large polysaccharide capsule that is type-specific *(10)*. Children under 24 months generally respond poorly to B-cell stimulation such as that induced by CPS thus explaining their poor antibody responses. These anticapsular antibodies are effective in promoting phagocytosis and killing of pneumococci only of the same serotype to which the patient becomes exposed either as upper respiratory flora or via infection. After infection, sufficient antibodies provide protection from subsequent challenge with homologous organisms. At the same time, preformed antibody interacting with CPS may initiate the complement cascade and thus contribute some to the pathology of the disease. Components of pneumococci other than the CPS, such as cell wall fragments, pneumolysin or other enzymes, or surface proteins, may contribute to the pathogenicity of the organisms *(10)*, but no such antibody has been described in humans which contributes a substantial degree of protection. However, defenses against several pneumococcal proteins protect against experimental disease across more than one serotype *(12–14)*.

In practical terms, therapy using horse or human serum containing high levels of specific anticapsular antibodies was used extensively in the past, but was complicated by reactions to horse serum, supplemented then supplanted by sulfa drugs and later by penicillin *(15,16)*.

Pneumococcal Vaccines

The first pneumococcal vaccines appeared shortly after the beginning of the twentieth century. They were comprised of killed whole cells of pneumococci, and by 1925, Avery and colleagues *(17)* had shown that serotype specificity was related to the capsular antigens present as complex polysaccharides. By 1945, MacLeod *(18)* had shown the success of a tetravalent pneumococcal vaccine that could prevent disease in military recruits. But the end of World War II, and the discovery and use of sulfas and then penicillin may have been a deterrent to the ultimate development of pneumococcal vaccines. In 1964, Austrian and Gold *(19)*, long after the first use of penicillin, once more pointed out the ongoing serious impact of pneumococcal disease in humans and encouraged the development of preventative measures such as pneumococcal vaccines.

Studies of the efficacy in gold miners in South Africa were carried out with a six-valent vaccine *(20)*; that study was large enough to show statistically significant protection provided by at least three of the six serotypes in the vaccine. It was also foundational to the vaccine licensure, which was based ultimately on additional data showing substantial levels of antibody to the remaining serotypes to be represented in the vaccine *(4)*.

Vaccines directed against the polysaccharide capsule of *S. pneumoniae* have been widely available in the US since 1977 *(Table 1)*. Manufactured by both Merck and Lederle, these polyvalent vaccines initially consisted of 14 individual capsular polysaccharides combined for use as a single injection, but by 1983, a 23-valent formulation (i.e., with 23 different capsular polysaccharides) was available *(4)*. In placebo-controlled efficacy studies, and in the licensed vaccines, equal quantities of all the individual polysaccharides were included without assurance of equivalent immunogenicity among serotypes. The 14-valent vaccines were designed to cover 80% of the serotypes responsible for bacteremic pneumococcal disease while the goal of the 23-valent vaccines was to cover 90% *(21)*. This illustrates very well the law of diminishing returns; if adding nine serotypes provided only 10% additional coverage in terms of prevalent disease in attempting to make a single universal vaccine, adding more serotypes could never be cost effective.

Some groups are at a higher risk of pneumococcal infection than are others *(Table 2) (2)*, in particular those who do not produce antibodies well. These will constitute the most appropriate candidates for vaccine use. Furthermore, responsiveness varies with age, i.e., children under 2 years of age and the elderly are said to respond less vigorously than patients in between these extremes *(22,23)*. However, recent data from a study that absorbed out the surface cell wall polysaccharide with the use of specific antibody was unable to confirm the decreasing antibody response with increasing age *(24)*.

Table 2. Recommendations for the Use of Pneumococcal Vaccine[a]

Groups for which vaccination is recommended[d]	Strength of recommendation[b]	Revaccination[c]
Immunocompetent persons[d]		
Persons aged ≥65 years	A	Second dose of vaccine if patient received vaccine ≥5 years previously and were aged <65 years at the time of vaccination.
Persons aged 2–64 years with chronic cardiovascular disease[e] chronic pulmonary disease,[f] or diabetes mellitus	A	Not recommended.
Persons aged 2–64 years with alcoholism, chronic liver disease,[g] or cerebrospinal fluid leaks	B	Not recommended.
Persons aged 2–64 years with functional or anatomic asplenia[h]	A	If patient is aged >10 years:single revaccination ≥5 years after previous dose. If patient is aged ≤10 years: consider revaccination 3 years after previous dose.
Persons aged 2–64 years living in special environments or social settings[i]	C	Not recommended.

Table 2 (continued). Recommendations for the Use of Pneumococcal Vaccine[a]

Groups for which vaccination is recommended	Strength of recommendation[b]	Revaccination[c]
Immunocompromised persons[d]		
Immunocompromised persons aged ≥2 years, including those with HIV infection, leukemia, lymphoma, Hodgkins disease, multiple myeloma, generalized malignancy, chronic renal failure, or nephrotic syndrome; those receiving immunosuppressive chemotherapy (including corticosteroids); and those who have received an organ or bone marrow transplant.	C	Single revaccination if ≥5 years have elapsed since receipt of first dose. If patient is aged ≤10 years: consider revaccination 3 years after previous dose.

[a]Taken from ref. 2.
[b]The following categories reflect the strength of evidence supporting the recommendations for vaccination: A = Strong epidemiologic evidence and substantial clinical benefit support the recommendation for vaccine use. B= Moderate evidence supports the recommendation for vaccine use. C = Effectiveness of vaccination is not proven, but the high risk for disease and the potential benefits and safety of the vaccine justify vaccination.
[c]Strength of evidence for all revaccination recommendations is "C."
[d]If earlier vaccination status is unknown, patients in this group should be administered pneumococcal vaccine.
[e]Including congestive heart failure and cardiomyopathies.
[f]Including chronic obstructive pulmonary disease and emphysema.
[g]Including cirrhosis.
[h]Including sickle cell disease and splenectomy.
[i]Including Alaskan Natives and certain American Indian populations.

161

Unfortunately the levels of antibody generated by vaccines that are necessary to protect against either pneumococcal pneumonia or invasive disease are unknown *(25)*; while a study to determine this level would be theoretically possible, such an undertaking with a multivalent in humans would be extraordinarily complex in design as well as unethical, since there is no animal model which closely parallels human responses to *S. pneumoniae* infection. In spite of the lack of knowledge of the exact level of protection required, the precise dose of each antigen which is necessary, the variation in responses from individual to individual, the duration of protection, and the precise mechanism of each aspect of pneumococcal disease, the use of the 23-valent vaccine has been moderately effective in preventing disease from serotypes represented in the vaccine *(21)*.

Rationale for New Vaccine Development

The 23-valent vaccines have not reached their full potential because of limited use in older immunocompetent adults. Even with this in mind, there are reasons to develop polyvalent vaccines with higher levels of protection. Case control studies of the CPS vaccines demonstrate efficacy rates from 56–81% *(2)*.

After natural infection, children under the age of 24 months do not usually produce antibodies well, but respond to some serotypes such as Type 3, beginning at about the age of 3 months *(26)*. However, for most of these children, the responses to the CPS of the infecting serotypes are not sufficiently brisk to confer the necessary protection *(27)* and are especially poor to types 6 and 14.

Because infants under the age of 24 months respond inadequately to most bacterial polysaccharides, including those from both *S. pneumoniae* and *H. influenzae (26,28)*, alternatives that would provide T-cell based immune responses have been in progress for a number of years *(29,30)*. In 1988, the first protein-conjugated vaccine against *H. influenzae* type b was released for use in the US. The technology that produced that conjugated haemophilus vaccine was utilized to produce conjugated vaccines against various strains of *S. pneumoniae* that are important in the causation of disease in children. A fortunate prospect for the future is that such vaccines will be available and may be successful in protecting against not only common non-life-threatening infections such as bacteria otitis media, but also in protecting against pneumococcal pneumonia and invasive pneumococcal disease such as bacteremia.

Of increasing importance as the wave of HIV infection continues, and the prospect of licensure and potential broader use of conjugated pneumococcal vaccines is realized, at least one study has concluded that one of the conjugated pneumococcal vaccines is more effective than a nonconjugated product among both HIV-infected and non-HIV-infected children who are 2 years or older *(31)*.

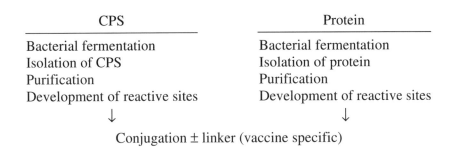

Fig. 1. Generalized schema for the production of conjugated vaccines.

Because it is generally accepted that HIV-infected patients should receive pneumococcal vaccine as soon as possible after their diagnosis *(32)*, it is important to continue studies to discern whether conjugated vaccines are necessary or whether the responses to pneumococcal polysaccharides per se will be adequate to provide protection to these patients.

Vaccine Development Issues

The issues discussed below regarding consistency of manufacture, lot size, mixing problems, and so forth, will hold for monovalent as well as multivalent vaccines, whether simple or conjugated. A pneumococcal vaccine with seven serotypes is not one vaccine, but seven different vaccines, the combination of which is threatened with all the complications and difficulties attendant with any other combination vaccine; the same is true to a greater extent for a 23-valent vaccine. But further complexities arise when a polyvalent conjugated vaccine is to be prepared because additional fermentation, purification, and chemical steps are required. A simplified schema of the production of a conjugated CPS vaccine is found in *Fig. 1*.

Preparation, Purification, and Production

The magnitude of this process for a monovalent vaccine is substantial; for a 7- to 11-valent vaccine it could become staggering, especially if one would try to optimize protein:polysaccharide ratios *(33)* for each conjugated component, then use a variety of polysaccharides with different chain lengths, test these in animals, and then test each in people to verify the utility of the animal model. Furthermore, one could choose to optimize the oligosaccharide or polysaccharide chain length, then study the effect of various "linkers," etc. *(34)*. In practice it is feasible to study these variables for one or two serotypes, but virtually impossible to study all of the variables for each CPS.

Table 3. Component Selection in Preparing Three Lots of a Trivalent Vaccine

Lot number	Component A	Component B	Component C
1	A_1	B_1	C_1
2	A_2	B_2	C_2
3	A_3	B_3	C_3

Four relevant issues will serve to illustrate the magnitude of the problems which confront the developer of these multivalent vaccines. The first, without respect to the regulations promulgated by the licensing agencies is the need to demonstrate manufacturing consistency. This is a rational step and one would want to manufacture at least three lots of a product for assuring the ability to consistently make the same product to reasonable standards. If, however, the proposed vaccine is a three-valent vaccine (e.g., a polyvalent vaccine with components A, B, and C), the issue becomes one of how many lots of each polysaccharide one should make and how many of the three lots of antigen A one would want to combine with those of antigen B and of antigen C and so forth. And when combined into a three-valent product, how many should be tested for possible interactions, whether chemical, physical, or immunological. Indeed, it would be conceivable that one should perform human dose-ranging studies on the intermediate products (i.e., the one-valent, the various two-valent) before going on to final mixing and formulation. The key issue to remember in this instance is that in an experiment in which one fails to hold at least variable constant, when a problem arises, one has no idea where to start to solve the problem. *Table 3* illustrates the possibilities: one could make three lots holding A constant, i.e., $A_1B_1C_1$, $A_1B_2C_2$, $A_1B_3C_3$, and so forth. The least useful approach is to hold no antigen constant, making $A_1B_1C_1$, $A_2B_2C_2$, $A_3B_3C_3$, but this approach makes problem solving almost impossible.

The second issue pertains to possible variation in lot sizes. For example, if one can consistently make a lot of antigen A at a size of 100 kg, while only being able to consistently make antigens B and C in lots no larger than 10 kg, it makes eminent sense to use a single lot of A to match with "consistently manufactured" lots of B and C. Surely the consistency with which one can divide the single lot of A is infinitely better in a biological system that the ability to manufacture consistently small lots of antigen A and antigen B!

The third consideration is that of mixing. A good rule of thumb, whether or not required by the licensing agency, is to mix the final product under manufacturing conditions in two different ways. The first makes the smallest and the largest possible mixed batches of final vaccine in the smallest mixing and filling equipment that will ever be used for the proposed product; the second repeats the procedure in the largest mixing and filling equipment one expects to use.

Finally, it is not unreasonable to say that since the entire process is for the purpose of putting an effective and safe vaccine into humans that is consistent from one vial to another and one lot to another, the entire process up to the point of mixing the individual antigens should be of no concern to the regulator rather than have it represent a real, perhaps impossible, challenge for the regulator to control. The real test is if the vaccine can be examined in the laboratory and shown to have consistency of manufacture, and the requisite safety and efficacy studies have been performed in humans, then how one gets to that place should be immaterial so long as all other requirements are met (e.g., good manufacturing practice).

Interference of one component on the response to another would be an additional complex issue if it were to occur in any combination vaccine. Fortunately, early studies showed a lack of interference of one serotype on another *(35)*. And it is presumed that any one conjugated CPS will not interfere with responses to other conjugated CPS. Because of the high degree of safety of older CPSs and of the newer Haemophilus conjugates, should there be suspicion or evidence of any interference, one would adjust the dose upward in a rationale increment until the desired level of response is achieved.

It is prudent to consider a system for combining these vaccines that is parallel to that used in diagnosing pneumococcal pneumonia before the universal availability of effective antibiotics such as penicillin. Polyvalent antisera containing antibodies against several serotypes were applied to pneumococci of undetermined type present in the sputum. If none of the serotypes were present as determined by the Quellung reaction (visible swelling of capsule seen under light microscopy), one ruled out these serotypes and moved on to the next polyvalent antiserum. By the process of elimination by groups, then by serotypes, one could define the antiserum needed to treat the patient.

Similarly, in developing multivalent conjugated CPS vaccines, this approach can be used; the first four serotypes (beginning with the least immunogenic CPS) could be studied in equal weight in the first vaccine. If reactions are minimal, one could move to the next set of four while waiting for the antibody responses. If tolerance is poor, one has four components to study, not nine or eleven, and progress can be made relatively easily.

By choosing the CPS with the lowest expected immunogenicity, it is possible to dose upwards as needed until either a putative protective level of anti-CPS antibody is reached or until tolerance becomes unacceptable. By studying the conjugated antigens in small groups, one accepts the possibility of the need to separate one or more out and study it alone. At the same time, one avoids the challenge of doing the impossible—fully studying each component (and its own variables) individually.

The value of this exercise is obvious; the process of developing a polyvalent vaccine today produces so many permutations and combinations that it is physically impossible to produce all the possible lots, conduct all the possible laboratory tests, or do all of the possible clinical studies which could be conceptualized. Therefore, what is required is a well thought out proposal of how each of these issues will be handled and such a plan should be done in advance, not in response to the first data which comes out of the clinical program.

At least three pneumococcal conjugate vaccines have advanced well into the clinical stages of development *(Table 1)*; the carriers used include diphtheria toxoid/ tetanus toxoid, CRM-197 (a derivative of diphtheria toxin) coupled to oligosaccharides rather than polysaccharides *(36)*, and an outer membrane protein complex (OMPC) derived from *Neisseria meningitis* type b *(37)*. Perhaps the most promising news for the conjugate programs is the responsiveness of 24-month-olds to conjugates of serotypes 6B and 14, to which young children usually respond poorly *(36,38)*.

Each of these three conjugates has been shown to induce antibodies to its component polysaccharides after three injections at 2, 4, and 6 months, as well as booster response at or after the age of 12 months *(30,33)*. One of these conjugate vaccines (CRM-197) has been shown to stimulate antibody in children who have failed, after the age of 24 months, to respond to the 23-valent polysaccharide vaccine *(39)*. However, in two studies using the CRM-197 oligosaccharide conjugate vaccine *(40,41)*, the authors were unable to show an advantage over currently licensed 23-valent polysaccharide vaccines in the immunization of healthy volunteers 60–80 years of age. The OMPC vaccine has been shown to reduce the nasopharyngeal carriage of certain vaccines serotypes (including penicillin-resistant strains) *(42)*; in another study the serotypes lost were replaced by nonvaccine serotypes *(43)*. All three of these vaccines use some type of alum in their formulations *(30)* and it is too early to say whether any more advanced adjuvants will improve responses to the current generation of pneumococcal polysaccharide vaccines.

Other approaches may become available to produce more highly effective vaccines against the pneumococcus. Among the most attractive would be one based on an antigen common to all virulent pneumococci; furthermore, were such an antigen found as a peptide, or protein, then either the so-called DNA technology or the embryonic somatic transgenic immunization *(44)* might provide the appropriate technology. However, at present we are confronted with the need to improve on the available CPS vaccines with all the complexity inherent in such.

Summary and Conclusions

Polyvalent pneumococcal vaccines with 23 antigens have been available since 1983 but have been unsuccessful in controlling invasive pneumococcal disease, especially in the very young and the elderly because of underutilization in adults and because children under 24 months respond poorly to B-cell stimulation. Since the pneumococcus remains an important killer of children and the elderly, and since resistance to penicillin has become increasingly important, there is a call for newer and more effective pneumococcal vaccines. Conjugation to any one of several proteins can convert the response in young children to a T-cell response; multivalent (7–11 serotypes) polysaccharide vaccines whose polysaccharides are linked to a diphtheria protein such as the CRM-197 moiety, to tetanus toxoid, or to the OMPC of *N. meningitidis* type b are in clinical trials and preliminary evidence suggests that they will be effective in reducing the amount of serious respiratory and invasive pneumococcal disease and perhaps that of pneumococcal otitis media *(45)*, an important cause of deafness worldwide.

Multivalent conjugated vaccines are a severe challenge to the most efficient and resourceful manufacturer and clinical investigator because of the potential permutations that one could consider in the manufacture and testing of these products. These people will have to become skilled in selecting the numbers of lots to produce at each step, how many lots of which combinations to test, when to test them in the clinic, and the art of applied statistics, or they will drown in the abyss of numbers with which they are presented.

References

1. Musher, D. M. (1993) *Streptococcus pneumoniae*, in *Principles and Practice of Infectious Diseases*, 4th ed. (Mandell, G. L., Douglas, R. G., and Bennett, J. E., eds.), Churchill Livingstone, New York, pp. 1811–1826.
2. Centers for Disease Control (1997). Recommendations of the advisory committee on immunization practices (ACIP). Prevention of pneumococcal disease. *MMWR* **46(No. RR-8)**, 1–24.
3. Leowski, J. (1986) Mortality from acute respiratory infection in children less than 5 years of age: global estimates. *World Health Stat. Q.* **39**, 138–144.
4. Austrian, R. (1989) Pneumococcal polysaccharide vaccines. *Rev. Infect. Dis.* **11(Suppl. 3)**, S598–S602.
5. Henrichsen, J. (1995) Six newly recognized types of *Streptococcus pneumoniae*. *J. Clin. Microbiol.* **33(10)**, 2759–2762.
6. Breiman, R. F., Butler, J. C., Tenover, F. C., Elliott, J. A., and Facklam, R. R. (1994) Emergence of drug-resistant pneumococcal infections in the United States. *JAMA* **271(23)**, 1831–1835.
7. Sniadack, D. H., Schwartz, B., Lipman, H., Bogaerts, J., Butler, J. C., Dagan, R., Echaniz-Aviles, G., Lloyd-Evans, N., Fenoll, A., Girgis, N. I., Henrichsen, J., Klugman, K., Lehmann, D., Takala, A. K., Vandepitte, J., Gove, S., and Breiman, R. F. (1995) Potential interventions for the prevention of childhood pneumonia: geographic and temporal differences in serotype and serogroup distribution of sterile site pneumococcal isolates from children-implications for vaccine strategies. *Pediatr. Infect. Dis. J.* **14**, 503–510.
8. Robbins, J. B., Schneerson, R., Anderson, P., and Smith, D. H. (1996) Prevention of systemic infections, especially meningitis, caused by *Haemophilus influenzae* type b. *JAMA* **276(14)**, 1181–1185.

9. Townsend, G. C. and Scheld, W. M. (1995) Clinically important trends in bacterial meningitis. *Infect. Dis. Clin. Pract.* **4(6),** 423–430.

10. Watson, D. A., Musher, D. M., and Verhoef, J. (1995) Pneumococcal virulence factors and host immune responses to them. *Eur. J. Clin. Microbiol. Infect. Dis.* **14(6),** 479–490.

11. Virolainen, A., Jero, J. Kayhty, H., Karma, P., Leinonen, M., and Eskola, J. (1995) Nasopharyngeal antibodies to pneumococcal capsular polysaccharides in children with acute otitis media. *J. Inf. Dis.* **172,** 1115–1118.

12. Klein, D. L. (1995) Pneumococcal conjugate vaccines: review and update. *Microb. Drug Resist.* **1(1),** 49–58.

13. McDaniel, L. S., Sheffield, J. S., Delucchi, P., and Briles, D. (1991) PspA, a surface protein of *Streptococcus pneumoniae*, is capable of eliciting protection against pneumococci of more than one capsular type. *Infect. Immun.* **59,** 222–228.

14. Paton, J. C., Lock, R. A., and Hansman, D. J. (1983) Effect of immunization with pneumolysin on survival time of mice challenged with *Streptococcus pneumoniae. Infect. Immun.* **40,** 548–552.

15. Finland, M. (1939) The use of serum, sulfanilamide and sulfapyridine in the treatment of pneumococci infections. *Med. Clin. North Am.* **23,** 1205–1209.

16. Casadevall, A. and Scharff, M. D. (1995) Return to the past: the case for antibody-based therapies in infectious diseases. *Clin. Infect. Dis.* **21,** 150–161.

17. Watson, D. A., Musher, D. M., Jacobson, J. W., and Verhoef, J. (1993) A brief history of the pneumococcus in biomedical research: a panoply of scientific discovery. *Clin. Infect. Dis.* **17(5),** 913–924.

18. MacLeod, C. M., Hodges, R. G., Heidelberger, M., et al. (1945) Prevention of pneumococcal pneumonia by immunization with specific capsular polysaccharides. *J. Exp. Med.* **82,** 445–465.

19. Austrian, R. and Gold, J. (1964) Pneumococcal bacteremia, with special reference to bacteremic pneomococcal pneumonia. *Ann. Int. Med.* **60,** 759–776.

20. Smit, P., Oberholtzer, D., Hayden-Smith, S., Koornhof, H. J., and Hilleman, M. R. (1977) Protective efficacy of pneumococcal polysaccharide vaccines. *JAMA* **238,** 2613–2616.

21. Shapiro, E. D., Berg, A. T., Austrian, R., Schroeder, D., Parcells, V., Margolis, A., Adair, R. K., and Clemens, J. D. (1991) The protective efficacy of polyvalent pneumococcal polysaccharide vaccine. *N. Engl. J. Med.* **325(21),** 1453–1460.

22. Koskela, M., Leinonen, M., Haiva, V., et al. (1986) First and second dose antibody responses to pneumococcal polysaccharide vaccine in infants. *Pediatr. Infect. Dis.* **5,** 45–50.

23. Roghmann, K. J., Tabloski, P. A., Bentley, D. W., et al. (1987) Immune response of elderly adults to pneumococcus: variation by age, sex, and functional impairment. *J. Gerontol.* **42,** 265–270.

24. Musher, D. M., Groover, J. E., Graviss, E. A., and Baughn, R. E. (1996) The lack of association between aging and postvaccination levels of IgG antibody to capsular polysaccharides of *Streptococcus pneumoniae. Clin. Infect. Dis.* **22,** 165–167.

25. Obaro, S. K., Monteil, M. A., and Henderson, D. C. (1996) The pneumococcal problem. *Br. Med. J.* **312(7045),** 1521–1525.

26. Peter, G. and Klein, J. (1997) *Streptococcus pneumoniae*, in *Principles and Practice of Pediatric Infectious Diseases* (Long, S., Pichering, L., and Prober, C., eds.), Churchill Livingstone, NY, pp. 828–835.

27. Hattotuwa, K. L. and Hind, C. R. K. (1997) Pneumococcal vaccine. *Postgrad. Med. J.* **73(858),** 222–224.

28. Stein, K. R. (1992) Thymus-independent and thymus-dependent responses to polysaccharide antigens. *J. Inf. Dis.* **(Suppl 1),** S49–S52.

29. Robbins, J. B. and Schneerson, R. (1990) Evaluating the *Haemophilus influenzae* type b conjugate vaccine PRP-D. *N. Engl. J. Med.* **323,** 1415,1416.

30. Eby, R. (1995) Pneumococcal conjugate vaccines. *Pharm. Biotechnol.* **6,** 695–718.

31. King, J. C. Jr., Vink, P. E., Farley, J. J., Parks, M., Smilie, M., Madore, D., Lichenstein, R., and Malinoski, F. (1996) Comparison of the safety and immunogenicity of a pneumococcal conjugate with a licensed polysaccharide vaccine in human immunodeficiency virus and non-human immunodeficiency virus-infected children. *Pediatr. Infect. Dis. J.* **15(3),** 192–196.
32. Rodriquez-Barradas, M., Musher, D., Lohart, C., Lacke, C., Groover, J., Watson, D., Baughn, R., Cate, T., and Crofoot, G. (1992) Antibody to capsular polysaccharides of *Streptococcus pneumonia* after vaccination of human immunodeficiency virus-infected subjects with 23-valent pneumococcal vaccine. *J. Inf. Dis.* **165,** 553–556.
33. Anderson, P. and Betts, R. (1989) Human adult immunogenicity of protein-coupled pneumococcal capsular antigens of serotypes prevalent in otitis media. *Pediatr. Infect. Dis. J.* **8,** S50–S53.
34. Steinhoff, M. C., Edwards, K., Keyserling, H., Thoms, M. L., Johnson, C., Madore, D., and Hogerman, D. (1994) A randomized comparison of three bivalent streptococcus pneumoniae glycoprotein conjugate vaccines in young children: effect of polysaccharide size and linkage characteristics. *Pediatr. Infect. Dis. J.* **13(5),** 368–372.
35. Riley, I. A. and Douglas, R. M. (1981) An epidemiologic approach to pneumococcal disease. *Rev. Infect. Dis.* **3,** 233–245.
36. Dagan, R., Zamir, O., Melamed, R., and Leroy, O. (1996) Immunogenicity of two tetravalent pneumococcal vaccines conjugated to either tetanus toxoid (Pnc-TT) or diphtheria toxoid (Pnc-D) in young infants and their boosterability by native polysaccharide (PS) antigens. Paper presented at the 36th Interscience Conference on Antimicrobial Agents and Chemotherapy, New Orleans, Louisiana, Sept. 15–18, American Society for Microbiology, Washington, DC, p. 151.
37. Anderson, E. L., Kennedy, D. J., Geldmacher, K. M., Donnelly, J., and Mendelman, P. M. (1996) Immunogenicity of heptavalent pneumococcal conjugate vaccine in infants. *J. Pediatr.* **128(5, Part 1),** 649–653.
38. Pichichero, M. E., Shelly, M. A., and Treanor, J. J. (1997) Evaluation of a pentavalent conjugated pneumococcal vaccine in toddlers. *Pediatr. Infect. Dis. J.* **16(1),** 72–74.
39. Javier, F. C. III, Leiva, L., Moore, C., Bradford, N., and Sorensen, R. U. (1997) Conjugate vaccine in children who failed to respond to the 23-valent polysaccharide vaccine. *J. Allergy Clin. Immunol.* **99(1, Part 2),** S426.
40. Powers, D. C., Anderson, E. L., Lottenbach, K., and Mink, C. M. (1996) Reactogenicity and immunogenicity of a protein-conjugated pneumococcal oligosaccharide vaccine in older adults. *J. Infect. Dis.* **173(4),** 1014–1018.
41. Shelly, M. A., Graves, B., Riley, G. J., and Treanor, J. J. (1995) Comparison of pneumococcal polysaccharide (PS) and CRM-197-conjugated pneumococcal polysaccharide (CRM-PS) vaccines in young and older adults. *Clin. Infect. Dis.* **21(3),** 789.
42. Dagan, R., Melamed, R., Muallem, M., Piglansky, L., Greenberg, D., Abramson, O., Mendelman, P. M., Bohidar, N., and Yagupsky, P. (1996) Reduction of nasopharyngeal carriage of pneumococci during the second year of life by a heptavalent conjugate pneumococcal vaccine. *J. Infect. Dis.* **174(6),** 1271–1278.
43. Obaro, S. K., Adegbola, R. A., Banya, W. A. S., and Greenwood, B. M. (1996) Carriage of pneomococci after pneumococcal vaccination. *Lancet* **348(9022),** 271,272.
44. Ulmer, J. B. (1997) Elegantly presented DNA vaccines. *Nat. Biotechnol.* **15,** 842,843.
45. Klein, J. (1994) Otitis Media. *Clin. Infect. Dis.* **19,** 823–833.

8 Rotavirus Vaccines

Paul A. Offit and H. Fred Clark

Introduction

There are two candidate rotavirus vaccines that consist of a combination of four or more viral strains. Each of the two candidate vaccines is made by genetically reassorting one animal rotavirus strain (i.e., simian or bovine) with each of several human rotavirus strains. The resultant reassortant strains retain the attenuated virulence characteristics of the animal strains and express one of the genes that encode the proteins that determine human rotavirus serotype. It is estimated that the simian × human reassortant rotavirus vaccine could be licensed by the Food and Drug Administration (FDA) and recommended for universal use in all infants by the Advisory Committee on Immunization Practices in 1998. Strategies used to formulate, construct, and combine animal × human rotavirus reassortant vaccines as well as selected aspects of rotavirus immunology, molecular biology, and pathogenesis will be described in this chapter. Since the rotavirus vaccine is itself a multivalent combination vaccine, issues related to the interactions among different serotype viruses will be discussed.

Disease Burden

Rotaviruses are the most common cause of severe dehydrating diarrhea in infants and young children throughout the world *(1,2)*. Almost all children are infected by the time they reach 2 to 3 years of age. In the United States, it has been estimated that rotavirus accounts annually for about 500,000 doctor visits, 50,000 hospitalizations, and 20–40 deaths of children with diarrhea *(3,4)*. In less developed countries, rotaviruses are also a common cause of disease and death in infants and young children *(5–7)*. Rotavirus is estimated to cause 480,000 to 640,000 deaths in children each year, approximately 20% of the estimated 2.4 to 3.2 million deaths from diarrhea *(8–11)*. The devastating worldwide impact of this disease has for many years stimulated interest in development of a safe and effective rotavirus vaccine.

From: *Combination Vaccines: Development, Clinical Research, and Approval*
Edited by: R. W. Ellis © Humana Press Inc., Totowa, NJ

Clinical Disease

Rotavirus disease is characterized by the sudden onset of watery diarrhea, fever, and vomiting *(12–15)*. Most disease is mild, but about 1 of every 50 children infected with rotavirus *(5,8)* will develop dehydration requiring admission to the hospital. For most children, fever and vomiting usually persist for 2–3 days and diarrhea for 4–5 days *(12–15)*.

The Virus

Rotaviruses have been detected in most species of domestic mammals and in birds. Although most human and animal rotaviruses share common antigens (group A rotaviruses) *(16)*, animal rotaviruses are distinguished from human strains by type-specific antigens located on the viral surface.

Rotaviruses are approx 70 nm in diameter and are a genus within the *Reoviridae* family. The virus contains three shells (an outer capsid, inner capsid, and core) that surround the genome of 11 segments of double-stranded RNA. Gene segments can be separated by migration in polyacrylamide gels. For the most part, each gene encodes a single viral protein. When two different rotavirus strains infect the same cell together, the gene segments may reassort independently, producing viral progeny of mixed parentage. Analysis of reassortant viruses has allowed for a determination of the relationship between the structure and function of rotavirus proteins. In addition, as described below, current candidate vaccines are reassortant viruses made by coinfection of cells with animal and human strains.

The outer shell of rotavirus contains two distinct proteins (vp4 and vp7), each of which elicits serotype-specific neutralizing antibodies *(17–19)*. Protein vp7 is encoded by gene segments 7, 8, or 9 in different rotavirus strains; protein vp4 is encoded by gene segment 4 *(20,21)*. The most highly represented viral structural protein is vp6, which is found in the internal capsid *(22,23)*. Three structural proteins (vp1, vp2, and vp3) form the viral core, and five other nonstructural proteins (NSP1, NSP2, NSP3, NSP4, and NSP5) are made during infection *(16)*.

Similar to the influenza viruses, rotavirus serotypes are classified on the basis of two surface proteins. The vp7 types are designated "G" types (because vp7 is a Glycoprotein) and the vp4 types are designated as "P" types (because Protease cleavage of vp 4 is essential for virus infectivity) *(24,25)*. Ten G types and seven P types have been found in rotavirus strains isolated from children worldwide, but four major G serotypes and two major P types predominate. P1aG1 appears to be the most common cause of disease worldwide. However, strains P1bG2, P1aG3, and P1aG4 also have been found to be important causes of rotavirus disease.

New Insights on Rotavirus Pathogenesis

Studies in humans and experimental animals found that rotavirus replicates in mature villous epithelial cells of the small intestine *(24–29)* and that replication progresses from the jejunum to the ileum *(27,30)*. Rotaviruses have never been detected consistently in the blood or sites distant to the intestine. Because inflammation in the lamina propria, Peyer's patch, or at the intestinal mucosal surface is not found after rotavirus infection *(24–29)*, it is unlikely that intestinal epithelial cell damage is mediated by the host immune response.

Recently one of the rotavirus nonstructural proteins (NSP4) was shown to act as an enterotoxin *(31)*. Suckling mice exposed to NSP4 developed diarrhea in an age-dependent, dose-dependent, and specific manner. Disease was caused by excess chloride secretion by a calcium-dependent signaling pathway. However, recent studies showed that diarrhea also could be induced by NSP4 in cystic fibrosis transmembrane conductance regulator knockout mice (CFTR –/–), suggesting that diarrhea is induced by an as-yet-unknown calcium-mediated chloride channel *(32)*.

The finding that NSP4 is associated with viral virulence is consistent with observations obtained by examining the genetics of virulence using reassortant rotaviruses generated from pathogenic and nonpathogenic strains *(33)*. These studies found that the genes that encoded vp3, vp4, vp7, and NSP4 were all required to reconstitute virulence.

Protection Afforded by Natural Infection

Immunologic Correlates of Protection Against Disease

Natural infection with rotavirus protects against moderate to severe, but not all disease associated with reinfection *(34–36)*. Studies of natural infection in infants and young children indicate that protection is mediated by the presence of virus-specific secretory immunoglobulin A (IgA) at the intestinal mucosal surface *(37,38)* and is predicted by the presence of virus-specific IgA in the serum or feces *(37–39)*.

Some children experience two episodes of rotavirus-induced diarrhea in successive years caused by the same serotype *(34,40–50)*. Children rarely develop symptomatic rotavirus infection twice within the same season *(37)*. These epidemiological observations are consistent with the fact that production of virus-specific secretory IgA (sIgA) at mucosal surfaces is usually short-lived. Indeed, rotavirus-specific IgA often is not detected at the intestinal mucosal surface one year after symptomatic infection *(38)*.

Although the presence of rotavirus-specific IgA in serum or feces predicts protection against symptomatic reinfection after natural infection, virus-specific IgA does not correlate with protection against disease in vaccine trials *(51–53)*. This phenomenon is explained in several possible ways. First, protection against disease following immunization with nonhuman rotaviruses may be mediated by virus-specific cytotoxic T lymphocytes (CTL). Some evidence supports the importance of CTL in protection against rotavirus disease in animals *(54–57)*. Alternatively, cytokines with antiviral activity may be associated with protection against challenge.

Importance of Serotype in Protection Against Disease

Both outer capsid proteins (vp4 [P type] and vp7 [G type]) contain epitopes that evoke both serotype-specific and crossreactive neutralizing antibodies *(58)*. Although infants and young children immunized with one rotavirus serotype are protected against challenge with different rotavirus serotypes (heterotypic protection) *(59)*, the relative importance of including both human P and G types in reassortant vaccine viruses containing animal rotavirus backgrounds remains undetermined. However, it is clear that following a primary natural rotavirus infection, infants develop virus-specific neutralizing antibodies in serum directed against the infecting G type at levels greater than those directed against other G types *(60–64)*. Similarly, children are more likely to be protected against disease following reinfection with a G type to which the child already has been exposed *(43)*. For these reasons, it may be of value for a rotavirus vaccine to contain all G types to which the child is likely to be exposed.

Goals for a Rotavirus Vaccine

The current goals for a rotavirus vaccine for human infants are based not on any a priori decision regarding what is desirable for public health, but rather the results of what seems possible with the most promising of the current vaccine candidates. Early hopes for a single dose vaccine of low cost given to the newborn infant were soon abandoned and replaced by more modest expectations.

A single-dose, orally administered, attenuated vaccine for rotavirus diarrhea of newborn calves was developed half a decade before human rotavirus was recognized *(65)*. However, early claims for effectiveness of this vaccine have never been substantiated in a controlled clinical trial. Consistent success in cattle has only been obtained with parenteral rotavirus vaccine given to the pregnant dam in a mixture with adjuvant *(66)* (a method clearly not feasible for human infants).

Hopes for early development of a vaccine to prevent all rotavirus infection and disease were modified after early experience with first generation animal origin (simian and bovine) vaccines. These products were irregularly effective, but even the most successful clinical trials were characterized by <100% protection *(59,67,68)*. In almost all trials in which vaccines were effective in preventing clinical disease, the vaccines did not cause a reduction in the rate of wild-type rotavirus infection. However, experience with even the least effective vaccines provided evidence that rotavirus vaccines selectively induce protection against the most severe dehydrating diarrhoeal disease *(67,69,70)*.

It is acknowledged that we do not now have the technical ability to design a completely protective rotavirus vaccine. This is not surprising given the fact that induction of completely protective immune responses against other diseases in which a mucosal surface is the target organ is notoriously difficult *(71)*. This challenge is compounded in rotavirus disease by the conflicting observations that nonimmune infants are susceptible to severe disease at a very early age (as young as gestational age zero *[72]*); yet maternally derived immunity may prevent "take," i.e., effective active vaccination, by an immunizing vaccine exposure in infants of ages up to 5 months old *(73)*.

Current expectations are related to the clinical experience with currently available "second generation" reassortant rotavirus vaccines which consistently have been at least partially (usually 50–70%) protective against all rotavirus disease *(74,75)*. These vaccines usually have provided >75% protection against severe dehydrating disease. This level of protection is clearly worthwhile against the disease expression that is associated with hospitalization and death. It is realistic to attempt to improve vaccines to a near 100% efficacy against the most severe disease before contemplating complete protection against all disease or a level of protection, which does not occur after natural disease.

A useful rotavirus vaccine must be given early enough to protect against a disease whose onset is a threat at any postpartum age. It must be utilized according to a schedule allowing simultaneous administration with other pediatric vaccines without impediment of the immune response to any of the immunizing antigens. Especially in developed countries where rotavirus is an infrequent cause of death, sequelae associated with vaccination must be minimal. A desirable vaccine must protect against all serotypes of rotavirus extant in the community. Because the greatest number of severe episodes and deaths occur in less developed nations, it is important that the vaccine be stable under adverse storage conditions of high temperature, preferably as a liquid formulation. For those nations that need it most, low cost is a necessity.

Protection Afforded by Immunization

Summary of Vaccine Development

Rotavirus vaccine development was and is handicapped by the failure to identify a single critical virion protective antigen. There have been extensive serological analyses of the antibody response to rotavirus infection and following immunization with candidate rotavirus vaccines. Assays used to measure antibody responses in serum and stool specimens that have been measured against each vaccine virus type have included neutralization and enzyme linked immunosorbent assay (ELISA) specific for IgG, IgM, or IgA. Nevertheless, a single component of the immune response that is unequivocally correlated with protection against rotavirus disease, i.e., an immunological correlate of efficacy, has not been identified.

It was noted early that there is a varying potential of rotaviruses to infect and to induce immune responses across species barriers and there are shared as well as strain-specific antigens among group A rotaviruses derived from different host species. It is now recognized that antigens (group) are most conserved upon the inner shell vp6 proteins. However, certain vp7 "G" surface protein serotypes also are found among several species of mammalian hosts.

Early studies in calves and piglets indicated a degree of cross-protection between bovine and human origin rotaviruses (76,77). In particular, Zissis et al. (77) demonstrated that piglets inoculated orally and/or parenterally with bovine virus developed resistance (characterized by reduced "days of fecal shedding") against challenge with human rotavirus of uncharacterized serotype. Such evidence led to the selection of bovine origin rotavirus as the first vaccine candidate for human use.

Initial human vaccine trials were performed with the bovine vaccine strain Nebraska calf diarrhea virus which was cultivated in primate cells and renamed strain RIT4237 as a human vaccine candidate (78). Highly attenuated and adapted by more than 150 passages in cell culture, RIT4237 was given in a dose of 10^8 TCID50 to infants as young as 1 month old. At this dosage level, no vaccine-associated adverse effects, fevers, or signs of gastrointestinal disease were ever detected (79). Rotavirus-specific serum binding antibody responses were characteristically induced in 70–90% of vaccinees, but virus neutralizing antibody responses were largely specific for bovine serotype G6 rotaviruses. Occasional increases in neutralizing antibody specific to human rotavirus serotypes were detected in infants with antibody evidence of exposure to human rotavirus prior to vaccination with the bovine rotavirus vaccine (80).

Efficacy trials of RIT4237 in Finland consistently revealed protection rates of 70% or more against human rotavirus disease that was predominantly of human serotype G1 (67,81). Infants were vaccinated at age 0–12 months. An advantage of two doses vs one dose was not clear. All infants were given oral buffer before vaccination. A principle was established that was to hold true for all rotavirus vaccine candidates: vaccine-induced protection measured by reduction in cases of clinically severe rotavirus diarrhea is nearly always greater than that measured by prevention of all cases of rotavirus diarrhea, which in turn is greater than the rate of reduction in infection (82).

After initial success in Finland, RIT4237 failed to protect in two clinical trials in Africa *(83,84)* and induced only about 50% protection in a trial in Peru *(85).* Further development was discontinued.

Additional clinical trials were subsequently performed with a bovine rotavirus strain designated WC3, isolated from a calf in Pennsylvania and evaluated as vaccine after only 12 passages in cell culture. Like RIT4237, this vaccine given at high dose (10^7 plaque-forming units [pfu]) to infants was extremely safe and induced mostly bovine rotavirus (G6) specific serum antibody responses in vaccinated infants *(73).* In an initial vaccine efficacy trial in Philadelphia, WC3 induced 76% protection against all cases of rotavirus disease *(59).* In subsequent trials WC3 vaccine was associated with 50% protection in Shanghai but minimal (<25%) protection in Cincinnati and in the Central African Republic *(70,86).* Development of WC3 vaccine was discontinued.

A simian origin rotavirus of serotype G3, strain RRV, isolated from a rhesus monkey with diarrhea was also evaluated as a vaccine for human infants *(87).* RRV differs from WC3 and RIT4237 in many aspects of its behavior in the human infant host. Not surprisingly, for a primate virus, administered at low (sixteenth) passage level in cell culture, RRV appears much better adapted to the human infant host than the bovine origin rotaviruses. It is also capable of better replication and more effective induction of immune responses in the newborn mouse than bovine origin rotavirus *(88).* RRV has an apparently unique capacity to spread systemically in mice causing hepatic infection and disease, leading to fatalities in SCID mice *(89).* However, no evidence of liver disease induction by RRV has been found in infants.

Unlike the bovine origin rotaviruses, RRV replicates in the human host in order to generate an antigenic mass that is immunogenic. Therefore, low doses are immunogenic (10^4–10^7 pfu), and evidence of replication is found in the fact that fecal shedding of RRV is detectable in most infant hosts, often in quantities great enough to be detected by ELISA *(90).* Apparently concomitant with replication of the virus in the infant gut, a clustering of febrile reactions (up to 20–30% or more of vaccinees) is observed 2–4 days after inoculation *(79,91).* Symptoms of gastroenteritis have followed vaccination in some Scandinavian trials *(69,79).* Vaccine reactions are most prominent in infants aged 6 months or more, when maternally-derived immunity has subsided *(79).* Reactions are reduced in younger infants (including newborns *[91]*) and in infants in less developed countries *(92).*

RRV induces detectable serum-antibody responses (ELISA IgA and neutralizing antibody of RRV specificity) in most infants. In a "head-to-head" comparison with RIT 4237 bovine rotavirus vaccine, RRV was more immunogenic (serum antibody) and more reactogenic *(79).*

Protective efficacy trials (one dose), originally performed in Finland, indicated <50% protection against all rotavirus disease, but higher levels of protection (67–80%) against severe rotavirus disease *(69,91)*. A series of efficacy trails in the United States gave efficacy values ranging from 0–65% *(69,93–95)*. An efficacy trial in Venezuela also gave 65% protection in a season when the natural challenge was of G3 specificity *(68)*. This observation was cited as proof that vaccine-induced protection against rotavirus disease is G serotype-specific, but in this trial, protection was in fact equally efficient against the lower prevalence non-G3 serotype disease episodes *(90)*. RRV was abandoned as a vaccine candidate because of inconsistent protective immunogenicity.

Other rotaviruses have had limited clinical trials or are in a much earlier state of development. A lamb origin rotavirus is being developed for human use in China (strain LLR *[96]*). It is reported to be safe in infants and to induce broadly cross-reactive serum antibodies of G1, G2, G3, and G4 specificity.

Early trials with cold-adapted human G1 and G9 rotaviruses revealed excellent attenuation but poor immunogenicity *(75)*. A "newborn strain" type P2G1 human origin rotavirus, strain M37, was also attenuated but poorly protective in infants *(97)*. Other naturally occurring "newborn" P2a strains including a P2aG10 strain widely prevalent in Bangalore, are in the early stage of evaluation as human vaccine candidates in India.

A human serotype 1 rotavirus recovered from an infant with gastroenteritis (strain 89–12) has been attenuated by serial passage in African green monkey cell culture and is now undergoing clinical trials. In Phase 1 studies the virus was nonreactogenic in infants but shed in feces. Serum IgA responses were induced in most infants, but less than 50% developed serum neutralizing antibodies to strain 89–12 *(98)*.

None of the human origin rotavirus candidates has yet been evaluated in clinical trials as extensive as those of RIT4237, WC3, or RRV animal origin viruses. Experience gained in clinical study of the bovine origin rotaviruses and the simian origin RRV is the basis of human × animal rotavirus reassortant vaccines (discussed later) that are currently the recipients of the most extensive development.

Importance of Serotype in Human Vaccine Development

Hoshino et al. *(99)* defined serotypes of major prototype isolates of rotaviruses early using parenterally hyperimmunized guinea pigs. These sera established serotypes based on the vp7 (G) viral surface protein. Different serotypes based upon the vp4 (P) viral surface protein were established later *(100)*. In studies of gnotobiotic pigs *(17)* and newborn mice, both anti-vp4 and anti-vp7 antibodies (in hyperimmunized dam's milk) were shown to protect against challenge *(19)*. Both the titer of antibody and the serotype specificity of the passively administered antibodies were shown to be highly correlated with protection *(101)*.

Unfortunately, the role of serotype in active protection by vaccine against subsequent virus challenge is less clear. What evidence exists is primarily based on G serotypes. Observations of vaccine include challenge studies in animals that have given both evidence of strong correlation and of no correlation of serotype-specific immunization and protection against virulent virus challenge *(102)*. Surprisingly, although several rotavirus G serotypes are prominent in disease of both cattle and swine, most commercial veterinary vaccines for these species have been univalent.

Epidemiological evidence suggests that both human G serotype-specific and cross-reactive immunity play a role in protection against disease. Thus, natural infection protects most efficiently against subsequent natural rotavirus infection of the homologous serotype, but the incidence of severe rotavirus gastroenteritis of any serotype is reduced after the first rotavirus infection *(103)*. Serotype-specific protection may not correlate perfectly with G-type specificity determined by the serum virus neutralization test. RRV has been shown repeatedly to be an inefficient inducer of serum neutralizing antibody to human prototype G3 rotavirus *(104,105)*, yet multivalent rhesus reassortant vaccine that contain RRV has been shown to protect against human G3 rotavirus disease more efficiently than does univalent G1 rhesus reassortant vaccine *(104,105)*.

Antigenic variation within the G1, G3, and G4 wild-type rotavirus population has also been shown *(106–108)*. but has not been correlated with success or failure of human vaccine candidates. In a large United States clinical trial of multivalent rhesus reassortant vaccine, wild-type G1 rotavirus recovered from disease in vaccinated infants was shown to be antigenically different than the G1 strain used in the reassortant vaccine. However, these G1 vaccine "breakthrough" isolates were identical to the wild-type G1 rotaviruses recovered from disease in placebo-inoculated infants *(106)*.

Similarly, the role of human P serotype specificity upon induction of immune protection is not clear. It has been reported that in Melbourne endemic hospital nursery infection with a P2G3 isolate protected against all rotavirus disease *(34)*. It has much more recently been suggested that the emergence as the dominant wild-type strain of a low pathogenicity P8[11]G10 strain in Bangalore, India, may have been responsible for the decline of rotavirus disease caused by all other serotypes *(109)*. Evidence from human vaccine studies is lacking. Only one efficacy study with a human P1 animal reassortant vaccine has been reported: the role of P1 protection could not be determined because three different serotype human G reassortants were included in the same vaccine *(110)*.

Therefore, there is clear evidence that rotavirus vaccine may induce protection against heterotypic wild-type rotavirus disease. Several animal origin rotaviruses have been protective in some, but not all, vaccine efficacy trials in infants. In a notable example of heterotypic protection, a univalent rhesus reassortant vaccine of serotype G2, evaluated in a Finnish efficacy trial, protected against wild-type human disease of serotype G1 etiology more efficiently than did a G1 univalent rhesus reassortant vaccine (111).

However, each animal origin rotavirus vaccine has had failures as well as successes in human clinical trials. The limited trials to date of laboratory or naturally attenuated human rotaviruses as vaccines have produced no evidence of efficacy. Inexplicably, the combination of a human rotavirus G surface protein and an otherwise predominantly RRV or WC3 bovine rotavirus genome has never failed to protect in a clinical efficacy trial, i.e., a human rotavirus surface protein on an animal rotavirus background seems to immunize humans more effectively than a human G surface protein on a human rotavirus genomic background.

How then, does one select the human G serotypes for inclusion in a rotavirus reassortant vaccine? The simple response has been to select serotypes G1, G2, G3, and G4 that have predominated worldwide from the time of first identification of G serotypes (112) and will certainly be included in the first generation of reassortant vaccines to be licensed in the United States and in Europe. Until recent years, type G1 predominated in most locations during most rotavirus seasons with occasional appearances of a G2 or G3 or rarely a G4 rotavirus season in selected locales. The reasons for fluctuation in serotype prevalence were unknown, given that disease occurs most prominently in seronegative infants encountering their first infection. However, it was most common for G1 rotavirus to predominate in one location year after year (although new predominant strains, as detected by RNA electropherotype, appeared within a given serotype during each successive year of study in a give locale).

Human infection with serotypes other than G1–G4 has been reported, but only very sporadically until recent years. In 1994, human infection with G5 rotavirus (predominantly found in swine) was reported in several Brazilian infants (113). More strikingly, strain G9 (first described in a single case from Philadelphia in 1985 [114]) has not only emerged as prominent in India, but has become the most common isolate in some Indian cities within the past decade (115). Since human rotavirus was discovered, this is the first suggestion that a non–G1–G4 serotype may emerge as a predominant pathogen. Clinical trials are now in the planning stages to determine whether multivalent G1–G4 rhesus rotavirus reassortant vaccine protects against rotavirus disease in an area where G9 virus predominates. If not, new vaccine viruses may need to be constructed. Certainly, worldwide surveillance for the identification of emerging new G serotypes will need to be greatly improved in comparison to the currently existing informal and incomplete data collection system.

At this time, it is uncertain whether human P surface proteins will be incorporated in multivalent reassortant rotavirus vaccine. If so, type P1a will undoubtedly be evaluated first. It is not known whether P1b and P2 serotypes are sufficiently antigenically different from P1a to justify their separate addition to multivalent vaccine; their utility will require extensive testing in clinical trials to justify their use. Furthermore, in terms of justifying the inclusion of additional P-type reassortants into a vaccine, the complexity of design and production of the vaccine increases as more types are added, thus creating a constraint on the pharmaceutical level.

Simian × Human Reassortant Rotaviruses

In an attempt to induce improved protective consistency, the rhesus rotavirus was modified by gene reassortant with human rotavirus strains to contain the single gene segment either for type G1, G2, or G4 antigenic specificity *(20,124)*. The expectation was that ten rhesus rotavirus segments would provide adequate attenuation. Although the vp7 gene has been shown to be one of four gene segments that apparently contribute to determination of virulence, there has been no evidence that addition of human rotavirus vp7 to the simian rotavirus increases the reactogenicity of the reassortant virus for human infants.

The expectation was that human vp7 rhesus reassortant rotavirus would induce a host immune response of a type-specificity characteristic of the human surface protein rather than that of the simian rotavirus parent. This goal was partially accomplished. When serum virus neutralizing antibody responses of orally-inoculated infants were evaluated, the incidence of immune responses to the human G parent virus was clearly enhanced. However, the number of infants with a detectable human G serotype-specific immune response was commonly <50% *(52,90,104,105,116)*. On the other hand, the rhesus reassortants with a human rotavirus G protein induced very efficient neutralizing antibody responses to rhesus rotavirus, represented by the P surface protein of the rhesus rotavirus. Serum binding IgG and IgA antibodies to rotavirus were also efficiently induced by the rhesus reassortants *(52,104,116)*.

As in the case of rhesus rotavirus, rhesus rotavirus reassortants were shed in the stools of many vaccinees, and there was an increased incidence of fevers in vaccinees compared to placebo recipients. The postvaccine fevers that occurred primarily 2–4 days after inoculation were normally observed in <20% of infants, and were reduced in frequency when the first dose was given at age <4 months (infants under the influence of maternal immunity).

Initial efficacy tests of rhesus reassortant vaccine were conducted with a univalent reassortant (D × RRV) of G1 type specificity. In an initial trial in Rochester, NY, this reassortant induced 77% protection against all rotavirus diarrhea. Surprisingly, in this trial rhesus rotavirus alone gave a similar degree of protection against predominantly G1 natural challenge *(51)*. In a second trial of univalent reassortant vaccines in Finland, both G1 and G2 reassortant vaccines each gave similar degrees of protection (67 and 66%) against rotavirus disease during a type G1 rotavirus season *(111)*.

Despite the facts that univalent vaccines were successful and it was unlikely in any given trial that vaccinees would be substantially challenged by non-G1 wild-type rotavirus, it was decided to proceed to a tetravalent vaccine to include protective antigens homotypic to the four major G types prevalent in the world at that time: G1–G4. A quadrivalent vaccine was formulated to contain three reassortants containing vp7 genes of either human serotype G1, G2 or G4. RRV served as the G3 antigen (although it was later determined to be a much less efficient inducer of neutralizing antibody to the human prototype G3 rotavirus [strain Price] than to RRV) *(104)*.

The rhesus rotavirus tetravalent vaccine (RRV-TV) has been administered to infants in doses ranging from 1×10^4 to 1×10^6 pfu of each component virus. Initial trials were performed at a combined dose of 4×10^4 to reduce reactogenicity; this dose was subsequently increased to a dose of 4×10^5 to enhance immunogenicity. A summary of observations of reactogenicity in these trials (in approx 2000 vaccinees *[117]*) indicates about a 15% excess of fevers (>38°C) following the first dose and a smaller excess of fevers >39°C after the first dose and >38°C after the second dose. Significantly increased incidence of decreased appetite (6% excess) and irritability (9% excess) were also observed after the first dose only. Doses of 4×10^4 and of 4×10^5 pfu have both been safely administered to infants as young as 2 days of age *(118)*.

Results of seven large (>400 infants) efficacy trials of RRV-TV have been reported. The pattern of protection observed has been very consistent in the four trials conducted in developed nations. In the two large multicenter trials conducted in the United States with the 4×10^4 and 4×10^5 doses respectively, the protection rates against all rotavirus disease were 57 and 49% respectively, while the protection rates against severe rotavirus disease were 82 and 80% respectively. Each of these trials encountered predominantly type G1 wild-type virus challenge *(52,116)*.

In a "developing nation environment" in a "developed nation," i.e., four American Indian reservations in the southwestern United States, the efficacy of RRV-TV (4×10^5 pfu/dose) was compared with that of the univalent G1 reassortant (4×10^5 pfu/dose). The natural challenge was almost exclusively (96%) serotype G3 rotavirus. Superior protection was associated with RRV-TV. Protection against all rotavirus disease was 50% for RRV-TV compared to only 29% for the univalent vaccine. Protection rates against severe rotavirus disease were 69 and 48% respectively. These data provide good evidence for the importance of homotypic protection by G3 in RRV-TV against natural challenge by serotype G3 *(105)*.

The highest rate of protection observed was detected in a Finnish trial in which there was 68% protection against all rotavirus disease and 91% protection against severe rotavirus disease. This trial was of sufficient size that 100% protection against hospitalization for rotavirus gastroenteritis in the study population could be demonstrated *(119)*.

Developing nation efficacy of RRV-TV was slightly less consistent. A low-dose (4×10^4 pfu) trial in Lima did not give significant protection against all rotavirus disease (24% overall) *(120)*. Another low-dose trial in Belem, Brazil, gave 57% protection against all rotavirus disease, but there was no greater protection against severe rotavirus disease *(121)*.

Greater success was obtained with RRV-TV in a high dose (4×10^5 pfu) trial conducted in Caracas. This trial was of a unique design such that exact comparison with other trials is not possible. As a "catchment trial," community infants were given either three doses of 4×10^5 pfu of RRV-TV or of placebo, and then passively monitored for protection as cases of rotavirus disease were presented at the hospital. Protection observed was 48% against the first case of rotavirus diarrhea, 88% against severe diarrhea and 75% protection against dehydrating diarrhea. This trial also revealed considerable "horizontal" spread of vaccine rotavirus. Vaccine strain virus infection was detected in association with infection with wild-type rotavirus disease in 15% of placebo infants with rotavirus disease and in 13% of vaccine recipients with "breakthrough" rotavirus disease. Indeed, vaccine strain rotavirus was present in stools of 5 of 23 tested cases of rotavirus dehydrating diarrhea in the placebo group. Thus, the secondary infection of infants with viruses of RRV-TV origin clearly does not alone protect them from severe rotavirus diarrhea, although these infections may have been of such a low titer that they could not initiate infection, hence protection, in contacts of vaccinees *(122)*.

Despite success in inducing protection with RRV-TV, attempts to identify the component of the infant immune response responsible for protection have been disappointing. Analysis of a "pivotal" United States efficacy trial of high dose RRV-TV compared with univalent RRV G1 reassortant indicated serum neutralizing antibody titers induced by RRV-TV at incidence ranging from 12–29% against the four human serotypes compared with 88% against rhesus rotavirus itself *(104)*. There were "associations" between antibody titers and protection, but protection was not preferentially associated with serotype-specific antibody. The investigators could only conclude that serum antibody responses to RRV-TV "are in some way related to protection." In this study, it was also determined that vaccine-induced antibody response titers were lower in originally seropositive infants and, similarly, that antibody responses to natural "breakthrough" rotavirus disease in vaccinees were of lower titer than those of naturally infected placebo infants. Unfortunately, local intestinal antibody responses to RRV-TV have not been reported.

INTERTYPIC INTERACTIONS
AMONG RHESUS REASSORTANT ROTAVIRUSES

The performance of several clinical efficacy trials in which RRV-TV was compared with univalent RRV provided an opportunity to evaluate possible interactions among the component viruses. Wright et al. *(123)* vaccinated infants with bivalent RRV containing G1 or G2 reassortants in two different ratios and determined that the neutralizing antibody response to either G1 or G2 rotavirus was significantly less following bivalent vaccine than after univalent vaccine only.

It was observed in early trials of RRV-TV in Venezuela that human G serotype specific antibody responses were less frequent than observed in earlier trials of individual reassortants *(122)*. In trials where "head-to-head" comparison was made of RRV-TV and RRV univalent G1 vaccine, respective G1 type antibody responses in tetravalent vs. univalent vaccine recipients were 19% vs 43% in the 1989–90 low dose multicenter trial *(52)*, 13% vs 34% (United States Multicenter trial 1991–92 *[127]*), and 24% vs 37% (United States "Native American" trial 1992–94 *[105]*). RRV-TV ratios of immune response to different vaccine component G types also varied from trial to trial. For example, immune responses to G4 in vaccinees were not significantly above placebo levels in the 1991–92 multicenter trial, in the Native American trial or in the Venezuela catchment trial. Yet, the incidence of G4 responses exceeded that of the G1 responses in the 1989–90 multicenter trial and in at least one United States consistency lot trial (ACIP) *(117)*.

Another measure of strain interaction in multivalent RRV vaccines may be reflected in the ratios of different vaccine component reassortants recovered from vaccinee stools, which presumably represents the relative efficiency of replication in the infant gut. Wright et al. *(123)* were surprised to discover that when G1 and G2 reassortants were given to infants in very different ratios (16:1 and 1:13), the relative frequency of viruses recovered from gut closely reflected the input ratio, despite the fact that it was assumed that several cycles of virus replication would have occurred in the interval between vaccination and collection of stools. Perez-Schael et al. *(90)* inoculated Venezuelan infants with RRV-TV at doses ranging from 0.25 to 1.0×10^4 pfu of each component reassortant; virtually all vaccinees shed vaccine virus recoverable by cell culture cultivation. Shedding of the RRV G2 reassortant and of RRV predominated. Of 20 infants given the lowest dose of RRV-TV, fecal shedding was identified as follows: any virus, 20 (100%); G2 20 (100%); RRV, 18 (90%); G1, 14 (70%); G4, 10 (50%) *(90)*.

In contrast, when United States infants were inoculated with a dose of 10^5 or 10^6 pfu of each component in RRV-TV, 95% of the recovered virus was RRV *(124)*.

Observations in the recent "catchment" RRV-TV trial in Caracas also suggested disproportionate horizontal dissemination of the RRV vaccine strain component in the community. In 29 infants in whom vaccine virus was associated with wild-type G1 virus in an episode of rotavirus gastroenteritis (11 vaccinated and 18 placebo infants), the vaccine virus strains recovered were exclusively RRV (28 infants) and the G4 reassortant (five infants, four in mixed infection with RRV) *(122)*.

The surprising observation that addition of a gene from a human strain rotavirus to a simian strain rotavirus confers a disadvantage for replication in the human host has not been explained. It is possible that components of the immune experience of the host are human rotavirus type-specific and contribute to this phenomenon. Alternatively, the human gene and its protein product are placed in the unnatural environment of 10 simian genes/proteins, hence the reassortant strain does not replicate as well as the simian strain *per se*.

Bovine × Human Reassortant Rotaviruses

Because the use of bovine rotaviruses as candidate vaccines in infants has been associated with efficient homologous serotype immune responses and with no fevers or other adverse effects, bovine rotavirus × human rotavirus reassortants have been constructed as vaccine candidates. Both bovine rotavirus-derived reassortant vaccines that have undergone clinical trials utilize bovine rotaviruses of type P7[5]. However, one bovine rotavirus was isolated in the United States (strain WC3) *(73)* and the other was isolated in the United Kingdom (strain UK) *(74)*.

WC3 REASSORTANTS

Several single gene or multigenic reassortants were developed having at least the vp4 of strain WC3 bovine rotavirus with an added gene or genes including the G protein of rotaviruses of serotypes 1, 2, 3, or 4 *(75,125)*. All reassortants except the G4 reassortant have been evaluated in infant clinical trials in which they were shown to retain the safety characteristics of the bovine strain WC3 parent virus. Infants inoculated with high doses (10^6–10^7 pfu) of these vaccines characteristically developed near 100% immune responses to WC3 rotavirus after two doses but lower rates of immune response to the human rotavirus parent. When reassortants containing human rotavirus origin P protein on a WC3 genome background were investigated in infant trials, they too exhibited the excellent safety profile characteristic of WC3. Surprisingly, they also induced immune responses to the WC3 parent rotavirus that were higher than those to the human rotavirus parent.

A double reassortant containing both human rotavirus P1a[8] and G1 proteins on a WC3 virus genome background was safe but induced very poor immune responses in infants. In contrast, a mixture of single gene reassortants of WC3 with only the P1a or G1 of human rotavirus was highly immunogenic (100% response to WC3, 71% response to G1 human rotavirus) while retaining an excellent safety profile *(110)*.

The G1 serotype reassortant has been evaluated in two or three doses in three efficacy trials in the United States. Protection rates ranged from 64–100% against all rotavirus disease and from 84–100% against severe rotavirus disease in predominantly G1 rotavirus seasons *(126,127)*. Serum neutralizing antibody responses in one, three dose trial were near 100% to WC3 and 70% to human G1 serotype rotavirus *(72)*.

A single multivalent clinical trial of WC3 reassortants has been completed. The vaccine included four reassortants bearing either human rotavirus type G1, G2, G3, or P1a protein. In a year when natural disease was primarily of G1 serotype, this vaccine provided 67% protection against all rotavirus disease and 69% protection against severe rotavirus disease. There was an 8% excess of mild diarrhea episodes in vaccinees compared to placebo controls after the first dose of vaccine *(128)*.

INTERTYPIC INTERACTION OF WC3 REASSORTANT VIRUSES

Multivalent and univalent WC3 reassortants have not been studied as separate cells in the same clinical trial. In the single multivalent trial of WC3 reassortants, serum neutralizing antibody responses to the G1 rotavirus parent were similar to those obtained with univalent G1 reassortant vaccine, but responses to G2 and G3 rotavirus parents were lower than expected (approx 30%). Approximately 8% of infants shed virus detectable by plaque assay of stool; the great majority of these infants shed the P1a reassortant indicating a selective propagation advantage for that virus in the infant gut. It has not yet been established whether the P1a reassortant alone or in association with other vaccine strains contributes to the slight excess of postvaccination episodes of diarrhea *(128)*.

UK REASSORTANTS

Single gene reassortants of UK bovine rotavirus have been developed incorporating the vp7 gene of either human serotype G1, G2, G3, or G4 rotaviruses. Phase 1 clinical studies of the G1 and G2 strain reassortants indicate that these reassortants induce immune responses in most infants after two oral doses while exhibiting the high safety profile characteristic of bovine rotavirus in infants *(129)*.

Clinical trials are continuing the study of the immunogenicity and efficacy of quadrivalent UK bovine rotavirus × human rotavirus reassortant vaccine.

Interaction of Oral Poliovirus Vaccine (OPV) with Rotavirus Vaccine

Practical considerations will demand that OPV may be coadministered with rotavirus vaccine, e.g., in the United States at six and fifteen months of age. There was an initial concern that use of this combination might lead to an impaired protective immune response to one or both of these vaccines. This concern is of diminishing importance in developed nations where use of OPV is rapidly being reduced. However, use of OPV may continue in some developing nations for an indeterminate length of time.

Some data support the hypothesis that responses to rotavirus vaccine may be inhibited by coadministration of the vaccine with OPV *(4)*. Several clinical studies indicated that coadministration of OPV with bovine rotavirus vaccine RIT 4239 led to a very significant inhibition of the rotavirus-specific immune response *(130,131)*. There have been no studies of the effect of coadministration with OPV upon the immune response to bovine strain rotavirus WC3 or to WC3 reassortant rotavirus vaccine.

Coadministration of OPV with RRV-TV at a dose of 10^4 pfu of each component in Bangkok was associated with very significant inhibition of the serum antibody titer to rotavirus after the first dose. Immune responses to rotavirus given with or without OPV were similar after the second and third dose, but mean antibody titers (serum neutralizing antibody to RRV) to rotavirus were still depressed after three doses of RRV + OPV *(132)*. A subsequent study of the effect of coadministration of OPV with monovalent RRV of serotype G1 or with RRV-TV at a 10^5 pfu dose indicated a slight inhibition of immune responses associated with OPV. However, final rates of seroconversion and protection did not appear to be affected by OPV *(133)*. In none of the above studies did there appear to be evidence of inhibition of the immune response to OPV attributable to coadministration with rotavirus vaccine. It is probable that RRV-TV when licensed will be recommended with no restrictions on coadministration with OPV or any other pediatric vaccines *(117)*.

Summary

The first rotavirus vaccines to reach the market will be "combination" vaccines in the sense that they contain several rotavirus reassortants, each of which uses a common animal rotavirus genome backbone to express a single surface protein of human rotavirus serotype. Each may be expected to give, with three oral doses, at least 50% protection against all rotavirus disease and a much greater level of protection against severe disease. First licensed will be RRV-TV containing four strains bearing vp7 surface antigens of human serotypes G1–G4 on a rhesus rotavirus genome background. This product will express a level of reactogenicity (fevers) characteristic of RRV. The use of four serotypes has been shown to reduce the efficiency of the G1 type-specific immune response characteristic of the G1 monovalent vaccine but to provide enhanced protection against natural challenge with G3 rotavirus.

The second candidate that has received extensive clinical trails (but less than RRV-TV) is comprised of rotavirus reassortants consisting of human rotavirus surface proteins vp4 (serotype P1a) and/ or vp7 (serotypes G1–G3) upon a bovine WC3 backbone. These reassortants have a safe level of reactogenicity characteristic of WC3 with the exception that the VP4 reassortant may contribute to postvaccination diarrhea. Protection achieved with a P1a, G1, G2, or G3 combination vaccine in a single trial was approximately 70% both against all rotavirus disease and against severe rotavirus disease.

Although other rotavirus vaccines are in earlier stages of development, there are as yet no reports of their clinical evaluation as multivalent combination vaccines.

In terms of vaccine interaction, small clinical trials of rotavirus given with OPV have revealed little effect of rotavirus vaccine upon the poliovirus-specific immune response. The OPV has been associated with a significant inhibition of immune responses elicited by bovine rotavirus vaccine RIT 4237 and much less inhibition of those elicited by RRV-based vaccine. Rotavirus vaccines to be licensed soon may be used extensively with OPV in the developed world. It also will be important to assess the interaction of rotavirus vaccine with licensed injected vaccines given simultaneously, e.g., DTP, Hib conjugate, and hepatitis B, even though one might not expect interference as readily as for another oral vaccine (OPV).

Limited experience indicates that polyvalent vaccines (for rotavirus G serotypes) possess advantage over monovalent vaccine. As all candidate rotavirus vaccines confer <100% protection, it may be predicted that evaluation of the ideal mixture of human rotavirus serotypes in vaccine (as well as different approaches for delivering serotype-specific immunogens) will be a continuing process.

References

1. De Zoysa, I. and Feachem, R. G. (1985) Interventions for the control of diarrhoeal diseases among young children: rotavirus and cholera immunization. *Bull. WHO* **63,** 569–583.
2. Kapikian, A. Z. and Chanock, R. M. (1996) Rotaviruses, in *Fields Virology,* 3rd ed., vol. 2 (Fields, B. N., Knipe, D. M., Howley, P. M., Chanock, R. M., Melnick, J. L., Monath, T. P., Roizman, B., and Straus, S. E., eds.), Lippincott-Raven, Philadelphia, pp. 1657–1708.
3. Glass, R. I., Kilgore, P. E., Holman, R. C., et al. (1996) The epidemiology of rotavirus diarrhea in the United States: surveillance and estimates of disease burden. *J. Infect. Dis.* **174(Suppl. 1),** S5–S11.
4. Kilgore, P. E., Holman, R. C., Clarke, M. J., and Glass, R. I. (1995) Trends of diarrheal disease-associated mortality in U. S. children, 1968 through 1991. *JAMA* **274,** 1143–1148.

5. Huilan, S., Zhen, L. G., Mathan, M. M., et al. (1991) Etiology of acute diarrhoea among children in developing countries: a multicenter study in five countries. *Bull. WHO* **69,** 549–555.
6. Levine, M. M., Losonsky, G., Herrington, D., et al. (1986) Pediatric diarrhea: the challenge of prevention. *Pediatr. Infect. Dis.* **5,** S29–S43.
7. Cook, S. M., Glass, R. I., LeBaron, C. W., and Ho, M.-S. (1990) Global seasonality of rotavirus infections. *Bull. WHO* **68,** 171–177.
8. Bern, C., Martines, J., deZoysa, I., and Glass, R. I. (1992) The magnitude of the global problem of diarrhoeal disease: a ten year update. *Bull. WHO* **70,** 705–714.
9. Murray, C. J. and Lopez, A. D. (1997) Global mortality, disability, and the contribution of risk factors: global burden of disease study. *Lancet* **349,** 1436–1442.
10. Walsh, J. A. and Warren, K. S. (1979) Selective primary health care. An interim strategy for disease control in developing countries. *N. Engl. J. Med.* **301,** 967–974.
11. Snyder, J. D. and Merson, M. H. (1982) The magnitude of the global problem of acute diarrhoeal disease: a review of active surveillance data. *Bull. WHO* **60,** 605–613.
12. Tallett, S., MacKenzie, C., Middleton, P., et al. (1977) Clinical, laboratory, and epidemiologic features of a viral gastroenteritis in infants and children. *Pediatrics* **60,** 217–222.
13. Carr, M., McKendrick, D., and Spyridakis, T. (1978) The clinical features of infantile gastroenteritis due to rotavirus. *Scand. J. Infect. Dis.* **8,** 241–243.
14. Kovacs, A., Chan, L., Hotrakitya, C., et al. (1987) Rotavirus gastroenteritis: clinical and laboratory features and use of the rotazyme test. *Am. J. Dis. Child.* **141,** 161–166.
15. Rodriguez, W., Kim, H., Arrobio, J., et al. (1977) Clinical features of acute gastroenteritis associated with human reovirus-like agent in infants and young children. *J. Pediatr.* **91,** 188–193.
16. Estes, M. (1996) Rotaviruses and their replication, in *Field's Virology,* 3rd ed., vol. 2 (Fields, B. N., Knipe, D. M., and Howley, P. M., eds.), Lippincott-Raven, Philadelphia, pp. 1625–1655.
17. Hoshino, Y., Sereno, M. M., Midthun, K., et al. (1985) Independent segregation of two antigenic specificities (vp3 and vp 7) involved in neutralization of rotavirus infectivity. *Proc. Natl. Acad. Sci. USA* **82,** 8701–8704.
18. Offit, P. A. and Blavat, G. (1986) Identification of the two rotavirus genes determining neutralization specificities. *J. Virol.* **57,** 376–378.
19. Offit, P. A., Clark, H. F., Blavat, G., and Greenberg, H. B. (1986) Reassortant rotaviruses containing structural proteins vp3 and vp7 from different parents induce antibodies protective against each parental serotype. *J. Virol.* **60,** 491–496.
20. Midthun, K., Greenberg, H. B., Hoshino, Y., et al. (1985) Reassortant rotaviruses as potential live rotavirus vaccine candidates. *J. Virol.* **53,** 949–954.
21. Kalica, A. R., Greenberg, H. B., Wyatt, R. G., et al. (1981) Genes of human (strain WA) and bovine (strain UK) rotaviruses that code for neutralization and subgroup antigens. *Virology* **112,** 385–390.
22. Larralde, G., Li, B., Kapikian, A. Z., and Gorziglia, M. (1991) Serotype-specific epitopes present on the vp 8 subunit of rotavirus vp 4 protein. *J. Virol.* **65,** 3213–3218.
23. Gorziglia, M. K. Y., Green, K., Nishikawa, K., et al. (1988) Sequence of the fourth gene of human rotaviruses recovered from asymptomatic or symptomatic infections. *J. Virol.* **62,** 2979–2984.
24. Mebus, C. A., Stair, E. L., Underdahl, N. R., and Twiehaus, M. J. (1974) Pathology of neonatal calf diarrhea induced by a reo-like virus. *Vet. Pathol.* **8,** 490–505.
25. Pearson, G. R. and McNulty, M. S. (1977) Pathological changes in the small intestine of neonatal pigs infected with a pig reovirus-like agent (rotavirus). *J. Comp. Pathol.* **87,** 363–375.
26. Snodgrass, D. R., Ferguson, A., Allan, F., et al. (1979) Small intestinal morphology and epithelial cell kinetics in lamb rotavirus infections. *Gastroenterology* **76,** 477–481.
27. Starkey, W. G., Collins, J., Wallis, T. S., et al. (1986) Kinetics, tissue specificity and pathological changes in murine rotavirus infection of mice. *J. Gen. Virol.* **67,** 2625–2634.

28. Holmes, I. H., Ruck, B. J., Bishop, R. F., and Davidson, G. P. (1975) Infantile enteritis viruses: morphogenesis and morphology. *J. Virol.* **16,** 937–943.
29. Suzuki, H., and Konno, T. (1975) Reovirus-like particles in jejunal mucosa of a Japanese infant with acute infectious non-bacterial gastroenteritis. *Tohoku J. Exp. Med.* **115,** 199–211.
30. Sheridan, J. F., Eydelloth, R. S., Vonderfecht, S. L., and Aurelian, L. (1983) Virus-specific immunity in neonatal and adult mouse rotavirus infection. *Infect. Immun.* **39,** 917–927.
31. Ball, J. M., Tian, P., Zeng, C. Q. Y., et al. (1996) Age-dependent diarrhea induced by a rotaviral nonstructural glycoprotein. *Science* **272,** 101–104.
32. Angel, J., Tang, B., Feng, N., et al. (1998) Studies of the role for NSP4 in pathogenesis of homologous murine rotavirus diarrhea. *J. Infect. Dis.* **177,** 455–458.
33. Hoshino, Y., Sereno, M. M., Kapikian, A. Z., et al. (1993) Genetic determinants of rotavirus virulence studied in gnotobiotic piglets, in *Vaccines '93*. Cold Spring Harbor Laboratory, pp. 277–282.
34. Bishop, R., Barnes, G., Cipriani, E., and Lund, J. (1983) Clinical immunity after neonatal rotavirus infection: a prospective longitudinal study in young children. *N. Engl. J. Med.* **309,** 72–76.
35. Bernstein, D. I., Sander, D. S., Smith, V. E., et al. (1991) Protection from rotavirus reinfection: 2-year prospective study. *J. Infect. Dis.* **164,** 277–283.
36. Ward, R. L. and Bernstein, D. (1994) Protection against rotavirus disease after natural infection. *J. Infect. Dis.* **169,** 900–904.
37. Matson, D. O., O'Ryan, M. L., Herrera, I., et al. (1993) Fecal antibody responses to symptomatic and asymptomatic rotavirus infections. *J. Infect. Dis.* **167,** 577–583.
38. Coulson, B., Grimwood, K., Hudson, I., et al. (1992) Role of coproantibody in clinical protection of children during reinfection with rotavirus. *J. Clin. Microbiol.* **30,** 1678–1684.
39. O'Ryan, M. L., Matson, D. O., Estes, M. K., and Pickering, L. K. (1994) Anti-rotavirus G type-specific and isotype-specific antibodies in children with natural rotavirus infection. *J. Infect. Dis.* **169,** 504–511.
40. Yolken, R., Wyatt, R., and Zissis, G. (1978) Epidemiology of human rotavirus types 1 and 2 as studied by enzyme-linked immunosorbent assay. *N. Engl. J. Med.* **299,** 1156–1161.
41. Black, R., Greenberg, H., Kapikian, A., et al. (1982) Acquisition of serum antibody to Norwalk virus and rotavirus in relation to diarrhea in a longitudinal study of young children in rural Bangladesh. *J. Infect. Dis.* **145,** 483–489.
42. Mata, L., Simhon, A., Urratia, J., et al. (1983) Epidemiology of rotaviruses in a cohort of 45 Guatemalan Mayan Indian children observed from birth to the age of three years. *J. Infect. Dis.* **148,** 452–461.
43. Chiba, S., Nakata, S., Urasawa, T., et al. (1986) Protective effect of naturally acquired homotypic and heterotypic rotavirus antibodies. *Lancet* **i,** 417–421.
44. Linhares, A., Gabbay, Y., Mascarenhas, J., et al. (1988) Epidemiology of rotavirus subgroups and serotypes in Belem, Brazil: a three-year study. *Ann. Inst. Pasteur./Virol.* **139,** 89–99.
45. Georges-Courbot, M., Monges, J., Beraud-Cassel, A., et al. (1988) Prospective longitudinal study of rotavirus infections in children from birth to two years of age in Central Africa. *Ann. Inst. Pasteur./Virol.* **139,** 421–428.
46. Friedman, M., Gaul, A., Sarov, B., et al. (1988) Two sequential outbreaks of rotavirus gastroenteritis: evidence for symptomatic and asymptomatic reinfection. *J. Infect. Dis.* **158,** 814–822.
47. Grinstein, S., Gomez, J., Bercovich, J., and Biscorn, E. (1989) Epidemiology of rotavirus infection and gastroenteritis in prospectively monitored Argentine families with young children. *Am. J. Epidemiol.* **130,** 300–308.
48. Reves, R., Hossain, M., Midthun, K., et al. (1989) An observational study of naturally-acquired immunity in a cohort of 363 Egyptian children. *Am. J. Epidemiol.* **130,** 981–988.

49. O'Ryan, M., Matson, D., Estes, M., et al. (1990) Molecular epidemiology of rotavirus in young children attending day care centers in Houston. *J. Infect. Dis.* **162,** 810–816.
50. DeChamps, C., Laveran, H., Peigue-Lafeville, J., et al. (1991) Sequential rotavirus infections: characterization of serotypes and electropherotypes. *Res. Virol.* **142,** 39–45.
51. Madore, H., Christy, C., Pichichero, M., et al. (1992) Field trial of rhesus rotavirus or human-rhesus rotavirus reassortant vaccine of vp7 serotype 3 or 1 specificity in infants. *J. Infect. Dis.* **166,** 235–243.
52. Bernstein, D., Glass, R., Rodgers, G., et al. (1995) Evaluation of rhesus rotavirus monovalent and tetravalent reassortant vaccines in United States children. *JAMA* **273,** 1191–1196.
53. Ward, R. and Bernstein, D. (1995) Lack of correlation between serum rotavirus antibody titers and protection following vaccination with reassortant RRV vaccines. *Vaccine* **13,** 1226–1252.
54. Offit, P. A. and Dudzik, K. I. (1989) Rotavirus-specific cytotoxic T lymphocytes appear at the intestinal mucosal surface after rotavirus infection. *J. Virol.* **63,** 3507–3512.
55. Offit, P. A. and Dudzik, K. I. (1990) Rotavirus-specific cytotoxic T lymphocytes passively protect against gastroenteritis in suckling mice. *J. Virol.* **64,** 6325–6328.
56. Dharakul, T., Rott, L., and Greenberg, H. B. (1990) Recovery from chronic rotavirus infection in mice with severe combined immunodeficiency: virus clearance mediated by adoptive transfer of immune CD8+ T lymphocytes. *J. Virol.* **64,** 4375–4382.
57. Franco, M., Tin,C., and Greenberg, H. (1997) CD8+ T cells can mediate complete short term and partial long term protection against reinfection by rotavirus. *J. Virol.* **71,** 4165–4170.
58. Matsui, S., Mackow, E., and Greenberg, H. (1989) Molecular determinants of rotavirus neutralization and protection. *Adv. Virus. Res.* **36,** 181–214.
59. Clark, H. F., Borian, F. E., Bell, L. M., et al. (1988) Protective effect of WC3 vaccine against rotavirus diarrhea in infants during a predominantly serotype 1 rotavirus season. *J. Infect. Dis.* **158,** 570–587.
60. Matson, D., O'Ryan, M., Pickering, L., et al. (1992) Characterization of serum antibody responses to natural rotavirus infections in children by vp7-specific epitope-blocking assays. *J. Clin. Microbiol.* **30,** 1056–1061.
61. Zheng, B., Han, S., Yan, Y., et al. (1988) Development of neutralizing antibodies and group A common antibodies against natural infections with human rotavirus. *J. Clin. Microbiol.* **26,** 1506–1512.
62. Puerto, F., Padilla-Noriega, L., Zamora-Chavez, A., et al. (1987) Prevalent patterns of serotype-specific seroconversion in Mexican children infected with rotavirus. *J. Clin. Microbiol.* **25,** 960–963.
63. Gerna, G., Sarasini, A., Torsellini, M., et al. (1990) Group- and type-specific serologic response in infants and children with primary rotavirus infections and gastroenteritis caused by a strain of known serotype. *J. Infect. Dis.* **161,** 1105–1111.
64. Clark, H., Dolan, K., Horton-Slight, P., et al. (1985) Diverse serologic response to rotavirus infection of infants in a single epidemic. *Pediatr. Infect. Dis.* **4,** 626–631.
65. Mebus, C. A., White, R. G., Bass E. P., and Twiehaus, M. J. (1973) Immunity to neonatal calf diarrhea virus. *JAVMA* **163,** 880–883.
66. Saif, L. and Fernandez, F. (1996) Group A rotavirus veterinary vaccines. *J. Infect. Dis.* **174,** S98–S106.
67. Vesikari, T., Isolauri, E., D'Hondt, E., et al. (1984) Protection of infants against rotavirus diarrhea by RIT 4237 attenuated bovine rotavirus strain vaccine. *Lancet* **1,** 977–980.
68. Flores, J., Perez-Schael, I., Gonzalez, M., et al. (1987) Protection against severe rotavirus diarrhea by rhesus rotavirus vaccine Venezuelan children. *Lancet* **1,** 882–884.
69. Gothefors, L., Wadell, G., Juto, P., et al. (1989) Prolonged efficacy of rhesus rotavirus vaccine in Swedish children. *J. Infect. Dis.* **159,** 753–757.

70. Georges-Coubot, M. C., Monges, J., Siopathis, M. R., et al. (1991) Evaluation of the efficacy of a low-passage bovine rotavirus (strain WC3) vaccine in children in Central Africa. *Res. Virol.* **142,** 405–411.

71. Ogra, P. L. (1996) Mucosal immunoprophylaxis: an introductory overview, in *Mucosal Vaccines* (Kiyono, H., Ogra, P. L., and McGhee, J. R., ed.), Academic, New York, NY, pp. 3–14.

72. Clark, H. F., Shrager, D., Lawley, D., Offit, P. A., and Ellis, R. Human-bovine G1 reassortant of rotavirus WC3: dose response patterns to vp7 (G1) and vp 4 (P5 [7]) are distinct. *Vaccine* (submitted for publication).

73. Garbag-Chenon, A., Fontaine, J.-L., Lasfargues, G., et al. (1989) Reactogenicity and immunogenicity of rotavirus WC3 vaccine in 5-12-month-old infants. *Res. Virol.* **140,** 207–217.

74. Kapikian, A., Hoshino, Y., Chanock, R., and Perez-Schael, I. (1996) Efficacy of a quadrivalent rhesus rotavirus-based human rotavirus vaccine aimed at preventing severe rotavirus diarrhea in infants and young children. *J. Infect. Dis.* **174,** S65–S72.

75. Clark, H. F., Offit, P., Ellis, R., et al. (1996) The development of multivalent bovine rotavirus (strain WC3) reassortant vaccine for infants. *J. Infect. Dis.* **174,** S73–S80.

76. Wyatt, R. G., Mebus, C. A., Yolken, R. H., et al. (1979) Rotaviral immunity in gnotobiotic calves: heterologous resistance to human virus induced by bovine virus. *Science* **203,** 548–550.

77. Zissis, G., Lambert, J. P., Marbehant, P., et al. (1983) Protection studies in colostrum-deprived piglets of a bovine rotavirus vaccine candidate using human rotavirus strains for challenge. *J. Infect. Dis.* **142,** 439–441.

78. Delem, A., Lobmann, M., and Zygraich, N. (1984) A bovine rotavirus developed as a candidate for use in humans. *J. Biol. Stand.* **12,** 443–445.

79. Vesikari, T., Kapikian, A., Delem, A., and Zissis, G. (1986) A comparative trial of rhesus monkey (RRV-1) and bovine (RIT 4237) oral rotavirus vaccines in young children. *J. Infect. Dis.* **153,** 832–839.

80. Vesikari, T., Isolauri, E., Delem, A., et al. (1983) Immunogenicity and safety of live oral attenuated bovine rotavirus vaccine strain RIT 4237 in adults and young children. *Lancet* **11,** 807–811.

81. Vesikari, T., Isolauri, E., Delem, A., et al. (1985) Clinical efficacy of the RIT 4237 live attenuated bovine rotavirus vaccine in infants vaccinated before a rotavirus epidemic. *J. Pediatr.* **107,** 189–194.

82. Vesikari, T. (1996) Trials of oral bovine and rhesus rotavirus vaccines in Finland: a historical account and present status. *Arch. Virol.* **12,** 177–186.

83. DeMol, P., Zissis, G., Butzler, J. P., et al. (1986) Failure of live, attenuated and rotavirus vaccine. *Lancet* **ii,** 108.

84. Hanlon, P., Hanlon, K., Marsh, V., et al. (1987) Trial of an attenuated bovine rotavirus vaccine (RIT 4237) in Gambian infants. *Lancet* **1,** 1342–1345.

85. Lanata, C. F., Black, R. E., deAguila, R., et al. (1989) Protection of Peruvian children against rotavirus diarrhea of specific serotypes by one, two, or three doses of the RIT 4237 attenuated bovine rotavirus vaccine. *J. Infect. Dis.* **159,** 452–459.

86. Bernstein, D. I., Smith, V. E., Sander, D. S., et al. (1990) Evaluation of WC3 rotavirus vaccine and correlates of protection in healthy infants. *J. Infect. Dis.* **162,** 1055–1062.

87. Kapikian, A., Midthun, K., Hoshino, Y., et al. (1985) Rhesus rotavirus: a candidate vaccine for prevention of human rotavirus disease, in *Molecular and Chemical Basis of Resistance to Parasitic, Bacterial, and Viral Diseases* (Lerner, R. A., Charnock, R. M., and Brown, F., eds.), Cold Spring Harbor Laboratory, Cold Spring Harbor, NY, pp. 357–367.

88. Bell, L. M., Clark, H. F., O'Brien, E. A., et al. (1987) Gastroenteritis caused by a human rotavirus (serotype 3) in a suckling mouse model. *Proc. Soc. Exp. Biol. Med.* **184,** 127–132.

89. Riepenhoff-Talty, M., Schaekel, K., Clark, H. F., et al. (1993) Group A rotaviruses produce extrahepatic biliary obstruction in orally inoculated newborn mice. *Pediatr. Res.* **33,** 394–399.
90. Perez-Schael, I., Garcia, D., Gonzolez, M., et al. (1990) Prospective study of diarrheal diseases in Venezuelan children to evaluate the efficacy of rhesus rotavirus vaccine. *J. Med. Virol.* **30,** 219–229.
91. Vesikari, T., Rautanen, T., Varis, T., et al. (1990) Rhesus rotavirus candidate vaccine. Clinical trial in children vaccinated between 2 and 5 months of age. *Am. J. Dis. Child.* **144,** 285–289.
92. Perez-Schael, I., Gonzalez, M., Daoud, N., et al. (1987) Reactogenicity and antigenicity of the rhesus rotavirus vaccine in Venezuelan children. *J. Infect. Dis.* **155,** 334–338.
93. Santosham, M., Letson, G. W., Wolff, M., et al. (1991) A field study of the safety and efficacy of two candidate rotavirus vaccines in a native American population. *J. Infect. Dis.* **163,** 483–487.
94. Christy, C., Madore, H. P., Pichichero, M. E., et al. (1988) Field trial of rhesus rotavirus vaccine in infants. *Pediatr. Infect. Dis. J.* **7,** 647–650.
95. Rennels, M. B., Losonsky, G. A., Young, A. E., et al. (1990) An efficacy trail of the rhesus rotavirus vaccine in Maryland. *Am. J. Dis. Child.* **144,** 601–604.
96. Dongmei, C., Zhisheng, B., Su, L., et al. (1994) Preliminary observation of reaction and serological efficacy of strain LLR-85-37 of oral rotavirus live vaccine. *Chinese J. Biol.* **7,** 53–56.
97. Vesikari, T., Ruuska, T., Koivu, H-P, et al. (1991) Evaluation of the M37 human rotavirus vaccine in 2- to 6-month-old infants. *Pediatr. Infect. Dis. J.* **10,** 912–917.
98. Bernstein, D. I., Smith, V. E., Sherwood, J. R., et al. (1998) Safety and immunogenicity of live, attenuated human rotavirus vaccine 89-12. *Vaccine* **16,** 381–387.
99. Hoshino, Y., Wyatt, R., Greenberg, H., et al. (1984) Serotypic similarity and diversity of rotaviruses of mammalian and avian origin as studied by plaque-reduction neutralization. *J. Infect. Dis.* **149,** 694–702.
100. Gorziglia, M., Larralde, G., Kapikian, A., et al. (1990) Antigenic relationships among human rotaviruses as determined by outer capsid protein VP4. *Proc. Natl. Acad. Sci. USA* **87,** 7155–7159.
101. Offit, P. A. and Clark, H. F. (1985) Maternal antibody-mediated protection against gastroenteritis due to rotavirus in newborn mice is dependent on both serotype and titer of antibody. *J. Infect. Dis.* **152,** 1152–1158.
102. Clark, H. F. and Offit, P. A. (1992) Rotavirus vaccines, in *Vaccines,* 2nd ed. (Plotkin, S. and Mortimer, E., eds.). W. B. Saunders, Philadelphia, pp. 809–822.
103. Velazquez, F. R., Matson, D. O., Clava, J. J., et al. (1996) Rotavirus infection in infants as protection against subsequent infections. *N. Engl. J. Med.* **335,** 1022–1028.
104. Ward, R. L., Knowlton, D. R., Zito, E. T., et al. (1997) Serologic correlates of immunity in a tetravalent reassortant rotavirus vaccine trial. *J. Infect. Dis.* **176,** 570–577.
105. Santosham, M., Moulton, L. H., Reid, R., et al. (1997) Efficacy and safety of high-dose rhesus-human reassortant rotavirus vaccine in Native American populations. *J. Pediatr.* **131,** 632–638.
106. Jin, Q., Ward, R. L., Knowlton, D. R., et al. (1996) Divergence of VP7 genes of G1 rotaviruses isolated from infants vaccinated with reassortant rhesus rotaviruses. *Arch. Virol.* **141,** 2057–2076.
107. Wen, L., Nakayama, M., Yamanishi, Y., et al. (1997) Genetic variation in the VP7 gene of human rotavirus serotype 3 (G3 type) isolated in China and Japan. *Arch. Virol.* **142,** 1481–1489.
108. Gerna, G., Sarasini, A., Matteo, A., et al. (1988) Identification of two subtypes of serotype 4 human rotavirus by using VP7 specific neutralizing monoclonal antibodies. *J. Clin. Microbiol.* **26,** 1388–1392.

109. Aijaz, S., Gowda, K., Jagannath, H. V., et al. (1996) Epidemiology of symptomatic human rotaviruses in Bangalore and Mysore, India, from 1988 to 1994 as determined by electropherotype, subgroup and serotype analysis. *Arch. Virol.* **141,** 715–726.
110. Clark, H. F., Welsko, D., and Offit, P. (1992) Infant responses to bovine WC3 reassortants containing human rotavirus VP7, VP4, or VP7 + VP4 [abstract], in *Program and abstracts of the 32nd Interscience Conference on Antimicrobial Agents and Chemotherapy* (Anaheim, CA). Washington, DC, American Society for Microbiology, p. 343.
111. Vesikari, T., Ruuska, T., Green, K. Y., et al. (1992) Protective efficacy against serotype 1 rotavirus diarrhea by live oral rhesus-human reassortant rotavirus vaccines with human rotavirus VP7 serotype 1 or 2 specificity. *Pediatr. Infect. Dis. J.* **11,** 535–542.
112. Hoshino, Y. and Kapikian, A. (1994) Rotavirus antigens. *Curr. Top. Microbiol. Immunol.* **185,** 179–227.
113. Gouvea, V., DeCastro, L., Timenitsky, M-CST, et al. (1994) Rotavirus serotype G5 associated with diarrhea in Brazilian children. *J. Clin. Microbiology* **32,** 1408,1409.
114. Clark, H. F., Hoshino, Y., Bell, L., et al. (1987) Rotavirus isolate WI61 representing a presumptive new human serotype. *J. Clin. Microbiol.* **25,** 1757–1762.
115. Cicerello, H. G., Das, B. K., Gupta, A., et al. (1994) High prevalence of rotavirus infection among neonates born at hospitals in Delhi, India: predisposition of newborns for infection with unusual rotavirus. *Pediatr. Infect. Disease J.* **13,** 720–724.
116. Rennels, M. B., Glass, R. I., Dennely, P. H., et al. (1996) Safety and efficacy of high-dose rhesus-human reassortant rotavirus vaccines—report of the national multicenter trial. *Pediatrics* **97,** 7–13.
117. National Communicable Diseases Centers (1997) Rotavirus vaccines for the prevention of rotavirus diarrhea in children: recommendations of the Advisory Committee on Immunization Practices (ACIP), U. S. Government Printing Office, Washington, D. C.
118. Dagan, R., Kassio, I., Sarov, B., et al. (1992) Safety and immunogenicity of oral tetravalent human-rhesus reassortant rotavirus vaccine in neonates. *Ped. Infect. Dis. J.* **11,** 991–996.
119. Joensuu, J., Koskenniemi, E., Pang, X., and Vesikari, T. (1997) Randomized placebo-controlled trial of rhesus-human reassortant rotavirus vaccine for prevention of severe rotavirus gastroenteritis. *Lancet* **350,** 1205–1209.
120. Lanata, C. F., Midthun, K., Black, R. E., et al. (1996) Safety, immunogenicity, and protective efficacy of one and three doses of the tetravalent rhesus rotavirus vaccine in infants in Lima, Peru. *J. Infect. Dis.* **174,** 268–275.
121. Linhares, A. C., Gabbay, Y. B., Mascarenhas, J. D. P., et al. (1996) Immunogenicity, safety, and efficacy of tetravalent rhesus-human, reassortant rotavirus vaccine in Belem, Brazil. *Bull. WHO* **74,** 491–500.
122. Perez-Schael, I., Guntinas, M. J., Perez, M., et al. (1997) Efficacy of the rhesus rotavirus-based quadrivalent vaccine in infants and young children in Venezuela. *N. Engl. J. Med.* **337,** 1181–1187.
123. Wright, P. F., King, J., Araki, K., et al. (1991) Simultaneous administration of two human-rhesus rotavirus reassortant strains of VP7 serotype 1 and 2 specificity to infants and young children. *J. Infect. Dis.* **164,** 271–276.
124. Kobayashi, M., Thompson, J., Tollefson, S. J., et al. (1994) Tetravalent rhesus rotavirus vaccine in young infants. *J. Infect. Dis.* **170,** 1260–1263.
125. Clark, H. F., Offit, P. A., Ellis, R. W., et al. (1996) WC3 reassortant vaccines in children. Brief review. *Arch. Virol.* **12,** 187–198.
126. Clark, H. F., Borian, F. E., and Plotkin, S. A. (1990) Immune protection of infants against rotavirus gastroenteritis by a serotype 1 reassortant of bovine rotavirus WC3. *J. Infect. Dis.* **161,** 1099–1104.

127. Treanor, J., Clark, H. F., Pichichero, M., et al. (1995) Evaluation of the protective efficacy of a serotype 1 bovine-human rotavirus reassortant vaccine in infants. *Pediatr. Infect. Dis. J.* **14,** 301–307.
128. Clark, H. F., White, C. J., Offit, P. A., et al. (1995) Preliminary evaluation of safety and efficacy of quadrivalent human-bovine reassortant rotavirus vaccine. *Ped. Res.* **37,** 172A.
129. Makhene, M., Midthun, K., Karron, R., et al. (1995) Safety and immunogenicity of human-UK bovine rotavirus reassortants in adults and pediatric subjects, in *Abstracts of the 5th Rotavirus Vaccine Workshop: Current Issues and Future Developments (Atlanta).* Atlanta: Centers for Disease Control and Prevention.
130. Vodopija, I., Baklaic, Z., Vlatkovic, R., et al. (1986) Combined vaccination with live oral polio vaccine and the bovine rotavirus RIT 4237 strain. *Vaccine* **4,** 233–236.
131. Giammanco, G., DeGrandi, V., Lupo, L., et al. (1988) Interference of oral poliovirus vaccine on RIT 4237 oral rotavirus vaccine. *Eur. J. Epidemiol.* **4,** 121–123.
132. Migasena, S., Simasathien, S., Samakoses, R., et al. (1995) Simultaneous administration of oral rhesus-human reassortant tetravalent (RRV-TV) rotavirus vaccine and oral poliovirus vaccine (OPV) in Thai infants. *Vaccine* **13,** 168–174.
133. Rennels, M. B., Ward, R. L., Mack, M. E., and Zito, E. T. (1996) Concurrent oral poliovirus and rhesus-human rotavirus vaccination: effects on immune responses to both vaccines and on efficacy of rotavirus vaccines. *J. Infect. Dis.* **173,** 306–313.

9   Combined Measles, Mumps, and Rubella Vaccines

Maurice R. Hilleman

Introduction

Combined measles–mumps–rubella vaccine (MMR) was made possible by the development of the individual vaccine components. Combined measles–mumps (MMVax), measles–rubella (MRVax), and mumps–rubella (Biavax) were also developed (all vaccines cited were developed by Merck & Co., Whitehouse Station, NJ). Hurdles in the development of the combined vaccines included achieving as good immune responses as with the individual vaccines alone, lack of increased reactogenicity, compatibility of formulation to assure stability of potency on drying and storage, and capability in quality control to quantify the infectivity (potency) of each viral component.

The benefits derived from measles, mumps, and rubella vaccines, singly or in combination, have been remarkable. Application in the United States led to reduction in the three diseases to inconsequential or near inconsequential levels within the decade following their introduction. All three viruses are of constant antigenic specificity, indicating that worldwide eradication is possible.

The development of combined vaccines is a long and tedious process that relies first, on the successful development of the individual vaccines and second on the achievement of safe and effective combination of the proved individual products. The development of combined measles–mumps–rubella (MMR) vaccine in our laboratories was the realization of a long-term plan *(1)* to create the monovalent vaccines and then to prepare single-dose bivalent and trivalent combinations of the three single vaccines. MMR was licensed in 1971. The only precedent for combined live viral vaccines was that of measles and smallpox that was licensed in 1967 *(2–4)*. Individual and combined vaccines are beset by specific problems that can be individual to each or collective to them all, and MMR serves as a cogent example.

From: *Combination Vaccines: Development, Clinical Research, and Approval*
Edited by: R. W. Ellis © Humana Press Inc., Totowa, NJ

Table 1. Special Problems in Development of Live Viral Vaccines

Selection of parent virus strains for vaccines.
  In the absence of animal models, judgment was substituted for animal data
    in assessing the likely reactogenicity and safety for man of attenuated measles,
    mumps, and rubella viruses.
  Inherent genetic incapability for favorable attenuation.
Eliminating indigenous viruses.
  Avian leukosis in chick embryo cell culture.
  Utilization of embryonated eggs from leukosis-free chicken flocks.

Collective Problems

Problems in Selection of Parent Virus Strains for Vaccines

Collectively, clinical studies of individual measles, mumps, and rubella
vaccines *(Table 1)* shared the lack of suitable animal models that would provide for reliable preclinical appraisal of safety and efficacy when given to
human beings. Hence, the vaccine development process was guided more by
judgment than data. Determination of the proper passage level to assure safety
in human subjects was made possible by the creation of numerous lots of
vaccine at sequential embryonated egg or cell culture passage levels (that were
presumed to correlate with increased attenuation) and their testing in human
volunteers. This was immensely difficult and costly since each test vaccine
was akin to a vaccine production lot that needed to comply with the rigorous
standards of the Federal Regulatory Authority (now the Food and Drug
Administration [FDA]) applied to commercially distributed products. The
largest problem was the need to make the judgment call as to what distant point
in the attenuation cycle would be appropriate to start first clinical tests. Once
total safety at a particular level was established, then sequential and progres-
sive workback for determining the optimal clinical reaction/efficacy relationship was more routine.

A second hurdle in vaccine strain development lay in the fact that different
clinical isolates of a particular virus may be different genetically, with many
failing to provide for the selectivity needed to achieve a satisfactory balance
between immunogenicity and attenuation. This was an especially difficult
problem for mumps vaccine *(see* ref. 5) because the virus attenuates rapidly in
chick embryos/cells and acceptability for a clinically useful product is confined to a very narrowly restricted passage history. A further contribution to
the research problem was that the laborious serum neutralization test alone
provided the sensitivity and reliability *(6)* needed to assess antibody responses
to vaccination.

Indigenous Viruses of Primary Chick Cell Cultures

A major problem in developing the Edmonston B measles virus vaccine in laboratories in 1961 *(7)* and its more attenuated successor (Moraten line) *(8)* was the ubiquitous occurrence in chick cells, in culture, of contaminating retroviruses of the avian leukosis complex, including leukemia, that were not detectable in in vitro tests. These viruses did not appear to cause untoward effects in man, based on many years of use of chick embryo-grown yellow fever virus vaccine. We were, however, restive and determined not to put the human population at possible or even remote risk to side effects as a result of presence of live leukemia virus.

An answer to the leukosis problem was provided by the development of the resistance-inducing factor (RIF) test *(9)* that permitted in vitro detection of viruses of the avian leukosis complex. Acting on the finding that eggs laid by hens that had antibodies against leukosis, Hughes et al. *(10)* developed experimental chicken flocks that were free of leukosis virus. Use of chick embryos from leukosis-free starter flocks to prepare cell cultures permitted laboratories to develop and to produce routinely measles vaccine that was free of leukosis viral contamination. Once leukosis-free chick cell cultures were available, it was also possible to develop and produce mumps as well as measles vaccines free of the contaminating avian leukosis agents.

Impediments and Solutions
in the Development of Individual Vaccines

Table 2 summarizes the major individual problems encountered with measles, mumps, and rubella vaccines and their solutions.

Measles

Enders' attenuated Edmonston B vaccine *(11)* was beset in the beginning with two significant problems, i.e.; that of excessive clinical reactogenicity, and that of universal gross avian leukosis contamination of chick embryo cell cultures used to grow the virus, as previously discussed. The initial solution to the problem of excess virulence was by coadministration of both standardized measles immune globulin and the vaccine injected into separate arms. Rubeovax, administered with immune globulin, was licensed in 1963. Immune globulin provided only an interim solution and it was essential to attenuate the virus further. This was accomplished by serial passage of the Edmonston virus in embryonated hens' eggs from which the Moraten line of more attenuated Enders' virus was derived. The vaccine was licensed in 1968 under the name of Attenuvax.

Table 2. Evolution and Impediments in Vaccine Development

Vaccine licensure	Hurdle	Solution
Measles		
1963—Rubeovax (Edmonston B)	Excessive virulence	Coadministration of immune globulin
1968—Attenuvax (Moraten)	Attenuate further	Adequately attenuated
Mumps		
1967—Mumpsvax (Jeryl Lynn)	Attenuation	Appropriate attenuation
Rubella		
(Merck Benoit duck)	Propagation and attenuation	Duck cell propagation Adequately attenuated
1969—Meruvax (HPV-77 duck)[a]	Excessive virulence— further attenuation	Attenuated in duck cells
1978—Meruvax II (RA27/3-MRC-5)	Reduce arthritis	Licensed in from the outside

[a]Also risk assessment for safety in pregnant women in contact with vaccinated children.

Mumps

The Jeryl Lynn strain of mumps virus, among a number of different viruses tested, was uniquely capable of appropriate attenuation. The Mumpsvax product was licensed in 1965. Expanded description of the research carried out on mumps vaccine is presented in a later section of this chapter.

Rubella

The licensed rubella virus vaccines were the sequel to pioneering studies with the Merck Benoit strain *(12–17)* of duck cell culture-attenuated virus isolated in our laboratories from a child named Benoit. The HPV-77 strain that was grown in bovine kidney cultures by Parkman and Meyer *(18)*, was substituted for the Benoit strain in order to respond to the perceived need and political pressures to concentrate on a single vaccine that could be developed more quickly than two separate vaccines, with the purpose of averting an anticipated rubella epidemic in the United States. The HPV-77 bovine virus *(18)* vaccine was excessively virulent and was never licensed. However, HPV-77 bovine cell strain was further attenuated in our laboratories to develop the HPV-77 duck cell line which was licensed (Meruvax®) *(16–20)* in 1989. Later, the HPV-77 duck cell vaccine was substituted by the RA27/3 human diploid cell grown virus *(21)* and was licensed under the name Meruvax® II in 1978 *(22,23)*. The latter virus was chosen because it appeared to cause fewer joint symptoms in adult women, and because it was shown to be superior in preventing subclinical infection and spread among vaccinees who were subsequently exposed to the virus in nature and developed inapparent infections.

A Major Problem

One major hurdle in the development of the first rubella vaccines was that of evaluation of safety for susceptible pregnant women in their first trimester who might have been exposed to susceptible children who had received the attenuated vaccine. There was no reason to expect a real problem since the vaccine was highly attenuated, and secretion of virus from vaccinees was minimal. The problem lay principally for spurious chance association between vaccine and spontaneous congenital defect of nonvaccine virus causation. The risk of such an event was calculated to be very small and a substantive clinical study was carried out without a problem. The vaccine has since been proved safe, even in infants born to mothers who inadvertently receive the vaccine during pregnancy.

Combined Vaccines

The development of the combined live virus vaccines against measles, mumps and rubella required establishment of evidences to show as good immune responses as with the individual vaccines given alone, lack of increased reactogenicity, compatibility of formulation to assure stability of potency on drying and on storage, and capability in quality control to quantify the infectivity (potency) of each viral component.

The excipients in the three individual vaccines were compatible in bivalent and trivalent formulations, and there was no alteration of stability in immunizing potency (infectivity titer) on long-term storage at 4°C. The principle hurdle lay with interference between the individual viruses in their competitive engagement of the host and induction of immune responses. The solution lay in adjusting the amount of each virus in the combinations to achieve satisfactory balance in content.

The means for determining balance lay with preparation of combined vaccines of varied quantitative viral content and testing them in susceptible children. In the same studies, susceptible children were given monovalent vaccines of standard formulation. By this mechanism, bivalent and trivalent formulations were achieved in which there was no reduction in immune response and no increase in reactogenicity. With such data, the bivalent *(24–26)* and trivalent *(23,27,28)* combinations were licensed for general distribution as summarized in *Table 3*.

MMR *(27,28)* and MMR II *(23)* were the final and successful culmination of long-term efforts and became both the driving force for immunization against measles, mumps, and rubella vaccines in the United States and the paradigm for

Table 3. Licensed Combined Measles-Mumps-Rubella Vaccines

1970	Biavax Combined Mumps (Jeryl Lynn) with Rubella (HPV-77 duck) vaccines.
1971	MRVax Combined Measles (Moraten) with Rubella (HPV-77 duck) vaccine.
1971	MMR Combined Measles (Moraten), Mumps (Jeryl Lynn), and Rubella (HPV-77 duck) vaccines.
1978	MMR II Combined Measles (Moraten) with Mumps (Jeryl Lynn) and Rubella (RA27/3) vaccines.

successful live virus vaccines that have been primarily used in the United States, Canada, and Europe, and are now being introduced into some developing countries. Measles vaccine was used worldwide shortly following its development, and was included in the six initial vaccines given in 1974 in the Expanded Program for Immunization (EPI) of the World Health Organization (WHO).

Special Consideration in Development and Use of Diverse Mumps Virus Vaccines

Some of the special problems in vaccine development and use, in general, are well exemplified by the experiences in efforts to create and use mumps virus vaccines. Detailed information of the experiences with the Jeryl Lynn strain live mumps vaccine (5) development are summarized here for illustrative purpose.

BACKGROUND

The earlier history of attempted development of both killed and live mumps virus vaccines has been marked by abortive and inconsequential efforts to evolve vaccines having the needed attributes of high-level protective efficacy, lasting duration, and apathogenicity (see refs. 29–31). The Jeryl Lynn strain live attenuated mumps virus vaccine (32,33), that was developed in our laboratories, has been unique in mumps vaccine development because of its desirable properties of clinical nonreactivity, high-level protective efficacy, and durable immunity, possibly lifelong, following but a single dose of vaccine (34,35).

Attenuated Jeryl Lynn Mumps Virus

Throat washings were taken on March 23, 1963 from a 5-year-old child (Jeryl Lynn) with mumps and were used to develop the Jeryl Lynn strain mumps vaccine (5,32,36–38). After a series of clinical tests, passage level A (collectively 12 passages in chick embryos and in chick embryo cell cultures) and level B (collectively 17 or 18 passages, 12 in chick embryos and 5 or 6 in cell culture) were selected for further clinical study. Table 4 presents (5) a synopsis of the findings. Clearly, both vaccines A and B were immunogenic, but only level B

Table 4. Clinical and Immunological Response
to Jeryl Lynn Mumps Vaccines A and B

| Passage level | Clinical[a] | | | Neutralizing[a] antibody response |
	Parotitis	Virus isolation	Serum amylase elevation	
A (12)	4/16	3/16	0/16	16/16
B (17)	0/14	0/14	0/14	14/14

[a]No children/total.

Table 5. Occurrence of Proved Mumps Cases
in Controlled Studies[a] for Protective Efficacy of Mumps Vaccine
in Children Who Were Exposed to Mumps Virus Infection

| Venue for exposure | Cases of proved mumps/total exposed | | Protective efficacy |
	Vaccinated	Nonvaccinated controls	
Classrooms	0/14	22/24	100%
Families	2/86	39/76	96%

[a]The total initially seronegative study population was 362 vaccinated and 505 controls.

vaccine caused no overt clinical reactions and was chosen for further investigations. Vaccine at collective passage level 27 was not adequately immunogenic and was not tested further. All vaccines were dried.

PROOF OF SAFETY AND EFFICACY

Studies to determine the safety and protective efficacy of the vaccine *(Table 5)* were carried out among 867 initially seronegative children, in families or in schools, who resided in the Havertown-Springfield area of Philadelphia *(37,38)*. Ninety-eight percent of vaccinated children developed neutralizing antibodies following vaccination. A synopsis presented in *Table 5* shows that the level of protective efficacy was about 98% and this correlated with the positive neutralizing antibody responses. The clinical reactions to vaccination were inconsequential and were limited mainly to local inflammation at the injection site.

Mumps Virus Quasi-species and Plurality Between and Within Clusters

Mumps virus *(30)* is placed in the genus Paramyxovirus and within the family Paramyxoviridae. The genetic order of the genome of mumps virus is shown in *Fig. 1*. Tentatively, there are seven genes separated by intergenic sequences as shown in *Table 6*. There are believed to be six structural proteins plus two

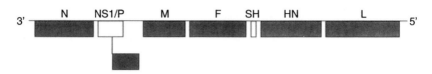

Fig. 1. Genomic map of mumps virus showing genes and intergenic sequences. Adapted from Rima, B. G., in *Encyclopedia of Virology*, Webster, R. G. and Granoff, A. (eds.), Academic Press, New York, 1994, p. 876.

Table 6. Proteins Encoded by the Mumps Virus Genome

N	Nucleocapsid	Structural
P	Phosphoprotein	Structural
M	Matrix	Structural
F	Fusion protein	Structural
HN	Hemagglutinin-neuraminidase	Structural
L	Large protein	Structural
NS1	Protein 1	Nonstructural
NS2	Protein 2	Nonstructural
SH	Small hydrophobic	Structural or nonstructural

nonstructural proteins, and the SH protein. The highly variable SH protein is hydrophobic and its structural or nonstructural status is unknown.

Viruses, especially RNA viruses belonging to any particular species, may differ greatly in their genetic composition. Individual strains of virus may vary substantively even within patients, and in in vitro culture. Individual viral isolates may be assembled into distinctive clusters based on the degree of genetic relatedness. Collectively, these differences are the basis for the designation of multiple quasi-species rather than strict species composition.

Based primarily on genetic analyses of the hypervariable SH region *(see Fig. 1)*, the Jeryl Lynn mumps virus was shown *(39)* to consist of two very similar but distinguishable quasi-species entities designated JL2 and JL5. It is not known whether these variants were present in the original patient or whether they arose on serial passage in chick embryos and in cell cultures during attenuation. It is also unknown how many such SH variants may be present in the Jeryl Lynn vaccine strain or in other mumps virus vaccines as well. The important matter is that variation in the SH region is without importance to the vaccine since it has no demonstrated effect either on its virulence or protective efficacy. With respect to vaccine safety, Afzal et al. *(39)* of the British regulatory authority have noted that the master seed-controlled passage system for production "ensures a consistently reproducible immunogenicity, safety, and tolerability profile" and "the product will remain consistent in quality and its excellent record of clinical safety and efficacy will be maintained."

Importantly, a number of attenuated and wild mumps viruses have been shown to fall into three *(39)* or four *(40)* distinctive clusters based on genetic composition. It is of importance that the Jeryl Lynn, the Russian Leningrad-3 *(41)*, and the Japanese Urabe *(42–48)* vaccine strains each reside in a different cluster. It is possible that the distinctive genetic profiles of these viruses may account for their differences in neurovirulence, as summarized below.

SUBSEQUENT STUDIES

In additional studies, the vaccine proved equally immunogenic and as nonreactogenic in adults as in children *(49)*. It was further determined *(50,51)* that the minimal amount of virus per dose required to immunize 97% or more of child or adult recipients was about 317 50% cell culture infectious units ($TCID_{50}$). Twenty thousand $TCID_{50}$ per dose are used routinely in the vaccine. The dried vaccine is stable on storage in the refrigerator *(32,52)* and there is no spread of virus by contact between vaccinated and susceptible children *(32)*. Immunity has proved durable and long lasting to the present *(34,35)*.

Little is known about subclinical reinfection on exposure to mumps and about the basis for immunity. Possible clinically discernible reinfection following natural infection has been reported, though with low frequency *(53)*. It may be conjectured, however, that as for measles and rubella, subclinical reinfection may occur and may be restricted to the respiratory mucosal cells. Virus neutralization by antibody may be presumed to be the principal mechanism for immunity. However, in most viral infections, reinfection is abortive and subclinical as a result of cytotoxic T-cell responses that rapidly clear away virus-infected cells. This is also probably true for mumps. It may be conjectured that long-term immunity is based on immunologic memory resident in memory B, T-helper, and cytotoxic T cells.

Central Nervous System Involvement in the Clinical Application of Certain Live Attenuated Mumps Vaccines

Native wild mumps virus is highly pantropic with respect to the organs and tissues it can infect *(31,54)*, but the principal clinical effects are on the parotids, the gonads, and the central nervous system. It was observed around the turn of the present decade that certain mumps virus vaccines used singly or in combination with measles and rubella viruses, were insufficiently attenuated and caused aseptic meningitis or meningoencephalitis. The Leningrad-3 strain was reported as early as 1986 *(55)* to be underattenuated, causing about one case of meningitis per 1000 vaccinated persons. Prime attention in western

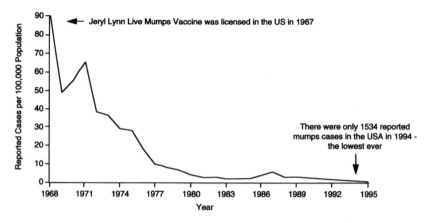

Fig. 2. Mumps cases, by year, in the United States, 1968–1994. Adapted from Summary of Notifiable Diseases, United States, 1994. Centers for Disease Control Reports, Morbidity and Mortality Weekely Report (MMWR) Supplement, vol. 43 (No. 53) Oct. 6, 1995, p. 42.

Europe *(42–45)*, in Canada *(46)*, and in Japan *(47,48)* was focused on the neuropathogenicity of the Urabe mumps strain-containing vaccines made by European and Japanese vaccine manufacturers. The WHO *(42,44)* estimated occurrence of about one case of meningitis per 4000 vaccinees. Identity of the Urabe vaccine strain in viral isolates from vaccinated patients was established by genetic sequencing of the viral nucleic acid. In Japan *(47,48)*, the attack rate for Urabe vaccine meningitis was about 1:400 to 1:1200. Also, there was one report of possible virus transmission from a vaccinated child to a suscep-tible sibling *(56)*. The high frequency of Urabe virus meningitis in Japan may have been associated with changes in the manufacturing process *(48)*. Use of the Urabe strain vaccine was discontinued in many countries *(40,45,46)* worldwide, even though the risk-to-benefit ratio from use of Urabe vaccine was still highly favorable considering the far greater severity of natural infection.

There is no definitive evidence to indicate that the Jeryl Lynn virus is ever causally associated with meningitis, and certainly no more than one case per million vaccinated persons. For this reason, the Jeryl Lynn vaccine has been frequently substituted, when available, for the Urabe product *(44,46)*.

The Legacy of Measles, Mumps, and Rubella Vaccines

The benefits from use of measles, mumps, and rubella vaccines, singly or in combination, are best illustrated in *Figs. 2–4* that show the reduction in occur-rence in the United States of the three diseases following introduction of vac-cines against them *(57)*. All measles, mumps, and rubella vaccines used in the United States have been exclusively of Merck source except for short-term use

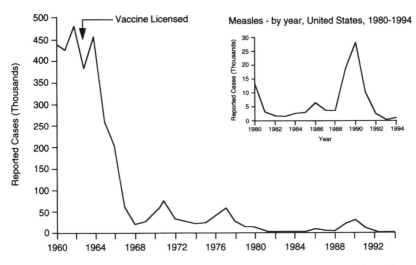

Fig. 3. Measles cases, by year, in the United States, 1960–1994. Adapted from Summary of Notifiable Diseases, United States, 1994. MMWR Supplement, vol. 43 (no. 53) Oct. 6, 1995, p. 40.

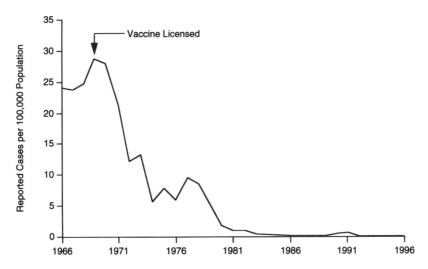

Fig. 4. Rubella cases, by year, in the United States, 1966–1994. Adapted from Summary of Notifiable Diseases, United States, 1994. MMWR Supplement, vol. 43 (no. 53) Oct. 6, 1995, p. 50.

of the Schwarz strain measles vaccine and the Cendehill strain rubella vaccine. It is seen that each of the three diseases has been reduced dramatically to inconsequential or near-inconsequential levels within the decade following its introduction. It is significant also that measles, mumps, and rubella are each caused by a single virus of constant immunologic specificity for protection. Therefore, all three diseases should be capable of worldwide eradication, especially through use of the combined vaccine and this may be a worthy target for the future. Protective immunity following proper initial response is of long if not permanent duration *(34,35)*.

References

1. Hilleman, M. R., Weibel, R. E., Buynak, E. B., and Villarejos, V. M. (1975) Practical aspects concerning combined live viral vaccines. *Schweiz. Rundschau. Med. (PRAXIS)* **64,** 12–24.
2. Kalabus, F., Sansarricq, H., Lambin, P., Proulx, J., and Hilleman, M. R. (1967) Standardization and mass application of combined live measles-smallpox vaccine in Upper Volta. *Am. J. Epidemiol.* **86,** 93–111.
3. Kalabus, F., Sansarricq, H., Lambin, P., Proulx, J., and Hilleman, M. R. (1967) Mass application by jet gun of combined measles-smallpox vaccine in Upper Volta. First International Conference on Vaccines Against Viral and Rickettsial Diseases of Man, Washington, DC, November 7-11, 1966. *Pan Am. Health Org. Sci. Publ.* **147,** 347,348.
4. Weibel, R. E., Stokes, J. Jr., Buynak, E. B., Leagus, M. B., and Hilleman, M. R. (1969) Clinical-laboratory experiences with a more attenuated Enders' measles virus vaccine (Moraten) combined with smallpox vaccine. *Pediatrics* **43,** 567–572.
5. Stokes, J. Jr., Weibel, R. E., Buynak, E. B., and Hilleman, M. R. (1967) Live attenuated mumps virus vaccine. II. Early clinical studies. *Pediatrics* **39,** 363–371.
6. Buynak, E. B., Whitman, J. E. Jr., Roehm, R. R., Morton, D. H., Lampson, G. P., and Hilleman, M. R. (1967) Comparison of neutralization and hemagglutination-inhibition techniques for measuring mumps antibody. *Proc. Soc. Exp. Biol. Med.* **125,** 1068–1071.
7. Hilleman, M. R., Stokes, J. Jr., Buynak, E. B., Weibel, R., Halenda, R., and Goldner, H. (1962) Enders' live measles virus vaccine with human immune globulin. 2. Evaluation of efficacy. *Am. J. Dis. Child.* **103,** 373–379.
8. Hilleman, M. R., Buynak, E. B., Weibel, R. E., Stokes, J. Jr., Whitman, J. E. Jr., and Leagus, M. B. (1968) Development and evaluation of the Moraten measles virus vaccine. *JAMA* **206,** 587–590.
9. Rubin, H. (1960) A virus in chick embryos which induces resistance in vitro to infection with Rous sarcoma virus. *Proc. Natl. Acad. Sci. USA* **46,** 1105–119.
10. Hughes, W. F., Watanabe, D. H., and Rubin, H. (1963) The development of a chicken flock apparently free of leukosis virus. *Avian Dis.* **7,** 154–165.
11. Katz, S. L. and Enders, J. F. (1959) Immunization of children with a live attenuated measles virus. *Am. J. Dis. Child.* **98,** 605–607.
12. Stokes, J. Jr., Weibel, R. E., Buynak, E. B., and Hilleman, M. R. (1967) Clinical and laboratory tests of Merck strain live attenuated rubella virus vaccine. First International Conference on Vaccines Against Viral and Rickettsial Diseases of Man, Washington, DC, November 7–11, 1966. *Pan Am. Health Org. Sci.* **147,** 402–405.
13. Buynak, E. B., Hilleman, M. R., Weibel, R. E., and Stokes, J. Jr. (1968) Live attenuated rubella virus vaccines prepared in duck embryo cell culture. I. Development and clinical testing. *JAMA* **204,** 195–200.
14. Weibel, R. E., Stokes, J. Jr., Buynak, E. B., Whitman, J. E. Jr., Leagus, M. B., and Hilleman, M. R. (1968) Live attenuated rubella virus vaccines prepared in duck embryo cell culture. II. Clinical tests in families and in an institution. *JAMA* **205,** 554–558.

15. Hilleman, M. R., Buynak, E. B., Weibel, R. E., and Stokes, J. Jr. (1968) Current concepts. Live, attenuated rubella-virus vaccines. *N. Engl. J. Med.* **279**, 300–303.
16. Hilleman, M. R., Buynak, E. B., Whitman, J. E. Jr., Weibel, R. E., and Stokes, J. Jr. (1969) Summary report on rubella virus vaccines prepared in duck embryo cell culture. *Symp. Series Immunobiol. Stand.* **11**, 349–356.
17. Weibel, R. E., Stokes, J. Jr., Buynak, E. B., and Hilleman, M. R. (1969) Live rubella vaccines in adults and children. HPV-77 and Merck-Benoit strains. *Am. J. Dis. Child.* **18**, 226–229.
18. Meyer, H. M. Jr., Parkman, P. D., and Panos, T. C. (1966) Attenuated rubella virus, II: production of experimental live-virus vaccine and clinical trial. *N. Engl. J. Med.* **275**, 575–580.
19. Hilleman, M. R., Buynak, E. B., Whitman, J. E. Jr., Weibel, R. E., and Stokes, J. Jr. (1969) Live attenuated rubella virus vaccines. Experiences with duck embryo cell preparations. *Am. J. Dis. Child.* **118**, 166–171.
20. Buynak, E. B., Larson, V. M., McAleer, W. J., Mascoli, C. C., and Hilleman, M. R. (1969) Preparation and testing of duck embryo cell culture rubella vaccine. *Am. J. Dis. Child.* **118**, 347–354.
21. Plotkin, S. A., Farquhar, J. D., Katz, M., and Buser, F. (1969) Attenuation of RA27/3 rubella virus in WI-38 human diploid cells. *Am. J. Dis. Child.* **118**, 178–185.
22. Weibel, R. E., Villarejos, V. M., Klein, E. B., Buynak, E. B., McLean, A. A, and Hilleman, M. R. (1980) Clinical and laboratory studies of live attenuated RA27/3 and HPV 77-DE rubella virus vaccines. *Proc. Soc. Exp. Biol. Med.* **165**, 44–49.
23. Weibel, R. E., Carlson, A. J. Jr., Villarejos, V. M., Buynak, E. B., McLean, A. A., and Hilleman, M. R. (1980) Clinical and laboratory studies of combined live measles, mumps, and rubella vaccines using the RA27/3 rubella virus. *Proc. Soc. Exp. Biol. Med.* **165**, 323–326.
24. Weibel, R. E., Stokes, J. Jr., Villarejos, V. M., Arguedas, G. J. A., Buynak, E. B., and Hilleman, M. R. (1971) Combined live rubella-mumps virus vaccine. Findings in clinical-laboratory studies. *JAMA* **216**, 983–986.
25. Villarejos, V. M. Arguedas, G. J. A, Buynak, E. B., Weibel, R. E., Stokes, J. Jr, and Hilleman, M. R. (1971) Combined live measles-rubella virus vaccine. *J. Pediatr.* **79**, 599–604.
26. Weibel, R. E., Villarejos, V. M., Hernández ,C. G., Stokes, J. Jr., Buynak, E. B., and Hilleman, M. R. (1973) Combined live measles-mumps virus vaccine. Findings in clinical-laboratory studies. *Arch. Dis. Child.* **48**, 532–536.
27. Hilleman, M. R., Weibel, R. E., Villarejos, V. M., Buynak, E. B., Stokes, J. Jr., Arguedas, G. J. A., and Vargas, A. G. (1971) Combined live virus vaccines. Proceedings of the International Conference on the Application of Vaccines Against Viral, Rickettsial, and Bacterial Diseases of Man, Washington, DC, December 14–18, 1970. *Pan Am. Health Org. Sci.* **226**, 397–400.
28. Stokes, J. Jr, Weibel, R. E., Villarejos, V. M., Arguedas, G. J. A., Buynak, E. B., and Hilleman, M. R. (1971) Trivalent combined measles-mumps-rubella vaccine. Findings in clinical laboratory studies. *JAMA* **218**, 57–61.
29. Cochi, S. L., Wharton, M., and Plotkin, S. A. (1994) Mumps vaccine, in *Vaccines* (Plotkin, S. A. and Mortimer, E. A. Jr., eds.), WB Saunders, Philadelphia, pp. 277–301.
30. Rima, B. K. (1994) Mumps virus in *Encyclopedia of Virology*, vol. 2 (Webster, R. G. and Granoff, A., eds.), Academic, London, pp. 876–883.
31. Wolinsky, J. S. and Waxham, M. N. (1990) Mumps virus in *Virology* (Fields, B. N. and Knipe, D. M., eds.), Raven, New York, pp. 989–1011.
32. Hilleman, M. R., Buynak, E. B., Weibel, R. E., and Stokes, J. Jr. (1968) Live, attenuated mumps-virus vaccine. *N. Engl. J. Med.* **278**, 227–232.

33. Hilleman, M. R. (1992) Past, present, and future of measles, mumps, and rubella virus vaccines. *Pediatrics* **90,** 149–153.
34. Weibel, R. E., Buynak, E. B., McLean, A. A., and Hilleman, M. R. (1979) Follow-up surveillance for antibody in human subjects following live attenuated measles, mumps, and rubella virus vaccines. *Proc. Soc. Exp. Biol. Med.* **162,** 328–332.
35. Weibel, R. E., Buynak, E. B., McLean, A. A., Roehm, R. R., and Hilleman, M. R. (1980) Persistence of antibody in human subjects for seven to ten years following administration of combined live attenuated measles, mumps and rubella virus vaccines. *Proc. Soc. Exp. Biol. Med.* **165,** 260–263.
36. Buynak, E. B. and Hilleman, M. R. (1966) Live attenuated mumps virus vaccine. 1. Vaccine development. *Proc. Soc. Exp. Biol. Med.* **123,** 768–775.
37. Weibel, R. E., Stokes, J. Jr., Buynak, E. B., Whitman, J. E. Jr., and Hilleman, M. R. (1967) Live, attenuated mumps-virus vaccine. 3. Clinical and serologic aspects in a field evaluation. *N. Engl. J. Med.* **276,** 245–251.
38. Hilleman, M. R., Weibel, R. E., Buynak, E. B., Stokes, J. Jr., and Whitman, J. E. Jr. (1967) Live, attenuated mumps-virus vaccine. 4. Protective efficacy as measured in a field evaluation. *N. Engl. J. Med.* **276,** 252–258.
39. Afzal, M. A., Pickford, A. R., Forsey, T., Heath, A. B., and Minor, P. D. (1993) The Jeryl Lynn vaccine strain of mumps virus is a mixture of two distinct isolates. *J. Gen. Virol.* **74,** 917–920.
40. Künkel, U., Driesel, G. Henning, U., Gerike, E., Willer, H., and Schreier, E. (1995) Differentiation of vaccine and wild mumps viruses by polymerase chain reaction and nucleotide sequencing of the SH gene: brief report. *J. Med. Virol.* **45,** 121–126.
41. Smorodintsev, A. A. and Klyachko, N. S. (1961) Mumps live vaccine in the U. S. S. R. : a summary of recent developments. *Prog. Med. Virol.* **3,** 273–286.
42. World Health Organization. (1992) Meningitis associated with measles-mumps-rubella vaccines. *Weekly Epidemiol. Record* **67,** 301,302.
43. Forsey, T., Bentley, M. L., Minor, P. D., and Begg, N. (1992) Mumps vaccines and meningitis. *Lancet* **340,** 980.
44. Miller, E., Goldacri, M., Pugh, S., Colville, A., Farrington, P., Flower, A., Nash, J., MacFarlane, L., Tettmar, R. (1993) Risk of aseptic meningitis after measles, mumps, and rubella vaccine in UK children. *Lancet* **341,** 979–982.
45. Schmitt, H-J., Just, M., and Neiss, A. (1993) Withdrawal of a mumps vaccine: reasons and impacts. *Eur. J. Pediatr.* **152,** 387,388.
46. Furesz, J. (1990) Vaccine-related mumps meningitis—Canada. *Can. Dis. Weekly Report* 16–50, 253,254.
47. Motegi, Y., Fujinaga, T. Tamura, H., and Kuroume, T. (1990) A survey of children with meningitis following measles, mumps, and rubella (MMR) immunization. *Pediatr. Res.* **27,** 95A (Abst. 558).
48. Yawata, M. (1994) Japan's troubles with measles-mumps-rubella vaccine. *Lancet* **343,** 105,106.
49. Davidson, W. L., Buynak, E. B., Leagus, M. B., Whitman, J. E. Jr., and Hilleman, M. R. (1967) Vaccination of adults with live attenuated mumps virus vaccine. *JAMA* **201,** 995–998.
50. Hilleman, M. R. (1970) Mumps vaccination, in *Modern Trends in Medical Virology* (Heath, R, B. and Waterson, A. P., eds.), Butterworths, London, pp. 241–261.
51. Buynak, E. B., Hilleman, M. R., Leagus, M. B., Whitman, J. E. Jr., Weibel, R. E., and Stokes, J. Jr. (1968) Jeryl Lynn strain live attenuated mumps virus vaccine. Influence of age, virus dose, lot, and γ-globulin administration on response. *JAMA* **203,** 9–13.

52. McAleer, W. J., Markus, H. Z., McLean, A. A., Buynak, E. B., and Hilleman, M. R. (1980) Stability on storage at various temperatures of live measles, mumps and rubella virus vaccines in new stabilizer. *J. Biol. Standard.* **8,** 281–287.
53. Gut, J-P., Lablache, C., Behr, S., and Kirn, A. (1995) Symptomatic mumps virus reinfections. *J. Med. Virol.* **45,** 17–23.
54. Nussinovitch, M., Volovitz, B., and Varsana, I. (1995) Complications of mumps requiring hospitalization in children. *Eur. J. Pediat.* **154,** 732–734.
55. Cizman, M., Mozetic, M., Furman-Jakopic, M., Pleterski-Rigle, D., Radescek-Rakar, R., and Susec-Michieli, M. (1986) Aseptic meningitis following combined vaccination with the Leningrad-3 strain of mumps virus and the Edmonston-Zagreb strain of measles virus. *Zdrav. Vestn.* **55,** 587–591.
56. Sawada, H., Yano, S., Oka, Y., and Togashi, T. (1993) Transmission of Urabe mumps vaccine between siblings. *Lancet* **342,** 371.
57. Summary of Notifiable Diseases, United States, 1994 (1995) *MMWR* (Suppl.), **43(53).**

10 Combination Vaccines
Regulatory Considerations for Developers

John R. Vose

Introduction

The objective of this chapter is to discuss the key regulatory issues that vaccine manufacturers must take into consideration during the development cycle of combination vaccines through to successful licensure. The discussion will consider a range of examples of such products, from those that contain multiple serotype antigens for protection against a specific disease ("multivalent", e.g., pneumococcal pneumonia, influenza) or multiple antigenic proteins (e.g., pertussis), to products that consist of a combination of several vaccines, each of which is protective against a specific disease ("multidisease"). Examples include acellular pertussis [aP] formulated with already licensed diphtheria (D), tetanus (T), and inactivated polio (IPV) used to reconstitute a lyophilized *Haemophilus influenzae* type *b* conjugate (Hib) vaccine. Another example is the combination vaccine formulated to protect against measles, mumps, and rubella (MMR); in this case there is a combination of live attenuated viruses.

It is also intended that comments made in this chapter regarding the examples named above will have some relevance to future combination vaccines now under development in research laboratories, such as combinations of cholera, typhoid, enterotoxigenic *Escherichia coli* (ETEC), *Shigella*, rotavirus and possibly *Campylobacter* and *Helicobacter* antigenic components against a spectrum of enteric diseases.

The Regulatory Environment

It is critical that in the development of this category of complex vaccines regulatory considerations be incorporated into the overall development plan early in the product life. Once the product concept has been delineated, often with strong input from marketing departments, the project team needs to develop a planning document that will define the various steps to be undertaken, iden-

From: *Combination Vaccines: From Clinical Research to Approval*
Edited by: R. W. Ellis © Humana Press Inc., Totowa, NJ

tifying potential regulatory issues to be addressed and resolved along the way in order to achieve the final goal. Clearly, the sooner such issues are identified, and the better and broader the range of the staff disciplines involved in the project team, the likelihood will be greater that all key issues are recognized. Once the planning phase has been completed, development work can be initiated with the goal of producing clinical lots for Phase I evaluation.

Many manufacturers find it helpful to organize a consultative meeting with a key regulatory authority before entering too deeply into the development program. In the United States, this may be in the form of a pre-investigational new drug application (IND) meeting; in Europe the procedure is currently more complicated, since face-to-face meetings are not easy to schedule with authorities.

With the introduction of new licensing procedures in Europe that started January 1, 1998, the focus is on two approaches. Biotechnology-derived products (i.e., developed using rDNA technology or using monoclonal antibodies) must be licensed via a centralized procedure (CP) managed from a London, UK, headquarters, known as the European Medicines Evaluation Agency (EMEA). Examples would include combination vaccines that contain rDNA-derived antigens such as hepatitis B (HB). In addition, manufacturers have the option of submitting other products for review by this procedure as long as the products are considered to be novel by the EMEA's committee of experts, known as the Committee for Proprietary Medicinal Products (CPMP). The definition of "novelty" remains vague, but it appears that the opportunity exists for having combination vaccines reviewed via this CP.

The second approach for licensing products in Europe is known as the mutual recognition procedure (MRP). As in the CP, a member state in the European Community is selected (uniquely in this case by the applicant; whereas in the CP the CPMP decides which member state will be given responsibility for review of the file) to be the key reviewer.

Currently in Europe there exists a complex and sometimes confusing set of options for asking technical questions about the development of a new vaccine product. In the CP, the choice of *Rapporteur* member state is made at a very late stage in the product development, generally 3–4 months prior to dossier submission. At this stage the product development is essentially completed. There is the possibility in this process for an applicant to submit a set of written questions concerning a new product for review by a group of experts designated by the CPMP. There is a proposed fee of about 60,000 ECU charged for this service, and the review may take several months to complete. Some manufacturers have found this service of considerable value, largely depending on the "quality" of the questions asked. However, this procedure does have the major drawback of not permitting direct interactions with experts such as is possible in the course of the FDA's pre-IND meetings. The drawback of the latter is that the advice received has an understandable United States-bias and may not be relevant to the rest of the world.

For the MRP, applicants may ask for informal meetings with the regulatory authorities of individual member states in order to discuss specific issues. These can be very helpful, but advice given by one member state may not be relevant to another. In addition budgetary pressures affect the capacity of many agencies to address the increasingly complicated set of regulations that authorities and Applicants must both interpret and implement. Limitations in staffing capabilities are of concern in Europe, owing to the increased number of filings that can be expected in the coming years and from the tendency to give priority to applications being reviewed by the CP.

A further difference between registration practices in the United States and Europe is that the former requires development of an Establishment License Application (ELA) in addition to the product license. In this respect, it is interesting to note that FDA has recently specifically excluded vaccines from the scope of their new rule entitled "Elimination of Establishment License Application (ELA) for Specified Biotechnology and Specified Synthetic Biological Products." Thus vaccines are exempt from the scope of the newly created biological license application (BLA) that would have incorporated the PLA with the ELA in a single document, i.e., similar to the European format. On the other hand, it is of interest that FDA has introduced the concept of the "well-defined biological" which, when applied to vaccines (with some difficulty for those products that are ill-defined in terms of purity of composition), could facilitate review of variations to the original license.

Although there is no specific establishment license in Europe, details of the facility must be included in Part II of the dossier. Inspections of facilities are required in all cases. Currently, vaccine manufacturers are faced with the possibility of multiple inspections from the FDA's Center for Biologics Evaluation and Research and Center for Drugs Evaluation and Research, from one or two European countries, from the World Health Organization (WHO) if the product is to be submitted for United Nations Children's fund tenders, and perhaps from other countries such as Japan, Australia, and Canada. Fortunately, new MRA are now being implemented between various countries. The most important of these is between the United States and Europe and should be completed by mid-2000. However, until this date, manufacturers will remain subject to multiple inspections.

In addition to asking technical questions of authorities, manufacturers are recipients of numerous points-to-consider guidance documents from both sides of the Atlantic. In April 1997, the FDA published its "Guidance for Industry for the Evaluation of Combination Vaccines for Preventable Diseases: Production, Testing and Clinical Studies" (1). The CPMP has also issued a guideline entitled

"Note for Guidance on Pharmaceutical and Biological Aspects of Combined Vaccines" *(2)*.

In addition to the above two "guideline" documents, the CPMP has developed another guidance document relating to preclinical toxicity requirements for biologicals including combination vaccines. This was published in 1998 and takes into account comments made by manufacturers who found the original draft excessive in its requirements. The WHO also produces "requirement" documents including some that are specific to combination vaccines (e.g., acellular pertussis (aP), DT, pneumococcal vaccines, and MMR). The newly created European Department for the Quality of Medicines (EDQM) in Strasbourg, France, which is responsible for the European Pharmacopoeia and also for coordinating batch release of biologicals in Europe, has issued its own documents covering some aspects of batch release. Its expert group (known as Group 15) focuses on developing vaccine monographs and plans to work on monographs for some combined vaccines (e.g., DTaP, DTaP plus HB, DTaP plus IPV, DTaP plus Hib, Hepatitis A [inactivated] plus HB). A monograph for aP (which may itself be considered as a multicomponent product) has also been prepared *(3)*.

During the development of new vaccines, including combination products, manufacturers have a number of other factors to consider in addition to taking into account comments and advice received from various governmental licensing authorities. These should include consideration of WHO recommendations and monographs when they exist for the individual components, especially important if the end-product is likely to be sold via UNICEF. In addition, ensuring that all materials used in the manufacture of these products meet the requirements of United States Pharmacopoeia, European Pharmacopoeia, and the Japanese Pharmacopoeia, as appropriate, is *sine qua non*. Any incompatibilities that may exist among these requirements must be explained in the dossier.

Finally, all biological products are subject to batch release (BR) regulations. Although these differ somewhat from region to region, developing a dialogue with CBER testing laboratories and with their equivalents in Europe (known as Official Medicine Control Laboratories, or OMCL) once the final formulation is known is essential.

Vaccine developers may need to create new tests to address the future requirements of BR; this may be best accomplished in collaboration with the above-named governmental official control laboratories. Both testing methodology and release criteria need to be modified to address the peculiarities that arise from the combination of, e.g., several "old established" antigens with new ones. An obvious example is the pertussis potency (Kendrick) test that involves an intracerebral challenge of live pathogen into the test animal. Although this method has been accepted for whole-cell pertussis vaccines, its use for the new generation of aP vaccines is questionable. Thus, new criteria are required with mouse immunogenicity models being favored by CBER and an aerosol-applied mouse lung challenge model being considered for Europe.

Standardization and harmonization of this and other test methods between the various testing laboratories is critical to ensure manufacturers will not have to face an array of differing BR test requirements from different countries. This is currently the situation even with some of the constituent antigens that may be used to formulate combination products. The activities of the International Congress on Harmonization's (ICH) Group M4 that is striving for harmonization to achieve a "Common Technical Dossier" may be helpful now that vaccines and other biologicals are to be included within the purview of their remit. There remains, however, a need to ensure WHO requirements for both "old" vaccines and new ones, including combination products, are in-line with those of licensing authorities in Japan, the United States, and Europe.

General Regulatory Issues to be Considered in the Development of Vaccines

In the development of a regulatory strategy for a combination vaccine intended for global markets, it is advisable that input from regulatory experts be built into the project team from an early stage in the product life-cycle, i.e., at the R&D phase. Although it is beyond the scope of this chapter to cover in detail the many regulatory issues that should be addressed during product development, several specific topics will be covered. These have been selected because they cover controversial items subject to changing legislation (or local preferences) that may (and are generally not) consistent from one country or continent, to another.

Transmissible Spongiform Encephalopathy (TSE)

Concern about this prion-associated disease has been largely based on the epidemic of bovine spongiform encephalitis (BSE) and the associated incidence of new variety Creutzfeldt-Jacob disease (nvCJD) primarily in the UK *(4)* and has been the subject of numerous scientific articles in recent months. From a regulatory point of view, the issue has been somewhat addressed in the United States Federal Register by a ruling on what substances are prohibited from use in animal feed *(5)*. However, of more concern to the pharmaceutical industry, and in particular the vaccine industry, is the recent European Commission decision "on the prohibition of the use of material presenting risks as regards Transmissible Spongiform Encephalopathies" authorized on July 30, 1997 *(6)*. This document takes a different position on the TSE problem from either FDA or the WHO in its press release *(7)*. It is anticipated that vaccines along with other medicinal products may be given a reprieve from the immediate impact of these requirements by which enforcement was delayed to January, 1999 together with a delay to January, 2000 if no alternative medicinal product is available at that time. Currently, debate continues at the level of the European Commission on this issue.

Further clarification on the interpretation of the rules is urgently required, but in the meantime many vaccine manufacturers are wisely pursuing strategies that will obviate the need for bovine, ovine, or caprine-derived materials in the manufacture of their products. This is, of course, an immense task that involves detailed audits of media and component suppliers to ensure total absence of all "specified risk materials." Maintenance of both antigen yield and, more importantly, functional characteristics (e.g., potency or stability) of these antigens is essential to the successful attainment of this goal. Equivalence needs to be demonstrated by both laboratory and clinical testing to the original vaccine and this could involve two years or more of effort with no assurance of successful results at the end of this period.

Choice of Preservative

Vaccines are presented in a number of ways, including vials (single or multidose), ampoules, and syringes (single or dual-chamber). The use of chemical preservatives has become standard practice for all such presentations with thiomersal, 2-phenoxyethanol, or phenol being commonly used. Incompatibilities of different preservatives with different antigens is well known, and the development of combination vaccines with their own possible inherent incompatibility problems further adds to these problems.

Not only are there technical problems associated with the selection of which preservative to use in vaccines, but some agencies in Europe have taken strong positions against the use of any preservative at all with concerns especially focused on thiomersal. This is based on a belief that manufacturers use preservatives in their vaccine formulation to compensate for any possible deficiencies in production standards, whereas, in fact, certain preservatives are also used for their stabilization effects. Nevertheless, manufacturers may be well-advised to review their manufacturing and especially filling operations with a view to introducing such high-quality standards that preservatives may not be required for their potential antimicrobial functionality. However, special consideration still need to be paid to those alum-adsorbed vaccines that are cloudy or turbid, whereby any changes resulting from contamination are difficult to observe. In addition, presentations in multidose vials present a separate problem owing to the possibility of contamination once the container is first opened. In such cases, an acceptable preservative must be used unless strong justification for their avoidance while maintaining sterility during usage is presented.

Use of Stabilizers

Ensuring long-term stability of vaccines either as combined or single valencies for periods up to three years is a requirement of all agencies. In addition, some release tests established by authorities require that products conform to specific stability standards when stressed at temperatures up to 37°C, i.e., at temperatures that may be experienced either in countries where cold-chain problems are linked with hot ambient temperatures or where vaccines are indeed purchased from pharmacies and transported under nonideal conditions prior to possible long-term storage in the family refrigerator before vaccination is requested by a medically qualified person. The latter is not the case in North America, but is practiced in some European countries.

Vaccines may lose potency over time through a variety of ways. Sometimes specific component antigens may become adsorbed to the glass of the container. This can be addressed by appropriate treatment of the glass itself, ensuring absence of any effect of the glass coatings on the purity (or concentration) of the vaccine itself. A more standard approach is to add a specific stabilizer to the vaccine formulation. This may be gelatin-based (ensuring no conflict with EC directives as noted above for TSE) or based on other proteins. Bovine serum albumin (BSA) or human blood plasma proteins have been successfully used in the past. Again, attention must be paid to the sourcing of such products in order to meet all relevant guidelines and directives. For human blood-derived products, exhaustive testing, including use of polymerase chain reaction (PCR) techniques, to demonstrate absence of several specified viral contaminants (e.g., Hepatitis A, B and C, HIV-1, and HIV-2) is required. In Europe, consideration also is being given to testing for parvovirus B19. For Europe, human plasma products must meet several additional rules concerning sourcing, including a specification that the donors must not have been paid for this services *(8)*. In Europe, a specific part of the Part II Pharmaceutical file (part II V) must describe all the steps taken to validate freedom from viral (and prion) contamination of the vaccine. Insufficient attention to this requirement will result in, at best, delays in review and, at worst, file rejection.

For licensing albumin, special attention needs to be given to the plasma source, donor exclusion and testing, pool testing, the manufacturing process (sterilization of final containers, kinetics of inactivation, validation details) in-process controls, product characterization, batch-to-batch control, and product stability details. It is necessary for the end-user of the albumin to ensure that the supplier complies with these requirements.

Preclinical Toxicity Testing Requirements

The European Commission has recently published a draft guideline outlining requirements for pre-clinical testing of biologicals (9). This is an important document as it aims to differentiate the full range of preclinical toxicity tests required for drugs from those indicated for biologicals, including vaccines. One important factor recognized by this document is that vaccines, unlike drugs, do not contain specific "active components." They consist instead of single or multiple antigens that exert their biological effect by stimulating production of humoral and/or systemic immune responses in the recipient. Also unlike drugs, vaccines are not given in a routine multidose manner, but rather are given as a single dose, or perhaps require a few additional doses but generally at intervals of months or even years. Another difficulty experienced in pursuing preclinical animal toxicity studies is that animals generally react to vaccines in a manner quite different from humans, thus putting in question the overall scientific rationale for such studies. For combination vaccines that include components with a long-established safety history in humans, the need for any preclinical toxicity testing should be questioned beyond some general safety testing in a minimal number of animals. Another argument against the value of chronic toxicity testing is that the immune response to the vaccine may neutralize the effectiveness of future doses and hence turn the test into a non-test. Finally, it is evident that the route of administration used in the animal model should resemble that proposed in the human. A vaccine intended for subcutaneous administration should be tested at the preclinical level using the same route, although this may prove difficult in some small animal species.

Nevertheless, it is evident that some carefully designed minimal tests can be helpful in determining the future safety and perhaps efficacy of new vaccine formulations. The scope of such testing needs to be well-argued in the dossier, for example in the preclinical toxicity Expert Report Part III of the European format dossier. Local tolerance in an appropriate model should also be considered in case the formulation of these "well-known" components has resulted in a combination that is more reactogenic than the individual components. In particular, interactions (e.g., degree of adsorption to aluminum-based adjuvants) may result in some changes in reactogenicity.

When combination vaccines are formulated with "new" aluminum-based adjuvants or are adjuvanted using new procedures to "old" aluminum-based adjuvants, it is evident that extensive animal testing will be required. Similarly, introduction of "new" antigenic components or "new" preservatives or other excipients will stimulate interest in conducting more animal-based tests.

It is essential that for European filings, the Expert Pre-clinical Toxicology Section be well-written, fully justifying the rationale for the approaches taken. Reducing wastage of animals because of unnecessary testing requirements should be an ongoing goal of both regulators and manufacturers. For this reason, reviews of current requirements by all concerned parties is helpful in identifying certain tests which may no longer be necessary. The need for monkey neurovirulence testing of viral strains such as rubella, for which the phenomenon of neurovirulence has never been determined in humans, is a case-in-point. In such situations, presentation of arguments to authorities can lead to revisions of the requirements. Such arguments of course must be supported by adequate scientific data. Cases of this nature are often best made through the activity of industry associations such as the European Vaccine Manufacturers (EVM) group of the European Federation of Pharmaceutical Industry Associations (EFPIA) or the U. S. Pharmaceutical Research and Manufacturers of America (PhRMA), or Japanese Pharmaceutical Manufacturers Association (JPMA). However, reaching a consensus on such issues between several competing companies may cause undue delays.

Introduction of Costly Test Procedures for Determining "Quality" of Vaccines

With the availability of sophisticated analytical equipment (e.g., matrix-assisted time-of-flight mass spectrometry [MALDI-TOF], fast atom bombardment mass spectrometry [FAB-MS], circular dichroism, and nuclear magnetic resonance spectrometry), control laboratories in both the United States and Europe are increasingly using such new methods to evaluate quality, including the consistency characteristics of vaccines. Although such methods can provide interesting data, the parameters they are evaluating are generally outside those upon which the original product license was obtained. Moreover, manufacturers may not all have access to such analytical tools or to the specific procedures adapted for the application to vaccines. Thus, it may be difficult for manufacturers to be able to respond to questions concerning new parameters or criteria of purity about which they have little or no information. Nevertheless, agencies are increasingly requiring such data which adds to the expense of vaccine development and also extends the time required to achieve licensure.

The use of polymerase chain reaction (PCR) technology for determining possible contamination of blood-derived products with specified viruses is also problematic, as it has the potential of introducing new possibly unachievable limits or indeed reaching misleading conclusions. As one example, a product-enhanced reverse transcriptase PCR (PERT) test has been applied to the assay of reverse transcriptase (RT) sequences in vaccines made using chicken embryo cells *(10)*. In this case, it is evident that such highly sensitive techniques can indeed determine trace amounts of sequences suggestive of RT activity. But it has now been determined by experts that the RT signal is not in fact indicative of the presence of infectious retrovirus. This signal is associated with noninfectious particles and is not transmissible to the many cell types tested so far. Clearly, although manufacturers need to be conscious of all components in their products that could affect the ultimate quality and safety of their vaccines, it is essential that too rapid conclusions not be drawn from the results of a single new analytical technique. Rather, a range of approaches is required to ensure the best scientific approach is taken and also to ensure that results are interpreted correctly.

Demonstration of Bioequivalence Data as Surrogate for Efficacy Data

A brief note on the importance of establishing bioequivalence using a broad range of analytical techniques is relevant in demonstrating that combination vaccines containing components made by a new process are equivalent to the same licensed product using older processes, and for which efficacy was established in the traditional sense. This principle of comparability for vaccines has now been accepted in principle by CBER (11) and represents a refreshing attitude to such issues. The concept is to have a product specific protocol, reviewed and approved by CBER (12), which would contain product specifications and a description of the additional testing and validation that would be required for any future manufacturing changes. Once the protocol is approved, the company may implement the change and simply report the data to CBER, lowering the level of the required review process by one category. This could allow companies to avoid placing products in quarantine while awaiting CBER review. This approach has not yet been as fully explored in Europe.

Need to Address Variable Global Vaccination Practices in Development of Clinical Trial Protocols

Although there has been some progress in the harmonization of various topics concerning vaccines, the plethora of schedules by which vaccines are administered remains a large issue.

Whereas in the United States and Canada, pediatric DTP vaccines are routinely administered at 2, 4, and 6 months of age followed by boosters at 15–18 months and then preschool doses. Other countries have chosen different approaches, all of which have to be taken into account in the development of new combination vaccines. For the WHO's Expanded Program of Immunization (EPI), the schedule is 3–5 weeks, 7–9 weeks, and 11–13 weeks; generally no booster is given. For Europe, the situation is further complicated by the existence of a variety of schedules ranged from accelerated (2, 3, 4 months) with either no booster (UK) or with booster doses (France), through 2, 4, 6 months with booster doses (Germany) to 3, 5, 12 months (Scandinavia and Italy).

Not only do the schedules vary from country to country, but the vaccination practices vary as well, thus requiring various studies to address concomitant vaccination requirements with HB, Hib, Polio (oral or inactivated, depending on the country) and MMR.

Vaccine developers therefore must design their clinical studies to address the above variances, taking into account the need to enroll subjects of various ethnic backgrounds (and perhaps age and weight variances, depending on the product) to cover off concerns that the product will be safe and efficacious in all target populations. Pre-IND type meetings with regulatory authorities may be helpful to reach a clinical trial strategy that adequately addresses all the above sensitivities for future global registration.

Specific Considerations for Combination Vaccines

Interference of Components on Immunogenicity

For the specific development of a combination vaccine, one of the prime concerns is that of interference with the immune response caused by the effect of one or more components on another antigen. Such interference may result in either a diminished or an increased response to individual components compared with when the specific component is administered alone.

Such interferences are generally immunological in nature and represent a poorly understood phenomenon involving:

1. Antigenic competition owing to intracellular competition among small T-cell epitopes for binding to major histocompatibility complex structures and their subsequent presentation on the cell surface to T-cells.
2. Adjuvant effects caused by (a) specific component(s) of the vaccine, e.g., whole-cell pertussis.
3. Adjuvant effect caused by differential adsorption of more than one component to the adjuvant.
4. Epitope-specific suppression.
5. Physical binding between or among vaccine components.

The potential problems with combined vaccines have been summarized as follows (13):

1. Enhanced reactogenicity through:
   a. excessive endotoxin load;
   b. excessive toxoid load;
   c. additive or synergistic effects;
   d. displacement of toxic factors from adsorption sites on the adjuvant;
   e. stimulation of toxic factors from adsorption sites on the adjuvant.

2. Suboptimal immunogenicity through:
   a. antigenic competition;
   b. epitope suppression;
   c. excessive antigen:adjuvant ratio.
3. Excessive batch-to-batch variation resulting from complex interactions of multiple components.
4. Suboptimal stability, e.g., from conjugate degradation through hydrolysis or through proteolysis.

It is therefore incumbent on the vaccine developer to ensure that these potential problems do not occur or are at least minimized to be of no clinical relevance. This is normally achieved during the formulation experimentation phase where changes in buffer, changes in the sequence of antigen adsorption to adjuvant, and changes in ionic strength can be adjusted to result in optimal product characteristics.

Different Presentations

For combination vaccines that involve a full-liquid presentation, these issues also must be considered in light of a two- to three-year shelf-life that must be demonstrated with both real-time and accelerated test conditions at a range of elevated temperatures. Other combination vaccines that involve reconstitution of lyophilized component(s) with a liquid combination vaccine may need testing of the final reconstituted product as well as demonstration of satisfactory performance of the individual components. The final product may have only a brief shelf-life of perhaps a few hours, but demonstration using laboratory tests of the sustained functionality of all components is required by some if not all Authorities. In such cases, compatibility studies also should be performed for presentations that use a by-pass or dual-chamber syringe in order to demonstrate absence of interference that may affect the clinical effectiveness of the vaccine. Correlating the results of such laboratory tests often using small animals with clinical data from human studies is not a simple matter and provides a challenge to both manufacturers and national control authorities.

Formulation Issues

The importance of the adjuvant selected for use in combined vaccines must not be underestimated. The various forms of adjuvant each demonstrate a different result when used with different combination of antigens. Aluminum hydroxide, aluminum phosphate, and calcium phosphate are all described in the European Pharmacopoeia. However, their use may be associated with differing adsorption capacities, perhaps including the phenomenon of desorption either rapidly or over the shelf-life of the product. Some authorities have suggested that such phenomena are indicative of product instability and that steps should be taken to eliminate such problems during the manufacturing process. In such cases, it is important to study whether or not such variations in adsorption have any impact on either vaccine stability or on the immunogenicity of a given component in humans before being required to make changes to the production protocol.

New adjuvants are increasingly being considered by manufacturers (e.g., detoxified lipid A, liposomes, microspheres, muramyl peptides, and saponins), and extensive testing must be done on any combination vaccines formulated to include them. These include demonstration of compatibility of the adjuvant with all antigens of the combination vaccine, evidence of efficient and stable adsorption, and provision of data showing safety of the adjuvant both alone and in the final combination formulation.

Stability Testing of Combination Vaccines

The annex to the ICH guideline *(14)* on stability testing of biotechnological/biological products provides a useful overview on regulator expectations for such studies. For combination vaccines, stability data are requested for each individual component before combination, after combination into bulk vaccine, and for the finished product. Data from at least three batches of each of the three manufacturing steps are required normally.

Consistency Testing of Combination Vaccines

The development of a combination vaccine containing a complex mixture of components, some of which may themselves be combinations of antigens (e.g., IPV or aP) requires demonstration that the final product can be manufactured in a consistent manner. In order to avoid numerous formulations that would cover all the mathematical permutations possible for multivalent or multidisease combinations, a more pragmatic approach should be sought. This approach would involve formulating and testing a logical defined subset of batches selected from the very large number of possible combinations. The first step is to demonstrate the consistency of each single component involving the testing of bulks from at least three consecutive production runs.

An approach for consistency testing of combined vaccines was developed by European Vaccine Manufacturers Regulatory Working Group and this has been adopted by the CPMP in their guideline.

The addition of one new valency *(Z)* to a combination vaccine base of well-established consistency represents a common situation, i.e., the addition of a new aP to DT. In this case, $D_1 T_1 aP_1 : D_1 T_1 aP_2$; and $D_1 T_1 aP_3$ should suffice to show consistency on the level of the final bulk. This may be shown in the case of a new component *(Z)* as follows:

$$A_1 B_1 C_1 \underline{\quad\quad} Z_1$$
$$A_1 B_1 C_1 \underline{\quad\quad} Z_2$$
$$A_1 B_1 C_1 \underline{\quad\quad} Z_3$$

In cases where more than one new valency (e.g., Y, Z) is to be added to a licensed combination vaccine, consistency could be shown with three consecutive final bulks as follows:

$$A_1 \, B_1 \, C_1 \, D_1 \underline{\quad\quad} Y_1 \, Z_1$$
$$A_1 \, B_1 \, C_1 \, D_1 \underline{\quad\quad} Y_2 \, Z_2$$
$$A_1 \, B_1 \, C_1 \, D_1 \underline{\quad\quad} Y_3 \, Z_3$$

An example of such a vaccine could be combining hepatitis A and hepatitis B with a licensed combination vaccine of DTaP-IPV for pediatric use.

The FDA "Guidance" document *(1)* also discusses the issue of demonstrating consistency. It recommends that lots for consistency studies ideally should be manufactured in the facility that corresponds to that indicated in the Establishment License Application. The equipment utilized for manufacture also should be the same, but the lots need not be made at full production scale. Release data for lots manufactured at full scale are normally required for European and United States registration purposes.

The FDA document indicates that each of the three consecutive manufacturing consistency lots should utilize a different bulk lot of each active component. Some easing of this requirement is indicated for cases where the components are already licensed; seeking guidance from CBER on a case-by-case basis is advised.

Overall the CBER approach is similar to that expressed in the draft CPMP guidelines, although their matrix indicates a difference in attitudes to this complex problem, i.e.,

$$X_1 + Y_1 + Z_1 \underline{\quad\quad} N_1 = \text{Final lot 1}$$
$$X_2 + Y_2 + Z_2 \underline{\quad\quad} N_2 = \text{Final lot 2}$$
$$X_3 + Y_3 + Z_3 \underline{\quad\quad} N_3 = \text{Final lot 3}$$

The FDA also recommends use of a random sampling procedure technique (using a random number generator) to aid in obtaining representative lot selections for formulation of the consistency batches.

From this, it is evident that some differences exist between United States and European attitudes to this issue. Obtaining "buy-in" to the plan is possible and deemed advisable by CBER, with such "buy-in" being currently more difficult to obtain in Europe owing to lack of structures analogues to FDA's review processes. Nevertheless, manufacturers need some indication that their proposals will be acceptable to all key regulatory agencies prior to embarking on a series of complex, time-consuming, and expensive formulation and consistency lot testing studies. Thus prior discussions with agencies to obtain their agreement to the proposed strategy are highly desirable.

References and Standards—
Potency Testing of Combination Vaccines

Potency testing as part of BR requirements raises problems as a result of possible interferences between various antigens. Traditionally, individual components used in formulating combination products are subject to potency testing by both manufacturers and national control agencies with the results compared to those of reference preparations of known potency. According to the FDA, the potency of each component should be similar to that found for the monovalent components "unless it can be determined that any reduction in potency due to interaction with other components of the combination product does not result in a lowering of efficacy in humans" *(1)*. In the case of a lyophilized vaccine (e.g., Hib reconstituted by a liquid combination vaccine, e.g., DTaP-IPV), demonstration of potency in the final reconstituted form is generally required in both United States and Europe.

The primary standard for such applications is the WHO International Standard. This is used for calibration of secondary reference materials and/or in-house references. In Europe, the secondary references are largely the responsibility of the European Pharmacopoeia in Strasbourg. Such references also may be used to calibrate national or in-house working reference preparations.

In addition to the above, for combination vaccines there may be a need for specific reference material ("in-house" or "homologous reference") that have been shown equivalent to a vaccine lot previously tested in clinical trials and have been shown satisfactory in man. Specifications stating the acceptable limits of the tests and their validation criteria should be developed by manufacturers in close consultation with the authorities. At present, this issue of selecting references and standards for combination vaccines remains somewhat unclear, yet it is essential clarification is achieved in the near future if combination vaccines are to successfully reach the market.

Animal Immunogenicity and Protection Studies
with Combination Vaccines

Both CBER and CPMP recommend use of animal immunogenicity and protection studies, where suitable animal models are available although it is not always evident that the available models have any relevance to the human situation. Such studies should be conducted early in the product life cycle. In addition, the new combination should be compared to the individual antigens in animals to determine any change in immunogenicity. Any protection studies, if deemed relevant to humans, should involve a challenge with a virulent strain(s) of each organism against which the vaccine is intended to protect.

Design of Clinical Studies for Combination Vaccines

Reference has already been made to the design of clinical studies that must address various schedules in order to meet global requirements plus take into account the ethnicity factor, age factors, local vaccination practices, and so forth.

One problem cited for combination vaccines is possible difficulties in the event of an adverse reaction in determining which of the many components could be responsible. Depending on the severity of the reaction, further doses may not be indicated. However, such action could deprive the subject of protection against certain diseases. This issue can be partly addressed by ensuring the ongoing supply of monovalent vaccines that could be available for use in such cases.

In many situations, the proof of efficacy of combination vaccines relies on historic data demonstrating the efficacy of the components, supported by comparative immunogenicity data plus results from animal protection models, where available. Where priming doses are to be followed by booster doses, multiyear studies for evaluation of both reactogenicity and immunogenicity after each dose will be required in order to support license claims. It may be possible for these data to be submitted post-licensure to enable amendment to the file permitting further booster doses. During these studies, compatibility with other vaccines (sometimes from other manufacturers) that may be given concurrently to the study vaccine will need to be addressed.

In the design of the clinical trials for a given combination vaccine, it is also important to ensure that the effect of various vaccination schedules recommended in different countries are adequately studied. For example, a vaccine tested at a 2-, 4-, 6-month schedule in North American infants may behave quite differently when given at 2-, 3-, and 4-months in the UK or France or at 3-, 5-, and 12-months as the primary series currently practiced in Scandinavia. Similarly, the practice of giving booster doses varies from country to country and should be studied in the development of the overall clinical trial strategy. The safety profile of a vaccine to be administered four, five, or even six times up to the age of puberty may need to be addressed in order to satisfy concerns of health authorities. This may be pursued post licensure but attention should be paid to ensuring long term follow-up of clinical trial subjects is feasible and acceptable.

Evidence of the stimulation of a humoral, and where useful, a systemic response will be demonstrated during clinical studies. Where there is a decline of antibody response following priming, evidence of a strong anamnestic response can be helpful in overcoming concerns that the priming was unsatisfactory in terms of long-term protection.

Finally, with respect to variable presentations of the same combination product in vials, ampoules, prefilled syringes, etc., it is important to recognize that each of these presentations may require submission of a complete new product application file with full supportive stability and clinical documentation, as appropriate. A further detail of note is the need to address different vaccination practices between United States and Europe. In the former, needles of 25-mm length are favored for adults. In France, UK, and Belgium 16-mm long needles are preferred, whereas Germany and Italy prefer longer needles. Thus for European dossiers it may be necessary to show that use of the short needles will not change the safety and immunogenicity profile of these vaccines compared with data obtained with longer needles. In this regard, special consideration needs to be given to sex, age, and above all, the weight range of the subjects in the clinical trials.

Conclusions

In summary, it is evident that vaccine manufacturers should not underestimate the complications inherent in the development of combination vaccines, recognizing the increasingly rigorous regulatory environment that creates conditions such products must meet. It would appear that today's environment is even more complex than that which existed during the period when older "combination" products such as DTP, MMR, IPV, OPV, Influenza or Pneumococcal vaccines were originally licensed. Indeed, the introduction of new requirements is now making it a challenge for manufacturers to maintain or upgrade these "old" products to meet today's regulations.

This chapter also pointed out the discrepancies that exist in regulatory requirements and vaccination practices from one country or region to another. The ICH procedure has contributed toward harmonization of some elements, although their focus has been primarily on issues of relevance to drug manufacture and less so on the needs of the biologics industry in general and the vaccine sector in particular. It is evident that much more effort toward harmonization of all these elements is required. The cooperative spirit developed through the ICH process among the regulators of the United States, Japan, Europe, and the industrial community that has led to progress in harmonization of so many regulations, will be an essential component in the next phases of the ICH process. This will focus on development of the Common Technical Dossier as a step toward the fabled "Global Dossier"—perhaps even electronically submitted using a universally accepted software.

In this regard, there is the ongoing need to train regulators in the new approaches endorsed in the ICH process in order to ensure their timely introduction in the review process.

Currently, outside of this ICH process, the lack of harmonization between the three major pharmacopoeias of Japan, the United States, and Europe remains an area of concern. Their monographs and requirements have the force of law in their respective territories, and where differences exist manufacturers must address them independently. This involves a waste of time and resources and may result in delays to the public in receiving products of significant public health value. Unfortunately, it appears to be very difficult for the various pharmacopoeial bodies to reach agreements in the same efficient manner as was achieved by ICH. Industry and regulatory agencies need to maintain and even strengthen their pressure on these organizations to work together to achieve harmonization of their existing requirements and to ensure new regulations are developed in a collaborative manner to avoid continued variations from one region to another.

A second example more specific to vaccines involves discrepancies that exist between the WHO requirements/vaccine monographs and the requirements, particularly for batch release, applied in Japan, the United States, and Europe. For those manufacturers who plan to sell their products outside of Japan, the United States, and Europe, e.g., via UNICEF tenders, it is considered important to demonstrate that the product passes the various WHO requirements.

The existence of so many differences between WHO requirements and those of Japan, the United States, and Europe raise a number of problems. The first is that WHO is not an official party to the ICH process but is involved with observer status. The second is that there is no current alternate process available that enables harmonization of WHO requirements with those other regions. This situation creates an opportunity for the vaccine industry individually or via its various associations to identify and prioritize the various items of concern and to participate in expert review groups involving the various Agency officials to reach a single set of requirements for vaccines including those involving mixtures of multiple antigens. This will likely be a lengthy process, and manufacturers will have to live with problematic discrepancies for some time to come.

It may be concluded that the development of combination vaccines and their successful passage through various differing regulatory hurdles is a daunting task. It requires a high level of sophisticated manufacturing and development capability, plus the existence of a global multitiered pricing system, to permit a sufficient overall return on the enormous investments necessary to meet the ever-increasing requirements that are involved in the development of such products on a worldwide basis. It is for these reasons that such complex multi-disease and multivalent combination vaccines are generally being developed only by large manufacturers. Indeed, the needs are so great that even these manufacturers are tending to collaborate through various forms of alliance or joint venture.

At the end of the day, however, manufacturers are slowly but inexorably succeeding in overcoming all the challenges provided by ever increasing regulatory hurdles and by the intrinsic complexity of the combination vaccine products themselves. Combination vaccines are now emerging into the marketplace, bringing with them the prospect of higher coverage rates, fewer vaccination needle jabs, greater protection against multiple diseases, and more efficient products in some cases using rDNA technology or sophisticated polysaccharide conjugation technology. In addition, new manufacturing techniques are being introduced, as are filling procedures that make the need for use of preservatives in certain presentations redundant. All these activities bode well for the future growth of the vaccine industry, sustained occupations for those who regulate, and most important of all, progress toward improved global public health by this very cost-effective process of preventative medicine known as "vaccinology."

References

1. Guidance for industry for the Evaluation of Combination Vaccines for Preventable Diseases: Production, Testing, and Clinical Studies. Food and Drug Administration, Center for Biologics, Evaluation, and Research, Bethesda, MD, April 1997.
2. Note for Guidance on Pharmaceutical and Biological Aspects of Combined Vaccines. Committee for Proprietary Medicinal Products/Biologicals Working Party/477/97 draft transmitted to interested parties, European Medicines Evaluation Agency, London, UK, June 1997.
3. European Pharmacopoeia Commission, Prepublication of texts adopted at November 1997 session, PA/PH/Exp.3/T(97)163DEF, pp. 485–490, Strasbourg, France.
4. Collee, J. G., Gerald, and Bradley, R. (1997) Bovine spongiform encephalopathy—a decade on, Parts 1 and 2. *Lancet* **349,** 636–641; 715–721.
5. *Federal Register* June 5, 1997, 21 Codex of the Federal Register part 589; Food and Drug Administration, Bethesda, MD, **62(108),** article 30936.
6. European Commission Decision 97/534 on the prohibition of the use of material presenting risks as regards transmissible spongiform encephalopathies, Brussels, Belgium, July 1997.
7. World Health Organization Press Release, Geneva, Switzerland. WHO/27, 27 March 1997. Spongiform Encephalopathies: New Recommendations on Medical Products.
8. European Commission Directive 89/381, Brussels, Belgium. Provisions for medicinal products derived from human blood or human plasma. Point 4, Article 3.
9. Note for guidance on pre-clinical pharmacological and toxicological testing of vaccines. Committee for Proprietary Medicinal Products/Safety Working Party/485/95, European Medicines Evaluation Agency, London, UK, February 1997.
10. Böni, J., Staider, J., Reigel, F., and Schüpbach, J. (1996) Detection of reverse transcriptase activity in live attenuated virus vaccines. *Clin. Diagn. Virol.* **5,** 43–53.
11. Food and Drug Administration guidance concerning demonstration of comparability of human biological products, including therapeutic biotechnology-derived products, Center for Biologics, Evaluation, and Research, Bethesda, MD, April 1996, pp. 1–9.
12. European Commission Regulation, 541/95 as modified by Regulation 1146/98, Variation to mutual recognition products, Brussels, Belgium. European Commission Regulation, 542/95 as modified by Regulation 1069/98, Variation to centralized products, Brussels, Belgium.
13. Corbel, M. J. (1994) Control testing of combined vaccines: a consideration of potential problems and approaches. *Biologicals* **22(4),** 353–360.
14. International Conference on Harmonization. Harmonized tripartite guideline: quality of biotechnological products: stability testing of biotechnological/biological products. Approved July 1997.

11 Testing and Licensure of Combination Vaccines for the Prevention of Infectious Diseases

*Lydia A. Falk, Karen Midthun,
Loris D. McVittie,
and Karen L. Goldenthal*

Introduction

Vaccines are exceptionally cost-effective agents for infectious disease prevention, control, and (potentially) eradication. Combination vaccines can reduce the number of immunizations required to achieve protection against multiple diseases and consequently can lead to increased vaccine coverage *(1,2)*. These advantages will become even more apparent as vaccines for new indications are approved *(3,4)*. The current Advisory Committee on Immunization Practices (ACIP) recommendations already necessitate that a large number of vaccines be given to infants within a short time interval *(5)*. The ACIP now recommends a sequential vaccination schedule of two doses of inactivated poliovirus vaccine (IPV) followed by two doses of oral poliovirus vaccine (OPV) for routine childhood vaccination *(6)*, anticipated to be an interim step before the implementation of an "all IPV" policy in the United States. Thus, the advantages of combination vaccines are especially evident for pediatric populations.

A combination vaccine consists of two or more vaccine immunogens in a physically mixed preparation intended to prevent multiple diseases (multidisease combination vaccine) or prevent one disease caused by different serotypes

Note: This paper represents the views of the individual authors and does not represent the official view of the US Food and Drug Administration.

From: *Combination Vaccines: Development, Clinical Research, and Approval*
Edited by: R. W. Ellis © Humana Press Inc., Totowa, NJ

(or serogroups) of the same organism (multivalent combination vaccine). The mixing can occur as a manufacturing step or can be performed by a health care professional following package insert instructions *(1,7)*. Any method of combining vaccines must be evaluated carefully to ensure that the final combination vaccine product is safe and effective.

There have been a number of examples where unexpected decreases in immune responses have been observed when antigens are combined, e.g., the decreased response to *Haemophilus influenzae* type *b* (Hib) conjugate vaccines in diphtheria and tetanus toxoids and acellular pertussis (DTaP) and Hib combinations *(8–12)*, and in a diphtheria and tetanus toxoids and whole cell pertussis (DTwP) and Hib combination *(13)*. In some cases, decreased immune responses have been attributed to a specific source, e.g., the detrimental effect of thimerosal (in DTwP preparations) on IPV potency in DTwP and IPV combinations *(14–16)* or the instability of pertussis antigens in DTwP and IPV combinations using benzethonium chloride (BEC) in the absence of thimerosal *(17,18)*. Thus, appropriate clinical trials for safety, immunogenicity, and (if applicable) efficacy, as well as relevant animal and laboratory studies, are needed even if the component vaccines are licensed *(1,7)*.

The focus of this chapter will be the Phase 1, 2, and 3 clinical studies of combination vaccines submitted to an Investigational New Drug Application (INDA). Assuming the new vaccine appears safe and effective, the results of these studies can be included in a Biologic License Application (BLA) to support approval for marketing in the US. This chapter will also cover some highlights of manufacturing and product testing, much of which would be addressed before IND studies begin; these results will also be submitted to the IND and, ultimately (usually in greater detail), to the BLA.

Manufacturing and Controls

Adequate manufacturing methods and production controls are important in establishing the safety and biologic activity of the product, as well as the consistency of the manufacturing process. Detailed information describing the source and quality of starting materials, characterization of seed stocks, adventitious agent testing, performance of manufacturing steps and process controls, potency, general safety, purity, and identity of the final product should be documented. Generally, the extent of documentation required by the Food and Drug Administration (FDA) will increase as clinical studies progress, as it is recognized that manufacturing refinements and improvements in test methods often occur during product development. The appropriate product testing and validation often depends on the type of product. Manufacturing and production controls apply to each component in the combination vaccine. In addition, changes in one component of the combination vaccine changes the final product. Genetic stability for recombinant constructs *(19,20)*, details on inactivation or attenuation methods for organisms or toxins *(21,22)*, and animal safety/toxicology of vaccines with novel adjuvants *(23,24)* are all examples of specific types of additional testing that may be appropriate depending on the type of vaccine being developed.

General Considerations for Product Characterization

DESCRIPTION OF MANUFACTURING

In addition to careful documentation of the source and quality of all materials used in the manufacture of the vaccine, detailed descriptions of the characterization of bacterial and viral master seeds and working seed stocks with regard to isolation, passage history, and growth characteristics should be provided. When utilizing seeds that have been modified by recombinant DNA technology, it is important to include information about the stability of the construct *(19,20)*. In the case of viral vaccines, cell substrate issues are critical safety concerns, therefore, information about the identity, source and passage history of cells, cell banking procedures, as well as thorough adventitious agent testing should be documented and the results of this testing provided *(25,26)*. In cases where either bacterial or viral organisms or toxins comprise the final vaccine product, the methods of attenuation, inactivation, or detoxification should be adequately described and validation data provided to support the safety of the vaccine *(21,22,27)*. Additionally, it is recommended that residual levels of nonorganism (i.e., cell substrate-derived) protein and DNA be measured or demonstrated to be cleared during production purification steps *(26)*.

FINAL FORMULATION TESTING OF COMBINATION VACCINES

The potency of a vaccine can be viewed as the ability of a product to effect a given result through either the use of laboratory tests or by controlled clinical data *(28)*. Quantitative potency tests are generally considered necessary to assess the biological activity of each active component of a combination vaccine and can also serve as one measure of product stability. A variety of potency assays may be acceptable. For example, potency tests may represent a serological evaluation or challenge test following vaccination of animals or may rely on physicochemical characterization, such as composition and molecular weight, as is the case for several polysaccharide vaccines. Ideally, the potency test should be predictive of the efficacy of the product in humans. In addition to potency, tests for product sterility and the absence of toxicity from extraneous contaminants, i.e., General Safety Test, should be provided *(29)*.

Situations have occurred where the combination of intermediate, single-component bulk materials compromised critical properties of other antigens in the final formulated product. Therefore, when evaluating the compatibility of the components, it is important to consider how excipients and other ingredients from the various monocomponent bulks will affect the activity and stability of the final product. In this evaluation, consideration should be given to the effects of adjuvant adsorption on previously nonadsorbed products, whether the rate of desorption is altered if a new buffer is introduced, and changes in the state of aggregation of individual components.

Potency and identity tests for each of the antigens in the final product should be established. Identity testing on the labeled final container may include immunological assays for vaccine antigens and serotyping of vaccine organism strains (29). The identity tests used for the final formulation may be the same as those used for testing intermediate bulks. It is important to demonstrate, however, that a potency or identity test used for an intermediate component performs reliably when combined into a complex mixture with possible addition of adjuvants, preservatives, buffers, or other additives.

When evaluating consistency of manufacture, it is important to demonstrate that the bulk intermediates and the final formulated combination vaccine can be manufactured reproducibly. In the US, the testing of at least three lots formulated using three different bulk lots for each antigen in the combination vaccine is usually recommended (7). However, as the number of antigens combined in the vaccine increases, alternative strategies for demonstrating consistency of manufacture may be appropriate. Lots selected for consistency testing should represent typical manufacturing lots with regard to product specifications.

STABILITY

Product stability testing is essential for selecting an appropriate dating period and for future extensions of the dating period. In most cases, all stability parameters are evaluated using real-time data under ideal conditions of storage (30). Appropriate storage periods may be established for intermediate bulks (and final formulated bulks if needed) such that final product dating is representative of component bulks that may have been held for any time during these defined storage periods. Stability protocols that specify which tests are to be performed at predetermined intervals should be initiated early in product development to ensure that sufficient sequential real-time data, often several years for the final container plus months to years for the bulks, are accumulated for lots representative of the final manufacturing process. Additionally, assessment of stability at other than ideal temperatures may provide useful supplemental information on stability of the product if improper storage conditions occur.

The tests to be performed may include physicochemical characteristics (e.g., pH, appearance, desorption in the case of adjuvanted vaccines, and free versus bound polysaccharide in the case of conjugate vaccines), sterility and the bioactivity of the combination product using animal models if available, and will depend on the features of the product susceptible to change during storage. Stability studies should be carried out on each presentation (e.g., single and multidose vials, prefilled syringes) of the final product.

If a vaccine is admixed just prior to administration, i.e., by a healthcare professional, it is recommended that the stability program evaluate the characteristics of the combination vaccine at several time points following mixing. These data may allow an estimate of the "window" between mixing and administration which can be definitively tested in a clinical trial. The evaluation of stability using several laboratory tests and animal models may allow for a better understanding of the potential positive and negative effects of combining monovalent components on the final combination vaccine formulation.

Specific Manufacturing Concerns for Combination Vaccines
INTERACTION OF ANTIGENIC COMPONENTS IN COMBINATION

When combining antigens, it may be necessary to re-evaluate the acceptability of tests being used preclinically for any component of the vaccine. For instance, the instability of pertussis antigens in wP vaccines when combined into a multicomponent vaccine has been reported *(17,18)*. These early reports suggested that the strain of mouse used in the pertussis potency test for DTwP had a lower capacity to respond when testing a combination vaccine containing the poliovirus vaccine *(17)*. These findings highlight the need for careful evaluation of release testing for the combination product and the re-evaluation of final release testing for each component as additional antigens are added to the multicomponent vaccine.

In addition, concern about the possible negative impact of using the same carrier protein for multiple polysaccharides has been raised *(31)*. This concern may apply to both combination vaccines and simultaneously administered vaccines. Specifically, the question is whether the vaccinated individual will be able to recognize and respond to these multiple stimuli equally, or whether there will be a reduction in the immune response to select immunogens, i.e., carrier suppression or epitope suppression. Although the validity of these concerns may be evaluated from clinical trial data, i.e., human immunogenicity data, an important goal of preclinical testing is to develop animal models to test this hypothesis. For example, one animal model being developed in an effort to mimic the immune response of infants to conjugate vaccines is the guinea pig model of Siber and coworkers *(32)*. This model evaluated the immune responses of guinea pigs to Hib conjugate vaccines when administered with vaccines (e.g., diphtheria and tetanus toxoids combination vaccine [DT], tetanus toxoid vaccine [T] and DTaP) containing antigens similar to those used as carriers in the conjugate vaccine.

With the addition of multiple antigens in creating more complex vaccines, the need for novel preclinical testing methods for each component has increased in importance, as has the goal of developing a validated animal model that can combine the potency testing of several antigens into a single animal model.

INTERACTION OF CONSTITUENTS IN COMBINATION

Evaluation of combination vaccines also includes determining the effects of excipients, adjuvants, and preservatives that might be used in the manufacture of intermediate bulk antigens or added to the formulation of the final product, on the potency of each antigen in the final combination product *(1,4,7,33,34)*. Studies with IPV have shown that the potency of the vaccine can be adversely affected by the choice of preservatives, i.e., the potency of poliomyelitis vaccine is decreased with the use of thimerosal *(14–16)*. In addition, in a combination of DTwP and IPV in which IPV contained the preservative BEC, decreased germicidal activity and reduced BEC levels were observed *(16)*. Thus, as a general rule, the actual concentration of a critical preservative in the final product should be measured.

In addition to deleterious effects on poliovirus vaccine potency following combination with other antigens, there have been reports of instability of pertussis antigens when combined into a multicomponent vaccine *(17,18)*. These early reports indicated that although DTwP vaccines were generally stable throughout the dating period, the addition of the poliovirus vaccine resulted in a rapid loss of potency under normal clinical conditions. These reports further illustrate the value of well-planned stability programs as an integral early part of the product testing program for combination products.

Clinical Evaluation of Combination Vaccines

Overview

Prelicensure clinical studies to evaluate the safety, immunogenicity and efficacy of combination vaccines should, in most cases, be randomized and well-controlled *(7,35)*. Randomization protects against systematic biases (including ones that may be difficult to identify), helps ensure balance for known and unknown prognostic factors, and facilitates the detection of small to moderate, but potentially clinically meaningful effects. It is also easier to interpret unexpected results if the study is randomized *(36,37)*. Comparisons to historical data, as opposed to a randomized control group, are less optimal because they may not account for factors such as population differences, immunological assay variability, simultaneous use of other vaccines, nuances of adverse event surveillance techniques, and so forth.

Nonblinded studies have been used to assess the safety and immunogenicity of new combination vaccines, especially in pediatric populations when the investigational and control groups receive different numbers of immunizations and/or immunization schedules. A potential for bias does exist with nonblinded safety and immunogenicity studies, but this appears to be less severe than that observed in some trial situations, e.g., infectious disease case ascertainment in an efficacy trial *(37)*.

Clinical Evaluation of Safety

The clinical development plan for new combination vaccines should be devised to provide an adequate safety database (as well as immunogenicity and, if applicable, efficacy data) to support licensure. In many situations, the new combination vaccines under development only contain components with already proven efficacy. For such new combination vaccines, comparative immunogenicity data may provide a sufficient basis to support efficacy, precluding the need for a large efficacy study (to demonstrate prevention of disease or infection). Specifically, comparative immunological data between the already licensed products and the respective components in the new combination vaccine may be used to support efficacy *(1,7,36,37)*.

As will be discussed later, adequate data to compare the immunogenicity of vaccines can usually be obtained with sample sizes of Phase 2 magnitude, e.g., several hundred, at most, per group. However, without the extensive clinical safety database that would have been obtained from a large double-blind, randomized efficacy trial(s) with thousands of individuals, additional prelicensure study(s) would be conducted to obtain an adequate safety database *(1)*. Thus, the design and sample size of such clinical studies to specifically evaluate safety are important topics for the development of such combination vaccines and is the focus of this section.

Prelicensure clinical studies to evaluate safety should, in most cases, be randomized and well-controlled. Typically, individuals in the control group receive the separate, simultaneously administered components (or already licensed combinations of components) contained in the new combination vaccine, as appropriate *(7,35)*. For example, in the investigation of a new DTaP and IPV combination vaccine, the control group may receive separate injections of already licensed DTaP and IPV vaccines. There are also situations where the safety of a new combination vaccine may be compared to a different manufacturer's licensed combination of the same immunogens, especially for Phase 3 safety studies.

When supplemental trials for safety are needed, data from one large multi-center safety study using one clinical protocol with consistent surveillance methods are more readily reviewed and interpreted than data from multiple, smaller safety studies. The most relevant safety data are those obtained from studies using the product at the dose, schedule and formulation intended for licensure.

Unequal randomization ratios (e.g., 3:1 or 2:1, with more persons in the new combination vaccine group) can be utilized to obtain more safety information on the new product. Use of unequal ratios requires a somewhat larger overall sample size; however, this scheme may result in more rapid recruitment of subjects if the new product involves fewer injections. Such unequal randomization ratios have been utilized, especially for expanded Phase 3 safety studies *(37)*.

Safety assessments should include active monitoring of subjects. Well-designed case report forms should query for specific events at preselected time points. These forms should also accommodate the recording of other events that are not specifically listed *(7)*. Selection of parameters for monitoring, as well as the frequency and duration of postvaccination follow-up, should take into consideration both the vaccine and the study population.

Phase 2 studies frequently provide data on common injection site reactions and systemic events and determine if the immunogenicity of the combination vaccine is equivalent to that of the same components in the control vaccines. Subsequently, a larger Phase 3 safety trial with a sample size suitable for the evaluation of less common adverse events is performed. For such larger trials, a simplified design may be acceptable where only a subset of subjects is assessed in detail for the more common events *(7)*. In order to obtain meaningful study results, an adequate monitoring system must be in place to detect and record the events of interest. The sample size should be based on the safety questions of interest, which will be influenced by factors such as the vaccine under study and the target population. The selection of less common but important event(s) for evaluation in a larger comparative safety trial is usually based on a consideration of the events observed in the available studies of the new combination vaccine, its separate components, and similar licensed products (if applicable).

A new combination vaccine using a different schedule from the one used for the individual components may predispose to the administration of an extra vaccine dose in clinical practice. For example, a combination product containing hepatitis B (HB) vaccine might be developed for administration at 2, 4, and 6 months of age. However, infants immunized with HB vaccine at or shortly after birth (a now common practice) followed by the three-dose series of the combination vaccine would receive a total of four doses of HB vaccine. Evaluation of the safety of an extra dose, if it is likely to occur, should be considered in prelicensure studies. A large safety trial (stratified at entry for balance) that enrolls both infants who did and did not receive HB vaccine at birth would be one way to obtain such data *(37)*.

The use of large Health Maintenance Organizations (HMO), with computerized databases on immunizations, medical outcomes, and potential confounders, can be helpful in ascertaining the incidence of uncommon events for both pre and postmarketing safety assessments *(38–40)*. Postapproval studies may be needed to assess the potential for rare but serious events.

Usually, the goal of comparative safety studies is to demonstrate similarity of the safety profile between the combination vaccine and the separately administered components. It has been suggested that these equivalence trials be designed and analyzed to reject a hypothesis of a difference, rather than the traditional null hypothesis of no difference *(41)*. Confidence intervals on the difference between the new combination vaccine and the separate components should accompany formal hypothesis tests or may themselves comprise the primary analysis.

Reactions to different immunizations received by the same individual are not considered independent observations. Thus, comparisons between the combination vaccine and the separate components for common adverse events should assess both by-injection and by-subject event rates. The pivotal analysis for injection site reactions is usually a comparison between the new combination vaccine injection site and the site of the most severe reaction observed for the component vaccines *(7)*. However, all component vaccine injection site reactions should be recorded per protocol for future reference. Point estimates and 95% confidence intervals should be provided for adverse event rates; this applies to both within and between comparator groups.

All safety trials will not require the same sample size; thus, the appropriate size will usually be determined not only by statistical but also by clinical and basic scientific judgments. Sample size calculations should be consistent with the null and alternative hypotheses to be tested, or may be based on confidence intervals if that is the planned method of evaluation.

The finding that a certain event is not observed, even in a large trial, should be considered from a statistical viewpoint *(37,42)*. It is still possible in this case to obtain an upper confidence limit on the rate of such an event for the target population. For a total of n subjects receiving the new combination vaccine, a 95% confidence interval for the true event rate can be estimated as $(0, 3/n)$, based on the "Rule of 3" *(42)*. For example, a safety data base of 4200 vaccinees among whom a particular adverse event did not occur would provide 95% confidence that the true rate for that event would not exceed 1 in 1400.

Clinical Evaluation of Immunogenicity

For new vaccines, efficacy is usually assessed in trials demonstrating prevention of disease or infection. However, for new combination vaccines with components consisting of previously licensed products and/or antigens with efficacy already demonstrated in clinical trials, serological endpoints may be adequate to substantiate efficacy for licensure.

For the evaluation of a new combination vaccine, the immune responses to the respective antigens in two or more products are compared. For example, the immune responses in a group of subjects receiving a new combination vaccine consisting of antigens X and Y, given as one injection, are compared to those observed for a different group receiving the two separately administered (usually already licensed) products with X and Y antigens, respectively.

The rationale for the use of serological endpoints is clearest when a previously accepted correlation between such serological endpoints and clinical efficacy already exists (*see* 21 Code of Federal Regulations 601.25(d)(2)). A serological correlate of protection for vaccine efficacy may be identified by analysis of results from a successful efficacy trial with clinical endpoints or may be inferred from other sources (e.g., protection afforded by a related hyperimmune globulin or observed in serological surveys of immunized populations) *(36)*.

Equivalence of immune response has also been used to evaluate new combination vaccines even when there is no clear correlate of protection. However, in the absence of an identified immune correlate of protection, or when the correlate is not well defined quantitatively, a decreased immune response for the new combination vaccine will be difficult to interpret, and it may not be possible to conclude that the new and old products are clinically comparable. The statistical hypothesis for the "acceptable differences" in these cases will be especially critical. In the case of acellular pertussis antigens, where there is no identified correlate(s) of protection, the pros and cons of using serological responses to evaluate new combinations have been discussed *(43–45)*.

Also, the use of serological endpoints is often important for a specific type of combination vaccine: multivalent products for a single etiological agent containing more than one antigen, e.g., 23-valent pneumococcal vaccine.

For such multivalent combination products, it may not be possible to show clinical efficacy for each distinct serotype in clinical trials because of problems such as low incidence of disease caused by certain serotypes. Thus, for a single etiologic agent for which an immunological correlate of protection has been determined for one or more of the serotypes (or serogroups), serological endpoints may be the basis for including the other serotypes in the formulation. For example, clinical efficacy was demonstrated only for the A and C components of the quadrivalent A-C-Y-W135 meningococcal capsular polysaccharide vaccine prior to licensure; efficacy was inferred for the less common serogroups Y and W135, each of which elicited high levels of bactericidal antibodies in immunized volunteers *(46)*.

Similar situations for multivalent vaccines may be anticipated in the future. For example, pneumococcal conjugate vaccines are under development to extend protection to infants. For epidemiological reasons, it may be useful to add new serotypes to a multivalent pneumococcal conjugate formulation with demonstrated efficacy. The addition of these serotypes may be evaluated on the basis of functional (bactericidal or opsonophagocytic) antibody responses that they induce *(47)*.

The following concepts are important when planning trials based on comparing the immune responses between (or among) groups *(36)*:

1. Detailed information about each assay intended to assess immune response should be provided to the IND in advance of using the assay, especially prior to the pivotal serological equivalence study(s).
2. The plan for statistical analysis of immunogenicity data should be submitted with the protocol. Again, this is particularly critical if the study will be the pivotal immunogenicity study to support licensure.
3. As noted earlier, it has been proposed that these equivalence trials be designed and analyzed to reject a hypothesis of a difference, rather than the traditional null hypothesis of no difference *(41)*. The comparisons of immune responses for the purpose of demonstrating efficacy should be statistically valid with an adequate sample size *(7,41,48,49)*. In particular, the conclusion that immune responses are equivalent cannot be made when the sample size is inadequate to identify meaningful differences.
4. The confidence limits on differences between groups being compared should be provided for the per-protocol critical immune response parameters, e.g., seroconversion rates and geometric mean titers (GMT).
5. Reverse cumulative distribution curves are a useful tool for comparing immune response data between groups, and are often of special interest for the low response part of the curves *(50)*.

Clinical Evaluation of Efficacy

Reviews of elements of prelicensure vaccine clinical efficacy trials such as design, sample size, blinding, selection of endpoints, statistical analyses, and consent forms are available *(36,51,52)*. This section will only focus on some specific combination vaccine topics.

Clinical efficacy testing of multivalent vaccines to support approval merits specific discussion. Because of the epidemiology of certain diseases, vaccines for these diseases (e.g., *S. pneumoniae* and rotavirus) are likely to be multivalent *(47,53)*. The primary endpoint of efficacy trials for multivalent products is often prevention of disease caused specifically by the serotypes (or serogroups) included in the vaccine. Depending on the epidemiology of the disease, it may also be possible to determine vaccine efficacy with reasonably narrow confidence limits for one or more individual serotypes in the vaccine. However, the clinical importance of preventing disease caused by the homologous vaccine serotypes should be put into perspective. Other outcomes of interest that would be analyzed, at a minimum, as secondary endpoints include prevention of disease caused by all serotypes (vaccine and nonvaccine serotypes), and prevention of a specific type of disease (pneumonia, otitis media, diarrhea, and so forth). While statistical significance may not be achieved for these secondary endpoints, it generally can be agreed upon that the findings should be consistent with a beneficial effect of the vaccine.

Although not a requirement for licensure, one goal of clinical efficacy testing is to identify an immunological correlate(s) of protection (53). Identification of quantitative correlate(s) of protection can make interpretation of data much easier for future studies that are based on assessment of immune responses. Examples include the previously mentioned situation of adding new serotype antigens to an existing vaccine, the interpretation of comparative immune response data to support the efficacy of new formulations or process changes, and the evaluation of immune responses among simultaneously administered vaccines.

Of note, many combination vaccines containing HB vaccine are developed for administration at 2, 4, and 6 months of age (or 2, 4, and 12–15 months of age) for infants who are born to HB surface antigen (HBsAg)-negative mothers. Questions may arise as to whether these vaccines can be used to complete the immunization series in infants who were born to HBsAg-positive mothers or mothers of unknown status, and who received HB vaccine and hyperimmune globulin at birth. Studies should be conducted to evaluate this special population (or cited, if available) if the goal is to include this indication in the labeling.

Simultaneous Use of Other Vaccines

New combination vaccines, especially for pediatric populations, are often administered on the same schedule as other vaccines that are currently licensed. If this is the case, the appropriate licensed vaccines should be administered simultaneously during trials of the new combination vaccine; this is especially relevant for Phase 2 and 3 studies (7) evaluating safety and immunogenicity, and, if applicable, clinical efficacy. Immune response assessments should be performed in statistically valid comparative studies (7) to show that subjects achieve acceptable immune responses to the combination vaccine and the simultaneously administered licensed vaccines. Ideally, such data that demonstrate adequate immune responses (for the new vaccine and simultaneously administered vaccines) should be available prior to proceeding to a large safety (or efficacy) study (7). This should help to avoid situations where large numbers of children need to be "rescued" with additional immunizations using licensed products.

Typically, the pivotal immunogenicity study will use one type of simultaneously administered vaccine per indication. For example, for a new DTaP and IPV vaccine, one type of simultaneously administered Hib conjugate vaccine will be used in the pivotal immunogenicity study *(7)*. The selection of the vaccine to be administered concurrently may be influenced by factors such as use of similar carrier proteins in conjugate vaccines. Data on simultaneous use of a new vaccine with other routinely administered vaccines is an important component of the package insert.

Conclusion

Careful planning will allow the appropriate preclinical, safety, immunogenicity and efficacy data (when applicable) to be obtained in a logical sequence to support licensure of a new combination vaccine in a time-efficient manner.

Acknowledgments

The authors would like to thank Drs. M. Carolyn Hardegree, Norman Baylor, Susan S. Ellenberg, Carl Frasch, and A. Dale Horne for helpful comments and Ms. Karen Chaitkin for her editorial assistance.

References

1. Goldenthal, K. L., Burns, D. L., McVittie, L. D., Lewis, B. P., and Williams, J. C. (1995) Overview—combination vaccines and simultaneous administration. Past, present and future, in *Combined Vaccines and Simultaneous Administration: Current Issues and Perspectives* (Williams, J. C., Goldenthal, K. L., Burns, D. L., and Lewis, B. P., Jr., eds.), *Ann. NY Acad. Sci.* **754,** xi–xv.
2. Mitchell, V. S., Philipose, N. M. and Sanford, J. P., eds. (1993) *The Children's Vaccine Initiative: Achieving the Vision.* Institute of Medicine, National Academy, Washington, DC.
3. Ellis, R. W. and Douglas, R. G., Jr. (1994) New vaccine technologies. *JAMA* **271,** 929–931.
4. Ellis, R. W. and Brown, K. R. (1997) Combination vaccines, in *Advances in Pharmacology* (August, J. T., Anders, M. W., Murad, F., and Coyle, J. T., eds.), Academic, San Diego, pp. 393–423.
5. Centers for Disease Control (1998) Recommended childhood immunization schedule— United States, 1998. *MMWR* **47,** 8–12.
6. Centers for Disease Control (1997) Poliomyelitis prevention in the United States: introduction of a sequential vaccination schedule of inactivated poliovirus vaccine followed by oral poliovirus vaccine. Recommendations of the ACIP. *MMWR* **46,** 1–25.
7. U. S. Food and Drug Administration, Center For Biologics Evaluation and Research. *Guidance for Industry for the Evaluation of Combination Vaccines for Preventable Diseases: Production, Testing and Clinical Studies* (April 1997).
8. Eskola, J., Olander, R. M., Hovi, T., Litmanen, L., Peltola, S., and Kayhty, H. (1996) Randomised trial of the effect of co-administration with acellular pertussis DTP vaccine on immunogenicity of *Haemophilus influenzae* type b conjugate vaccine. *Lancet* **348,** 1688–1692.
9. Greenberg, D. P., Wong, V. K., Partridge, S., Howe, B. J., Jing, J. and Ward, J. I. (1995) Evaluation of a new combination vaccine that incorporates diphtheria-tetanus-acellular pertussis (DTaP), hepatitis B (HB) and *Haemophilus influenzae* type B (Hib) conjugate (PRP-T) vaccines [abstract no. G70], in *Program and abstracts of the 35th Interscience Conference on Antimicrobial Agents and Chemotherapy (San Francisco).* American Society for Microbiology, Washington, DC, p. 170.

10. Schmitt, H. J. (1995) Immunogenicity and reactogenicity of 2 Hib tetanus conjugate vaccines administered by reconstituting with DTPa or given as separate injections [abstract no. G63], in *Program and abstracts of the 35th Interscience Conference on Antimicrobial Agents and Chemotherapy (San Francisco)*. American Society for Microbiology, Washington, DC, p. 169.

11. Shinefield, H., Black, S., Ray, P., Lewis, E., Fireman, B., Hohenboken, M., and Hackell, J. G. (1995) Safety of combined acellular pertussis DTaP-HbOC vaccine (Lederle-Praxis) in infants [abstract no. G72], in *Program and abstracts of the 35th Interscience Conference on Antimicrobial Agents and Chemotherapy (San Francisco, CA)*. American Society for Microbiology, Washington, DC, p. 171.

12. Pichichero, M. E., Latiolais, T., Bernstein, D. I., Hosbach, P., Christian, E., Vidor, E., Meschievitz, C., and Daum, R. S. (1997) Vaccine antigen interactions after a combination diphtheria-tetanus toxoid-acellular pertussis/purified capsular polysaccharide of *Haemophilus influenzae* type b-tetanus toxoid vaccine in two-, four- and six-month-old infants. *Pediatr. Infect. Dis. J.* **16,** 863–870.

13. Ferreccio, C., Clemens, J., Avendano, A., Horwitz, I., Flores, C., Avila, L., Cayazzo, M., Fritzell, B., Cadoz, M., and Levine, M. (1991) The clinical and immunologic response of Chilean infants to *Haemophilus influenzae* type b polysaccharide-tetanus protein conjugate vaccine coadministered in the same syringe with diphtheria-tetanus toxoids-pertussis vaccine at two, four and six months of age. *Pediatr. Infect. Dis. J.* **10,** 764–771.

14. Sawyer, L. A., McInnis, J., Patel, A., Horne, A. D., and Albrecht, P. (1994) Deleterious effect of thimerosal on the potency of inactivated poliovirus vaccine. *Vaccine* **12,** 851–856.

15. Davisson, E. O., Powell, H. M., MacFarlane, J. O., Hodgson, R., Stone, R. L., and Culbertson, C. G. (1956) The preservation of poliomyelitis vaccine with stabilized merthiolate. *J. Lab. Clin. Med.* **47,** 8–19.

16. Pivnick, H., Tracy, J. M., and Glass, D. G. (1963) Studies of preservatives of poliomyelitis (Salk) vaccine I. *JAMA* **52,** 883–888.

17. Pittman, M. (1962) Instability of pertussis-vaccine component in quadruple antigen vaccine. *JAMA* **181,** 25–30.

18. Gardner, R. A. and Pittman, M. (1965) Relative stability of pertussis vaccine preserved with merthiolate, benzethonium chloride, or the parabens. *Appl. Microbiol.* **13,** 564–569.

19. International Conference on Harmonisation (1996) *Draft Guideline for Industry; Quality of Biotechnological Products; Analysis of the Expression Construct in Cells used for Production of r-DNA Derived Protein Products. Fed. Reg.* **61,** 7007–7008.

20. U. S. Food and Drug Administration, Center For Biologics Evaluation and Research (1992) Supplement to the Points To Consider in the production and testing of new drugs and biologics produced by recombinant DNA technology: nucleic acid characterization and genetic stability, 9 pp.

21. U. S. Department of Health and Human Services. U. S. Food and Drug Administration, Center For Biologics Evaluation and Research (1947). *Minimum Requirements: Diphtheria Toxoid,* 7 pp.

22. U. S. Department of Health and Human Services. U. S. Food and Drug Administration, Center for Biologics Evaluation and Research (1952) *Minimum Requirements: Tetanus Toxoid,* 19 pp.

23. Gupta, R. K. and Siber, G. R. (1995) Adjuvants for human vaccines-current status, problems and future prospects. *Vaccine* **13,** 1263–1276.

24. Goldenthal, K. L., Cavagnaro, J. A., Alving, C. R., and Vogel, F. R. (1993) Safety evaluation of vaccine adjuvants. *AIDS Res. Hum. Retrovir.* **9,** S47–S51.

25. International Conference on Harmonisation (1997) Draft guideline on quality of biotechnological/biological products: derivation and characterization of cell substrates used for production of biotechnological/biological products. *Fed. Reg.* **62,** 24,312–24,317.

26. Points to consider in the characterization of cell lines used to produce biologics. (1993) *Fed. Reg.* **58,** 42,974–42,975.

27. Viral and rickettsial vaccines; proposed implementation of efficacy review. (1980) *Fed. Reg.* **45,** 25,652–25,758.

28. Habig, W. H. (1993) Potency testing of bacterial vaccines for human use. *Vet. Microbiol.* **37,** 343–351.

29. U. S. Code of Federal Regulations (1997) Title 21, parts 610. 11 and 610. 14 Washington DC, U. S. Government Printing Office.

30. International Conference on Harmonisation (1996) Draft guideline for industry; quality of biotechnological products: stability testing of biotechnological/biological products. *Fed. Reg.* **61,** 36,466–36,469.

31. Corbel, M. J. (1994) Control testing of combined vaccines: a consideration of potential problems and approaches. *Biologicals* **22,** 353–360.

32. Gupta, R. K., Anderson, R. Cecchini, D., Rost, B., Griffin, Jr., P., Benscoter, K., Xu, J., Montanez-Ortiz, L., and Siber, G. R. (1994) Development of a guinea-pig model for potency/immunogenicity evaluation of diphtheria, tetanus acellular pertussis (DTaP) and *Haemophilus influenzae* type b polysaccharide conjugate vaccine. *Dev. Biol. Stand.* **86,** 283–296.

33. Insel, R. A. (1995) Potential alterations in immunogenicity by combining or simultaneously administering vaccine components, in *Combined Vaccines and Simultaneous Administration: Current Issues and Perspectives* (Williams, J. C., Goldenthal, K. L., Burns, D. L., and Lewis, B. P., Jr., eds.), *Ann. NY Acad. Sci.* **754,** 35–47.

34. Elliot, A. Y. (1995) Manufacturing issues for multivalent vaccines, in *Combined Vaccines and Simultaneous Administration: Current Issues and Perspectives* (Williams, J. C., Goldenthal, K. L., Burns, D. L., and Lewis, B. P., Jr., eds.), *Ann. NY Acad. Sci.* **754,** 23–26.

35. Decker, M. D. and Edwards, K. M. (1995) Issues in design of clinical trials of combination vaccines, in *Combined Vaccines and Simultaneous Administration Current Issues and Perspectives* (Williams, J. C., Goldenthal, K. L., Burns, D. L., and Lewis, B. P., Jr., eds.), *Ann. NY Acad. Sci.* **754,** 234–240.

36. Goldenthal, K. L. and McVittie, L. D. (1997) The clinical testing of preventive vaccines for infectious disease indications, in *Biologics Development: A Regulatory Overview*, 2nd ed. (Mathieu M., ed.), Parexel, Waltham, MA, pp. 123–139.

37. Midthun, K., Horne, A. D., and Goldenthal, K. L. (1998) Clinical safety evaluation of combination vaccines. *Dev. Biol. Stand.,* **95,** 245–249.

38. Black, S. and Shinefield, H. (1995) Comprehensive evaluation of vaccine safety: Assessment of local and systemic side effects as well as emergency and hospital utilization, in *Combined Vaccines and Simultaneous Administration: Current Issues and Perspectives* (Williams, J. C., Goldenthal, K. L., Burns, D. L., and Lewis, B. P., Jr., eds.), *Ann. NY Acad. Sci.* **754,** 364–367.

39. Wassilak, S. G. F., Glasser, J. W., Chen, R. T., Hadler, S. C., and The Vaccine Safety Datalink Investigators (1995) Utility of large-linked databases in vaccine safety, particularly in distinguishing independent and synergistic effects, in *Combined Vaccines and Simultaneous Administration: Current Issues and Perspectives* (Williams, J. C., Goldenthal, K. L., Burns, D. L., and Lewis, B. P., Jr., eds.), *Ann. NY Acad. Sci.* **754,** 377–382.

40. Chen, R. T., Glasser, J. W., Rhodes, P. H., Davis R. L., Barlow, W. E., Thompson, R. S., Mullooly, J. P., Black, S. B., Shinefield, H. R., Vadhein, C. M., Marcy, S. M., Ward, J. I., Wise, R. P., Wassilak, S. G., Hadler, S. C., and the Vaccine Safety Datalink Team (1997) Vaccine safety datalink project: a new tool for improving vaccine safety monitoring in the United States. *Pediatrics* **99,** 765–773.

41. Blackwelder, W. C. (1995) Similarity/equivalence trials for combination vaccines, in *Combined Vaccines and Simultaneous Administration: Current Issues and Perspectives* (Will-

iams, J. C., Goldenthal, K. L., Burns, D. L., and Lewis, B. P., Jr., eds.), *Ann. NY Acad. Sci.* **754,** 321–328.

42. Hanley, J. A. and Lippman-Hand, A. (1983) If nothing goes wrong, is everything all right? Interpreting zero numerators. *JAMA* **249,** 1743–1745.

43. Granoff, D. M. and Rappuoli, R. (1997) Are serological responses to acellular pertussis antigens sufficient criteria to ensure that new combination vaccines are effective for prevention of disease? *Dev. Biol. Stand.* **89,** 379–389.

44. Granoff, D. M. (1996) Challenges for licensure of new diphtheria, tetanus, acellular pertussis (DTaP) combination vaccines: point. *Pediatr. Infect. Dis. J.* **15,** 1069–1070.

45. Edwards, K. M. and Decker, M. D. (1996) Challenges for licensure of new diphtheria, tetanus toxoid, acellular pertussis (DTaP) combination vaccines: counterpoint. *Pediatr. Infect. Dis. J.* **15,** 1070–1073.

46. Zollinger, W. D. (1991) Meningococcal Meningitis, in *Vaccines and Immunotherapy* (Cruz, S. J. Jr., ed.), Pergamon, New York, pp. 113–126.

47. Paradiso, P. R. and Lindberg, A. A. (1996) Glycoconjugate vaccines: future combinations. *Dev. Biol. Stand.* **87,** 269–275.

48. Horne, A. D. and Goldenthal, K. L. *Clinical and Statistical Considerations for Evaluating Preventive Vaccines: Selected Current Topics.* (submitted for publication).

49. Horne, A. D. (1995) The statistical analysis of immunogenicity data in vaccine trials. A review of the methodologies and issues, in *Combined Vaccines and Simultaneous Administration Current Issues and Perspectives* (Williams, J. C., Goldenthal, K. L., Burns, D. L., and Lewis, B. P., Jr., eds.), *Ann. NY Acad. Sci.* **754,** 329–346.

50. Reed, G. F., Meade, B. D., and Steinhoff, M. C. (1995) The reverse cumulative distribution plot: A graphic method for exploratory analysis of antibody data. *Pediatrics* **96(Suppl),** 600–603.

51. O'Neill, R. T. (1988) On sample sizes to estimate the protective efficacy of a vaccine. *Stat. Med.* **7,** 1279–1288.

52. Fast, P. E., Sawyer, L. A., and Wescott, S. L. (1995) Clinical considerations in vaccine trials with special reference to candidate HIV vaccines. *Pharm. Biotechol.* **6,** 97–134.

53. Henchal, L. S., Midthun, K., and Goldenthal, K. L. (1996) Selected regulatory and scientific topics for candidate rotavirus vaccine development. *J. Infect. Dis.* **174(Suppl 1),** S112–S117.

12 Issues for Health Practitioners in the Use of Combination Vaccines

*Kathryn M. Edwards
and Michael D. Decker*

Introduction

For many years, the vaccine schedule for infants and young children in the United States had remained essentially unchanged. Parenteral combination diphtheria and tetanus (DT) toxoids and whole-cell pertussis vaccine had been administered since the late 1940s and oral poliovirus vaccines had been introduced in the 1960s. For over 30 years, parents and health care professionals alike were accustomed to an infant vaccination schedule that required a single parenteral injection at 2, 4, and 6 months of age. Then, in the late 1980s, the *Haemophilus influenzae* type *b* (Hib) vaccines were found to be effective and were routinely recommended, first for toddlers and later for infants, increasing the number of parenteral injections to two for each of the scheduled infant vaccination visits. When targeted immunization programs for hepatitis B (HB) in the early 1990s did not prove effective in reducing rates of hepatitis B among selected high-risk populations, routine immunization of all infants with hepatitis B vaccine was endorsed. With this change, three injections were needed at each visit at 2, 4, and 6 months of age. Most recently, with the recommendation in 1997 that the first two doses of oral poliovirus vaccine (OPV) be replaced with parenteral enhanced inactivated poliovirus vaccine (IPV) to reduce the possibility of vaccine-acquired paralytic polio (VAPP), the number of injections delivered at routine infant visits increased to four. Parents and practitioners expressed concern that children had become "pincushions," *(1)* and indeed, resistance in the community to the IPV recommendation was engendered more by concern over increasing the number of injections than by fundamental disagreement with the strategy of sequential IPV-OPV. Moreover, numerous other vaccines suitable for infants

From: *Combination Vaccines: Development, Clinical Research, and Approval*
Edited by: R. W. Ellis © Humana Press Inc., Totowa, NJ

and children are under development or becoming available, suggesting that the problem of vaccination schedule congestion and multiple injections may not pass quickly.

In this chapter, the practical considerations for the development and use of combination vaccines will be the focus. Some of the unique difficulties which combination vaccines pose in the development and licensure process will be briefly reviewed; suggestions on how practitioners can deal with an ever-increasing supply of combination products from different manufacturers will be provided; practical concerns with the use of combination vaccines, such as interchangeability, delivery of unneeded antigens, and tracking of immunization status will be discussed; and the various social, economic, and scientific issues that should guide selection of vaccine candidates to be licensed will be addressed. For example, could the lack of currently licensed multivalent combination products interfere with the timely immunization of children? Is it appropriate to license combination products of somewhat reduced immunogenicity? Are such reductions relevant to clinical protection? If they are, is some reduction in protection an acceptable tradeoff in order to avoid a deterioration in immunization rates associated with the refusal to administer multiple vaccines at the same visit? Finally, practical suggestions for implementation of the use of combination vaccines in individual physicians' practices will be given.

It should be noted that the term "combination vaccines" in this chapter refers to multidisease combinations and not to multivalent combinations directed against the same pathogen.

The Need for Combination Vaccines

One simple but ultimately self-defeating strategy to reduce the number of injections given at a single visit is to defer one or more injections until another clinic visit. However, Ball and Serwint recently demonstrated that deferring one or more immunizations until another visit, termed an "acknowledged missed opportunity," resulted in 25% of the deferred children never returning for the indicated vaccine (2). The measles epidemic of 1989–1991 demonstrated that "missed opportunities" for vaccine delivery resulted in poor immunization rates against measles and led to uncontrolled disease (3). Clearly, the best solution to overcome the resistance of parents and providers to the large number of injections required at a single immunization visit is to combine multiple antigens into a single parenteral vaccine.

The administration of multiple vaccine antigens to the global birth cohort of 125 million children has been recognized to be of intense international interest. The Children's Vaccine Initiative (CVI) was established at the World Summit for Children in New York City in 1990 (4). Endorsed by multiple governmental and policy-making bodies, the CVI advanced the view that the ideal vaccine would consist of a single dose (preferably oral) containing multiple antigens, effective when administered near birth, heat-stable, and affordable to the world's children. The Institute of Medicine supported the complete participation of the United States in the CVI in 1993 *(5)*. Currently, the CVI is working closely with the World Health Organization (WHO) Global Programme for Vaccines and Immunization and with the United Nations International Children's Emergency Fund (UNICEF) to propose solutions to some of the obstacles identified in the generation of combination vaccines. In concert with developmental agencies, governments, donors, commercial and public sector vaccine manufacturers, vaccine researchers, and national immunization program managers, the CVI is attempting to facilitate production of combination vaccines for all of the world's children. The long-term goal of the CVI is the administration of a mucosal vaccine that would eliminate the necessity of parenteral injections, but this goal is acknowledged to be one that is not attainable in the short term. The short-term solution to the problem of multiple injections is the development and use of combination parenteral vaccines, in which multiple vaccine antigens are combined in a single vial or syringe.

History

The combining of several related or unrelated antigens into a single product is not a new idea; combination vaccines have long been the backbone of our pediatric and adult immunization programs. Combination vaccines commonly used include diphtheria and tetanus toxoids, produced alone (DT or Td) or with whole-cell (DTP) or acellular (DTaP) pertussis vaccine; trivalent inactivated or live attenuated oral poliovirus vaccine (OPV); and measles and rubella vaccine, produced alone (MR) or with mumps vaccine (MMR). In November 1945, the first combination vaccine was licensed in the United States, the trivalent influenza vaccine *(6)*. The second combination product was a hexavalent pneumococcal vaccine, licensed in 1947 *(6)*. Although DTP was developed in 1943, it was not licensed until March 1948. IPV was licensed in 1955, and the individual OPV serotypes were licensed in 1961–62. Difficulties in overcoming the interference seen when three live vaccines were administered simultaneously delayed licensure of trivalent OPV until June 1963. MMR and MR were licensed in April 1971, and quadrivalent meningococcal vaccine in 1978. Combination vaccines currently under development incorporate newer components such as conjugate *Haemophilus influenzae* type *b* (Hib), acellular pertussis (aP), or hepatitis B (HB) antigens. Vaccine manufacturers are developing additional combination vaccines that protect against many more pathogens, in keeping with the ultimate goal of combining all the antigens recommended for routine immunization into a single multivalent product *(see Table 1)*.

Table 1. Pediatric Combination Vaccines Presently Licensed or Under Development[a]

| Combination vaccine[b] | Producers or vendors of licensed vaccines | | Under development[c] |
	Licensed in US	Licensed outside US	
Td/IPV		PMC-Fr, PMC-Ca	
DT/IPV		PMC-Ca	
DT/HB		PMC-Fr	
DTP/IPV		PMC-Ca, PMC-Fr	
DTP/Hib	PMC-US, WL	PMC-Ca, PMC-Fr, SB, WL	
DTP/Hib/IPV		PMC-Ca, PMC-Fr	
DTP/HB		SB	
DTP/Hib/HB		SB	Yes
DTaP/IPV		NAVA, PMC-Ca, PMC-Fr, SB	
DTaP/Hib	PMC-US[d]	PMC-Fr, SB	Yes
DTaP/IPV/Hib		PMC-Ca, PMC-Fr, SB	Yes
DTaP/HB		SB	
DTaP/IPV/HB			Yes
DTaP/Hib/HB			Yes
DTaP/Hib/IPV/HB			Yes
DTaP/Hib/IPV/HB/HA			Yes
HB/Hib	Merck		
HB/HA		SB	
MMR-V			Yes
PnC/MnC			Yes
PnC/MnC/Hib			Yes

Abbreviations: aP, acellular pertussis vaccine; D, diphtheria toxoid vaccine; HA, hepatitis A vaccine; HB, hepatitis B vaccine; Hib, conjugate *Haemophilus influenzae* type *b* vaccine; IPV, enhanced inactivated trivalent poliovirus vaccine; MMR-V, measles, mumps, rubella, and varicella vaccine; MnC, meningococcal conjugate vaccine; NAVA, North American Vaccine; P, whole-cell pertussis vaccine; PMC, Pasteur Mérieux Connaught (Ca, Canada; Fr, France; US, USA); PnC, pneumococcal conjugate vaccine; SB, SmithKline Beecham; T, tetanus toxoid vaccine; WL, Wyeth Lederle Vaccines and Pediatrics.

[a]Products combining only multiple serotypes of a single pathogen are excluded, as are DT, DTP, DTaP, OPV, IPV, and MMR. Only those manufacturers who distribute their products globally are listed; other manufacturers may produce some products (e.g., DTP/IPV) for local or regional use. Some products represent components derived from, or joint efforts of, more than one manufacturer; in such cases, their principal distributor is shown.

[b]No discrimination is made between products distributed in combined form and those distributed in separate containers, for combination at the time of use.

[c]Indicated vaccines may be under development by more than one company.

[d]Licensed for the fourth (booster) dose only (as of July 1998).

Development and Licensure of Combination Vaccines

Background

Customarily, each of the individual vaccines comprising a candidate combination product has been previously licensed, either as a separate product or as part of a simpler combination, based on data demonstrating its safety, immunogenicity, and efficacy. For a new combination vaccine to be licensed, there must be confidence that the new combination will not be substantially more reactive, less immunogenic, or less efficacious than the simpler, previously accepted product (7–9).

For most combination vaccines, safety studies of moderate size have not found that giving the vaccines in combination resulted in increased local or systemic reactions compared to giving the same antigens separately (10,11). Maintaining immunogenicity has been more challenging; it has not been uncommon to find that one or more components of a candidate combination vaccine induced significantly lower levels of antibody compared to the same components given alone (12,13). However, in the past such problems almost always have been overcome by further development work, often involving adjustment of the relative proportions of each component or changes in "inactive" components of the vaccine. For example, decreased immunogenicity has been noted with products combining DTaP and conjugate Hib vaccines, delaying the licensure of these combination vaccines for use in infants in the United States (although they have been licensed in Canada and elsewhere) (11). Similar problems are being addressed by the developers of MMR-varicella combinations.

Typically, separate efficacy trials have not been required for licensure of candidate combination products; rather, licensure has been granted based on demonstration of immunogenicity comparable to that of the components given individually (or in previously licensed combinations). Such licensure decisions would seem to be relatively straightforward for vaccines with established correlations between serologic responses and protection, such as hepatitis A (HA), HB, and Hib, but difficulties do arise. For example, what should be done when the immunogenicity of a component is sharply reduced when given in combination, yet antibody responses nonetheless remain above protective levels? When recently faced with such a situation involving a DTaP-Hib combination, the Food and Drug Administration (FDA) declined to grant licensure for infant use, despite the fact that the combination produced mean Hib antibody levels that equalled or exceeded those produced by another licensed Hib vaccine (14–16). There is no doubt that the FDA and the advisory bodies must be assured that a candidate combination vaccine will not afford less protection against disease than the licensed component vaccines administered separately. However, it is equally important that licensure of combination vaccines not be denied because of reduced immunogenicity that has no biologic relevance. The requiring of efficacy trials in such situations is not likely to be a viable solution; given the high cost of such trials, manufacturers might well elect to forego the combination vaccine and focus on marketing their already licensed component vaccines.

Evaluation of Combination Products

Trials of combination vaccines should be prospective, randomized, double-blinded, and have appropriate comparison (control) groups (7–9). Defining the comparison arms can be difficult when evaluating a multicomponent vaccine. If no previous data are available and if one wishes to determine reduced immunogenicity of any component in the combination vaccine, the number of study arms required for complete evaluation of an n-component vaccine is 2^n, based on the possible combinations alone. Moreover, other variables may further increase the number of study arms required. For example, the order of administration of certain antigens may play an important role in immunogenicity. It has been shown that the response to some Hib vaccines may depend on previous or concurrent administration of DTP. Evaluation of such factors may require study arms that receive the antigens in different sequences.

Another complicating aspect is that decreased antibody levels to one component of a combination vaccine could be due to interactions that would happen even if the antigens were injected at different sites during the same visit. They might be a result of chemical or physical interactions that occur only when the antigens are combined in a single injection; the need to differentiate these two possibilities would require more study arms. Ethical concerns also may complicate study design, because vaccines that are recommended for routine use in the study population cannot be withheld in order to study vaccine interactions, although they could be administered at intervening visits.

The complex issues of evaluating the combination products are further increased by the availability of multiple vaccine preparations designed for protection against the same pathogen. Although this concern does not increase the number of arms required for study of one particular combination vaccine, it remarkably increases the number of potential combination vaccines to be evaluated. Considering only the three Hib conjugate vaccines, two HB vaccines, and three acellular pertussis vaccines presently licensed in the United States for use in infancy, there could, in theory, be as many as 18 DTaP/Hib/HB combination vaccines. Each such combination would be unique: demonstration that one combination performed as well as its component antigens given singly would be no assurance that any other combination would behave in a similar way.

With all of these factors contributing to increase the number of study arms in combination vaccine trials, what approaches could be used to ease these design problems and enable studies of reasonable size *(7–9)*? Multicenter studies allow larger numbers of patients and more study arms to be evaluated than would be feasible at a single institution. When the trial is appropriately designed with standardized protocols, this can be an effective way to evaluate multiple vaccines or multicomponent products, as shown by the Multicenter Acellular Pertussis Trial (MAPT) *(17)*. The Swedish and Italian DTaP efficacy trials, with their coordinated protocols and control vaccines provide another excellent example *(18,19)*.

One straightforward and attractive solution to the combination vaccine study design dilemma is to ensure that earlier studies have laid an appropriate foundation for study of a combination vaccine, by evaluating predecessor vaccines that differ from the new combination only by lacking a single component *(7–9)*. A study then can compare the new combination to its predecessor plus the new component, given separately. An alternative solution is to compare the new combination against each of its components given alone, deferring study of the sub-combinations in the hope that no interference will be observed.

Finally, it may be possible to streamline study of a combination vaccine by administering a previously studied vaccine to one of the comparison arms in order to allow comparison of the current results to those obtained in an earlier study. This bridging technique has been used in the Swedish acellular pertussis efficacy trials to compare the results from each trial *(18,20,21)*. The risks of this approach can be decreased through cooperative efforts to assure the comparability of serologic and reaction data gathered for similar vaccines in separate studies. With sufficient standardization, inclusion of a previous study arm as a comparison arm in the current study could allow comparison with the results obtained in the other arms of the prior study.

Interchangeability of Combination Products

When multiple combination vaccines are available from several different manufacturers, practitioners will question whether the vaccines can be used interchangeably *(22)*. This question can be difficult to answer even for monocomponent vaccines. Definitive answers for each of the different multicomponent vaccines will be nearly impossible. For example, several years ago a study was conducted to evaluate interchangeability of the three conjugate Hib vaccines indicated for the infant primary series *(23)*. Of the 27 theoretically possible permutations of three vaccines and three injections, five were evaluated. It was reassuring that all of the sequential combinations evaluated generated antibody responses that equalled or exceeded those produced by giving a single vaccine for all three doses. However, one alternative that was not evaluated has recently become relevant. PRP-OMPC was selected as the predominant

Hib vaccine in the Vaccines for Children program in 1998, making it probable that, early in the year, some children received PRP-OMPC for their third dose after having been given another vaccine for the first two doses. Despite the lack of data regarding the immunogenicity of this specific regimen, there is little doubt of its acceptability. However, this circumstance illustrates how restricted are our abilities to completely investigate all questions of interchangeability. Once we are faced with multiple, distinct DTaP, DTaP/Hib, DTaP/Hib/IPV (and so on) vaccines, the likelihood shrinks that any particular substitution will have been explicitly studied. Indeed, it has been suggested that the cost of evaluating all potential schedules using several different combination vaccines from different manufacturers would be $5–15 billion (24).

The evaluation of the interchangeability of combination vaccines produced by different manufacturers is further complicated by the fact that manufacturers may be reluctant to evaluate the products of other companies for liability reasons, or may believe that demonstration of the interchangeability of various vaccines might decrease their share of that market. Thus, funding for the conduct of these "mix-and-match" studies may not be viewed as a high priority by the manufacturers. Nonetheless, this is an important topic, and it is to be hoped that the National Institutes of Health (NIH) and others will continue to fund studies of vaccine interchangeability. Lack of such data can have unfortunate consequences. First, as noted previously, a vaccination deferred often becomes a vaccination missed; any deferral owing to unavailability of, or confusion regarding, the vaccines previously administered is to be deplored. Second, an inability to interchange vaccines may lead to exclusive purchase of vaccines from only one company and discourage competition among the vaccine manufacturers. This would be regrettable, because competition provides an incentive to improve the products and assures that the vaccine supply of the nation is not dependent on a single source.

Recommendations

In this day of bulk vaccine purchase through competitive bidding by large health maintenance organizations (HMOs) and the government, it is unrealistic to presume that the same vaccine will always be available for each child at the time of each vaccination. The situation is further complicated by the fact that 25% of children see at least two different health care providers during the course of their vaccination series, and that the average time for a child to remain in a publicly funded health-care plan is 10 months. Different practitioners are likely to stock different combination vaccines. Although each office practice or clinic must maintain a suitable selection of vaccines in order to comply with the current recommended United States vaccination schedule (Fig. 1), it is neither feasible nor necessary to stock all brands of each type of licensed monovalent or combination vaccine.

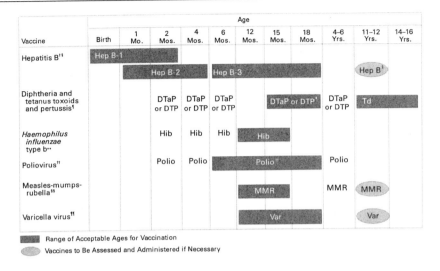

Fig. 1. Recommended childhood immunization schedule–United States, January–December 1998. Reprinted from *Recommended Childhood Immunization Schedule—United States, 1998*. MMWR 1998;47:8–12.

*This schedule indicates the recommended age for routine administration of currently licensed childhood vaccines; vaccines are listed under the ages for which they are routinely recommended. Catch-up immunization should be done during any visit when feasible. Some combination vaccines are available and may be used whenever administration of all components of the vaccine is indicated. Providers should consult the manufacturers' package inserts for detailed recommendations.

† Infants born to hepatitis B surface antigen (HBsAg)-negative mothers should receive 2.5 m g of Merck vaccine (Recombivax HB ®) or 10 m g of SmithKline Beecham (SB) vaccine (Engerix-B ®). The second dose should be administered at least 1 month after the first dose. The third dose should be administered at least 2 months after the second but not before 6 months of age. Infants born to HBsAg-positive mothers should receive 0.5 mL hepatitis B immune globulin (HBIG) within 12 hours of birth, and either 5 m g of Merck vaccine (Recombivax HB ®) or 10 mg of SB vaccine (Engerix-B ®) at a separate site. The second dose is recommended at age 1–2 months and the third dose at age 6 months. Infants born to mothers whose HBsAg status is unknown should receive either 5 m g of Merck vaccine (Recombivax HB ®) or 10 m g of SB vaccine (Engerix-B ®) within 12 hours of birth. The second dose of vaccine is recommended at age 1 month and the third dose at age 6 months. Blood should be drawn at the time of delivery to determine the mother's HBsAg status; if it is positive, the infant should receive HBIG as soon as possible (no later than age 1 week). The dosage and timing of subsequent vaccine doses should be based on the mother's HBsAg status.§ Children and adolescents who have not been vaccinated against hepatitis B in infancy may begin the series during any visit. Those who have not previously received three doses of hepatitis B vaccine should initiate or complete the series during the routine visit to a health-care provider at age 11–12 years, and unvaccinated older adolescents should be vaccinated whenever possible. The second dose should be administered at least 1 month after the first dose, and the third dose should be administered at least 4 months after the first dose and at least 2 months after the second dose.¶ Diphtheria and tetanus toxoids and acellular pertussis vaccine (DTaP) is the preferred vaccine for all doses in the vaccination series, including completion of the series in children who have received one or more doses of whole-cell diphtheria and tetanus toxoids and pertussis vaccine

(DTP). Whole-cell DTP is an acceptable alternative to DTaP. The fourth dose (DTP or DTaP) may be administered as early as age 12 months, provided 6 months have elapsed since the third dose and if the child is unlikely to return at age 15–18 months. Tetanus and diphtheria toxoids, adsorbed, for adult use (Td), is recommended at age 11–12 years if at least 5 years have elapsed since the last dose of DTP, DTaP, or diphtheria and tetanus toxoids, adsorbed, for pediatric use (DT). Subsequent routine Td boosters are recommended every 10 years.

** Three Haemophilus influenzae type b (Hib) conjugate vaccines are licensed for infant use. If Haemophilus b conjugate vaccine (meningococcal protein conjugate) (PRP-OMP) (PedvaxHIB ® [Merck]) is administered at ages 2 and 4 months, a dose at age 6 months is not required.

†† Two poliovirus vaccines are currently licensed and distributed in the United States: inactivated poliovirus vaccine (IPV) and oral poliovirus vaccine (OPV). The following schedules are all acceptable to the ACIP, AAP, and AAFP. Parents and providers may choose among these options: 1) two doses of IPV followed by two doses of OPV; 2) four doses of IPV; or 3) four doses of OPV. ACIP recommends two doses of IPV at ages 2 and 4 months followed by a dose of OPV at age 12–18 months and at age 4–6 years. IPV is the only poliovirus vaccine recommended for immunocompromised persons and their household contacts.

§§ The second dose of measles-mumps-rubella vaccine (MMR) is recommended routinely at age 4–6 years but may be administered during any visit, provided at least 1 month has elapsed since receipt of the first dose and that both doses are administered beginning at or after age 12 months. Those who have not previously received the second dose should complete the schedule no later than the routine visit to a health-care provider at age 11–12 years.

¶¶ Susceptible children may receive varicella vaccine (Var) at any visit after the first birthday, and those who lack a reliable history of chickenpox should be vaccinated during the routine visit to a health-care provider at age 11–12 years. Susceptible children aged ≥13 years should receive two doses at least 1 month apart.

The Advisory Committee on Immunization Practices (ACIP) has recognized certain vaccines as interchangeable, including DTP (and its individual components), IPV, OPV, and HB *(25)*. The conjugate Hib vaccines are also considered interchangeable, as long as three doses are given (although recent reports of increased Hib colonization and disease in Alaska may support a preference for initiating Hib immunization with PRP-OMPC in that population, with its exceptionally high risk of invasive Hib disease) *(26,27)*.

For those vaccines lacking data regarding interchangeability of licensed products, such as DTaP *(28)* and the newer combination vaccines *(22)*, the ACIP has recommended that the same product be used throughout the primary series. However, if the identity of the product previously used is not known, or if the product is not available at the time of the child's visit, then any licensed product appropriate to the child's immunization status and requirements may be used. The authors concur strongly. Although specific data would be desirable, we know of no reason to anticipate that interchange of vaccines would produce a less than satisfactory outcome, and the imperative remains: do not miss a vaccination opportunity.

Ad-Hoc Combinations

Providers should not produce extemporaneous combination vaccines by mixing separate vaccines in the same syringe absent published evidence establishing the stability, safety, and immunogenicity of the resultant combination (and if there were such evidence, one would expect it to be reflected in the package inserts).

Alternative Backbones for Combination Vaccines

The preceding discussion of interchangeability implicitly presumed that the vaccines to be interchanged contained similar antigens. However, it is clear that the market will offer combination vaccines based on various "backbones." For example, both DTaP/Hib and HB/Hib combinations are presently on the market. If any DTaP/Hib combinations become licensed for infant use, then one practice might stock a Hib-HB combination and monovalent vaccines for IPV and DTaP, whereas another routinely used a DTaP-Hib combination along with monovalent IPV and HB vaccines. Complications will escalate as more antigens are added to these combinations. These inconsistencies pose questions not only for children who change providers, but also within a single practice. Consider, for example, a practice that immunizes children at birth for HB and that wishes to make use of the Hib-HB combination thereafter to reduce needlesticks. If a child is given HB at birth and the Hib-HB combination (containing PRP-OMPC) at 2 months of age, must they be given PRP-OMPC as a single agent at 4 months of age, or can they again be given the Hib-HB combination (even though they do not require another dose of HB at this time)?

Extra Doses of Vaccine

As new vaccines become available that combine different antigens, physicians increasingly will discover that the least complicated (and even, the most economical) alternative will be to use a combination vaccine that will deliver an antigen that the patient has already received in the recommended quantity and timing for their age. Fortunately, for many vaccine antigens it has been shown that an extra dose may be given without adverse effects. In fact, Hib, IPV, HB, and most live viral vaccines are of low reactogenicity, and administration of superfluous doses has not been found to be problematic (22). There are some antigens for which increased local reactions are seen with too-frequent administration; diphtheria toxoid, tetanus toxoid, and pneumococcal polysaccharide vaccines are among the most prominent in this category (29–31). However, given current combination vaccine development efforts, it is unlikely to be necessary to give these particular antigens with undue frequency; rather, it will be the low-reactogenicity antigens that occasionally will be administered superfluously.

It appears likely that the ACIP will support the use of a combination vaccine containing some antigens that are not necessary at that time for the child, when products that contain only the needed antigens are not readily available or their use would result in extra injections *(22)*. We concur with this approach.

Cost Considerations

Most of the newer vaccines, such as DTaP and Hib conjugate, are more expensive to produce than DTP, OPV, and other traditional vaccines. Although costs will not limit the use of these vaccines in the United States, it is a major concern in some parts of the world. For example, DTP is produced locally at low cost in many countries, and its replacement with DTaP would not be a sensible use of healthcare resources. On the other hand, some other relatively expensive vaccines, such as HB or Hib, offer such clear benefits that they are being used in many developing countries. If a country has decided to use, e.g., Hib conjugate vaccine, it is probable that a combination that also provides other, relatively inexpensive, antigens (e.g., a DTP/IPV/Hib combination) can be purchased for less than the cost of purchasing the component vaccines individually. Furthermore, use of such a combination vaccine would offer additional savings in administration costs, by decreasing the number of products that must be stored, shipped, tracked, and injected.

Safety Concerns

Some parents groups concerned with vaccine adverse reactions have been critical of the administration of multiple vaccine antigens simultaneously and have suggested that doing so is unsafe. However, reviews of the reactions associated with simultaneous administration of multiple antigens have demonstrated a remarkable safety record *(10)*. Nonetheless, as new combination vaccines are licensed it will be necessary for practitioners to be diligent about reporting adverse events. Before administering a subsequent dose of any vaccine, practitioners should inquire about adverse events associated with the previous vaccination. Since prelicensure studies cannot uncover all contingencies, it is important that adverse reactions or deviations from the expected responses to all newly developed and licensed vaccines be promptly reported. Unexpected events occurring soon after vaccination, especially if severe enough to require medical attention, always should be reported.

The Vaccine Adverse Event Reporting System (VAERS)

The National Childhood Vaccine Injury Act requires health care providers and manufacturers to report serious adverse events after vaccination to the Department of Health and Human Services (DHHS). DHHS has directed that the

Vaccine Adverse Event Reporting System (VAERS) *(32)* be established to provide a single system for collection and analysis of reports of all adverse events associated with vaccine. DHHS has determined that the CDC and the FDA implement VAERS. In November 1990, VAERS became fully functional for reporting vaccine adverse events in the country. Certain events were mandated for reporting, such as encephalopathy after DTP or MMR, or paralytic polio after OPV. Persons also were encouraged to report all other clinically significant adverse events following the administration of any licensed vaccine in all age groups, on the possibility that the adverse event might be causally associated with the vaccination. The written VAERS report is designed to permit description of the adverse event, the type of vaccine received, the timing of the vaccination and the adverse event, demographic information about the recipient, concurrent medical illnesses or medication, and the prior history of adverse events following vaccine. The form is preaddressed and postage-paid and is mailed directly to VAERS. These forms are mailed each year to those physicians likely to administer vaccines. In addition, a 24-hour toll-free telephone number is available to answer questions, to provide additional forms, or to assist in completing the forms. The adverse events are assigned a code, similar to the International Classification of Diseases (ICD) code, and entered into a computer data base. A letter of receipt is sent to the reporter and follow-up clinical status is determined at 60 days and one year after the report.

Once the VAERS data are entered into the computer database, they are reviewed by teams of investigators, including pharmacists, physicians, and statisticians. Reports that are serious, including death, permanent disability, hospitalization, prolongation of hospitalization, or life-threatening events are given additional attention. The data are monitored continually to detect clusters of events by vaccine type, manufacturer, and lot of vaccine. Reports may trigger additional investigation. Unfortunately, since the VAERS reports are nonrandom clinical reports, they are useful for generating hypotheses but not for testing them. Large, linked databases may be able to provide the data needed to test hypotheses of causation after an association is noted by VAERS. Health care providers perform an important function by reporting all clinically significant adverse events to VAERS, particularly as they relate to new combination vaccine products.

Improving Immunization Records

As the number and variety of combination vaccines proliferates, it becomes increasingly unlikely that a practitioner will be able to deduce the precise vaccination history of a new patient by parental history alone. Parents often do not bring immunization records with them at the time of scheduled appointment. In one reported survey, 73% of the children attending a public clinic did not have their immunization records available at the time of the clinic visit *(33)*. In repeated attempts to obtain records on these children, records could never be found for 11% of the children. Although legislation has mandated since March 1988 that medical records of vaccination should contain the identity of the vaccine manufacturer, the date of administration, and the lot number of the vaccine given, the completeness and accuracy of these data still remain a problem *(34)*. A recent study compared the actual vaccine data recorded in the patients' medical record with what was recorded in the computerized data base and found the 40% of the records did not agree *(35)*. The optimal solution would be a national vaccination history database, which not only would provide practitioners with individual vaccination histories and health planners with a comprehensive measure of the vaccination status of the community, but also would greatly facilitate postmarketing surveillance of vaccine efficacy and safety. The implementation of such a system awaits increased governmental funding and continued assurance that the confidentiality of the patient can be maintained. One possible way to achieve this system would be by access via a computer card or vaccine credit card that the parent would have with them at all times. Such a system was recently reported to provide up-to-date immunization information at each clinic visit for 80% of the participants in the pilot program *(36)*.

Pending availability of one large centralized database for all, postmarketing surveillance and evaluation of vaccine use can be facilitated by use of the large linked pharmacy, provider, and hospital databases maintained by some commercial healthcare organizations or the integrated data information systems of some states' Medicaid programs.

Methods also are needed to improve the accuracy and convenience of recording and transferring vaccine information from the vaccine vial to the medical record. Particularly difficult are the names of the combination products that differ in only one or two syllables. One attractive alternative to copying the information from the vaccine package to the chart would be detachable stickers, indicating the type and lot of the vaccines, that could simply be peeled off and attached to the patient's chart. Another attractive alternative would be to include machine-readable bar codes on each dose of vaccine, which could be read into a centralized vaccination system to facilitate electronic transfer of information. The ability to monitor immunization programs for vaccine safety, coverage, and efficacy is of paramount importance to the vaccination program in this country. Such monitoring requires the ability to determine which vaccine was administered to each child. However, VAERS and the Vaccine Safety Dataline, an active surveillance system, have detected error rates exceeding 10% in recording of vaccine information *(22)*. If we are to maintain public confidence in our vaccination system, accurate records are needed and must be the focus of continued efforts.

Preference for Combination Vaccines

The ultimate goal of immunization is the eradication of disease, while the immediate goal is the prevention of disease. There are three central issues to attaining these goals: maintaining timely immunization, conducting intensive disease surveillance, and instituting vaccination and treatment in the face of identified outbreaks of disease. Recent surveys of healthcare providers suggest that they do not like to administer multiple injections of different vaccine antigens at one visit *(1,37–40)*. Many defer one or more injections for a later visit; this practice obviously interferes with the timely immunization of children. In addition, each vaccine deferral increases the likelihood that when the child returns, invalid contraindications to vaccination will prohibit immunizations. Such invalid contraindications include a mild acute illness, such as upper respiratory infections, otitis media, or diarrhea; current antimicrobial therapy or the convalescent phase of an illness; recent exposure to an infectious disease; pregnancy of the mother or other household contact; breast-feeding; a history of nonspecific allergies; or a history of relatives with adverse reactions to vaccine components *(41)*. In fact, reviews of contraindications to vaccinations indicate that only 4% of the contraindications to vaccination listed in the physicians' records were definite; the remainder of the contraindications were not valid and contributed to untimely vaccination *(41)*. The opportunity to administer multiple antigens at a single visit circumvents the problems associated with deferred immunizations and the attendant risks of missed opportunities.

From the parental point of view, the major barriers to timely immunization include cost, employment conflicts, lack of transportation, difficulty understanding the complex vaccination schedules, failure to recognize the importance of the disease being prevented, forgetting appointments, and inflexible office schedules with long waits *(42)*. Administration of combinations that deliver multiple vaccines at the same visit will eliminate many of these concerns.

Harmonized Vaccination Schedules

There are three bodies that are prominent in offering vaccination recommendations: the Red Book Committee of the American Academy of Pediatrics (AAP), the ACIP of the Centers for Disease Control (CDC), and the American Academy of Family Practitioners (AAFP). Happily, in recent years these three groups have coordinated their recommendations so as to produce a harmonized recommended childhood vaccination schedule for the United States. The harmonized schedule is published each January in the medical journals of the AAP, AAFP, and CDC (and reprinted widely), reaching the majority of health care providers *(26)*. The 1998 schedule *(Fig. 1)* differs from the 1997 schedule in offering further flexibility in timing of certain vaccinations: the first OPV dose in the sequential IPV-IPV-OPV-OPV regimen now can be given beginning at 6 months and the second dose of MMR at 4–6 years of age. Increased attention is given to the visit at age 11–12, to ensure that two doses of MMR have been administered as well as HB and varicella vaccine.

The Future

Barry Bloom stated, "There are few fields in all of biomedical science in which the reciprocity between basic and applied science is as great as it is in immunology and vaccines. The realization that one can study basic principles of immunology equally well using HIV, leishmania, or any antigens derived from pathogens represents a paradigm shift that effectively blurs the distinction between basic and applied research and brings a new appreciation that everyone has something to contribute. We will be increasingly dependent on knowledge of basic science, mechanisms of pathogenesis, mechanisms and thresholds of protection, and ultimately on the development of new and useful surrogate end points for protection. Reciprocally, the development and testing of new candidate vaccines and vehicles will undoubtedly generate new knowledge about human immune function and capability that cannot be gleaned in any other way"(43).

Given the explosion in the knowledge of basic immunology and pathogenesis of infectious disease in the past decade, it is difficult to know what vaccines will be developed and what novel methods of delivery will be available in the years ahead. However, by fostering collaboration between basic scientists and clinical researchers and by continuing support for basic and clinical research, we can continue to work toward the goal of comprehensive immunization of the world's children with one safe, effective, and affordable vaccination.

References

1. Woodin, K. A., Rodewald, L. E., Humiston, S. G., Carges, M. S., Schaffer, S. J., and Szilagyi, P. G. (1995) Physician and parent opinions: are children becoming pincushions from immunizations? *Arch Pediatr. Adolesc. Med.* **149,** 845–849.
2. Ball, T. M. and Serwint, J. R. (1996) Missed opportunities for vaccination and the delivery of preventive care. *Arch Pediatr. Adolesc. Med.* **150,** 858–861.
3. National Vaccine Advisory Committee (1991) The measles epidemic. *JAMA* **266,** 1547–1552.
4. Children's vaccine initiative [news] (1992) World Health Forum **13,** 93.
5. Mitchell, V. S., Philipose, N. M., and Sanford, J. S. (1993) *The Children's Vaccine Initiative: Achieving the Vision.* National Academy Press, Washington, DC, 221 pp.
6. Grabenstein, J. D. (1995) *Immunofacts: Vaccines and Immunologic Drugs.* Facts and Comparisons, St. Louis.
7. Edwards, K. M. and Decker, M. D. (1994) Combination vaccines: hopes and challenges. *Pediatr. Infect. Dis. J.* **13,** 345–347.
8. Decker, M. D. and Edwards, K. M. (1995) Issues in design of clinical trials of combination vaccines, in *Combined Vaccines and Simultaneous Administration: Current Issues and*

Perspectives (Williams, J. C., Goldenthal, K. L., Burns, D. L., and Lewis, B. P. Jr, eds.) *Ann. NY Acad. Sci.* **754**, 234–240.

9. Edwards, K. M. and Decker, M. D. (1997) Combination vaccines consisting of acellular pertussis vaccines. *Pediatr. Infect. Dis. J.* **16(4 Suppl)**, S97–S102.

10. King, G. E. and Hadler, S. C. (1994) Simultaneous administration of childhood vaccines: an important public health policy that is safe and efficacious. *Pediatr. Infect. Dis.* **13**, 394–407.

11. Decker, M. D. and Edwards, K. M. Combination vaccines, in *Vaccines*, 3rd ed. (Plotkin and Orenstein), in press.

12. Gold, R., Scheifele, D., Barreto, L., Wiltsey, S., Bjornson, G., Meekison, W., Guasparini, R., and Medd, L. (1994) Safety and immunogenicity of *Haemophilus influenzae* vaccine (tetanus toxoid conjugate) administered concurrently or combined with diphtheria and tetanus toxoids, pertussis vaccine and inactivated poliomyelitis vaccine to healthy infants at two, four and six months of age. *Pediatr. Infect. Dis. J.* **13**, 348–355.

13. Baker, J. D., Halperin, S. A., Edwards, K., Miller, B., Decker, M., and Stephens, D. (1992) Antibody response to *Bordetella pertussis* antigens after immunization with American and Canadian whole-cell vaccines. *J. Pediatr.* **121**, 523–527.

14. Decker, M. D., Edwards, K. M., Bradley, R., and Palmer, P. (1992) Comparative trial in infants of four conjugate *Haemophilus influenzae* type b vaccines. *J. Pediatr.* **120**, 184–189.

15. Greenberg, D. P., Lieberman, J. M., Marcy, S. M., Wong, V. K., Partridge, S., Chang, S. J., Chiu, C. Y., and Ward, J. I. (1995) Enhanced antibody responses in infants given different sequences of heterogeneous *Haemophilus influenzae* type b conjugate vaccines. *J. Pediatr.* **126**, 206–211.

16. Capeding, M. R., Nohynek, H., Pascual, L. G., Kayhty, H., Sombrero, L. T., Eskola, J., and Ruutu, P. (1996) The immunogenicity of three *Haemophilus influenzae* type B conjugate vaccines after a primary vaccination series in Philippine infants. *Am. J. Trop. Med. Hyg.* **55(5)**, 516–520.

17. Edwards, K. M., Meade, B. D., Decker, M. D., et al. (1995) Comparison of 13 acellular pertussis vaccines: overview and serologic response. *Pediatrics* **96**, 548–557.

18. Gustafsson, L., Hallander, H. O., Olin, P., Reizenstein, E., and Storsaeter, J. (1996) A controlled trial of a two-component acellular, a five-component acellular, and a whole-cell pertussis vaccine. *N. Engl. J. Med.* **334**, 349–355.

19. Greco, D., Salmaso, S., Mastrantonio, P., et al. (1996) A controlled trial of two acellular vaccines and one whole-cell vaccine against pertussis. *N. Engl. J. Med.* **334**, 341–348.

20. Ad Hoc Group for the Study of Pertussis Vaccines (1988) Placebo-controlled trial of two acellular pertussis vaccines in Sweden—protective efficacy and adverse events. *Lancet* **1**, 955–960.

21. Olin, P., Rasmussen, F., Gustafsson, L., Hallander, H. O., and Heijbel, H., for the Ad Hoc Group for the Study of Pertussis Vaccines (1997) Randomised controlled trial of two-component, three-component, and five-component acellular pertussis vaccines compared with whole-cell pertussis vaccine. *Lancet* **350**, 1569–1577.

22. Centers for Disease Control and Prevention ( ) Combination Vaccines for Childhood Immunization. Recommendations of the Advisory Committee on Immunization Practices ACIP), the American Academy of Pediatrics (AAP), and the American Academy of Family Physicians (AAFP), in press.

23. Anderson, E. L., Decker, M. D., Englund, J. A., Belshe, R. B., Anderson, P., and Edwards, K. M. (1995) Interchangeability of conjugated *Haemophilus influenzae* type b vaccines in infants. *JAMA* **273**, 849–853.

24. Halsey, N. A. (1995) Practical considerations regarding the impact on immunization schedules of the introduction of new combined vaccines, in *Combined Vaccines and Simultaneous Administration: Current Issues and Perspectives* (Williams, J. C., Goldenthal, K. L., Burns, D. L., and Lewis, B. P. Jr, eds.), *Ann. NY Acad. Sci.* **754**, 250–254.

25. Centers for Disease Control and Prevention (1994) General Recommendations on Immunization: Recommendations of the Advisory Committee on Immunization Practices (ACIP). *MMWR* **43(No. RR-1)**.

26. American Academy of Pediatrics, Committee on Infectious Diseases (1998) Recommended childhood immunization schedule-United States, January–December 1998. *Pediatrics* **101,** 154–157.

27. Galil, K., Singleton, R., Levine, O., Fitzgerald, M., Ajello, G., Bulkow, L., and Parkinson, A. (1997) High prevalence of Haemophilus influenzae type b (Hib) carriage among Alaska natives despite widespread use of Hib conjugate vaccine. *Abstracts of the 35th Annual Meeting of the Infectious Diseases Society of America,* San Francisco, September 1997.

28. Centers for Disease Control and Prevention (1997) Pertussis vaccination: use of acellular pertussis vaccines among infants and young children—recommendations of the Advisory Committee on Immunization Practices (ACIP). *MMWR* **46(No. RR-7),** 19.

29. Centers for Disease Control and Prevention (1991) Diphtheria, tetanus, and pertussis: recommendations for vaccine use and other preventive measures. Recommendations of the Immunization Practices Advisory Committee (ACIP). *MMWR* **40(No. RR-10),** 1–28.

30. Centers for Disease Control and Prevention (1997) Prevention of pneumococcal disease. Recommendations of the Advisory Committee on Immunization Practices (ACIP). *MMWR* **46(No. RR-8),** 1–24.

31. Rennels, M. B., Deloria, M. A., Pichichero, M. E., Edwards, K. M., Anderson, E. L., Englund, J. A., and Steinhoff, M. C. (1998) Entire thigh swelling after 4th dose of 10 different DTaP vaccines: relationship to other reactions and to vaccine contents. *Pediatr. Res.* Abstract 901. Pediatric Academic Societies. May 1–5, 1998, New Orleans, LA.

32. Chen, R. T., Rastogi, S. C., Mullen, J. R., Hayes, S. W., Cochi, S. L., Donlon, J. A., and Wassilak, S. G. (1994) The Vaccine Adverse Event Reporting System (VAERS). *Vaccine* **12,** 542–550.

33. Watson, M. A., Feldman, K. W., Sugar, N. F., Commer, C. J., Thomas, E. R., and Lin, T. (1996) Inadequate history as a barrier to immunization. *Arch. Pediatr. Adolesc. Med.* **150,** 135–139.

34. Centers for Disease Control (1988) National Childhood Vaccine Injury Act (1988) Requirements for permanent vaccination records and for reporting of selected events after vaccination. *MMWR* **37,** 197–200.

35. Shaw, J. S., Samuels, R. C., and Bernstein, H. H. (1998) Vaccine registries are useful despite data entry errors. *Pediatr. Res.* Abstract 110. Pediatric Academic Societies. May 1–5, 1998, New Orleans, LA.

36. Suara, R. O., Collins, M., Scales, C., Lagoc, A., and Michols, A. (1998) Decreasing missed opportunities: use of credit card immunization record. *Pediatr. Res.* Abstract 694. Pediatric Academic Societies. May 1–5, 1998, New Orleans, LA.

37. Askew, G. L., Finelli, L., Lutz, J., DeGraat, J., Siegel, B., and Spitalny, K. (1995) Beliefs and practices regarding childhood vaccination among urban pediatric providers in New Jersey. *Pediatrics* **96,** 889–892.

38. Madlon-Kay, D. and Harper, P. (1994) Too many shots? Parent, nurse, and physicians attitudes toward multiple simultaneous childhood vaccinations. *Arch Fam. Med.* **3,** 610–613.

39. Melman, S. T., Chawla, T., Kaplan, J. M., and Anbar, R. D. (1994) Multiple immunizations: Ouch! *Arch Fam. Med.* **3,** 615–618.

40. Zimmerman, R. K., Bradford, B. J., Janosky, J. E., Mieckowski, T. A., DeSensi, E., and Grufferman, S. (1997) Barriers to measles and pertussis immunization: the knowledge and attitudes of Pennsylvania primary care physicians. *Am. J. Prev. Med.* **13,** 89–97.

41. McMonnochie, K. M. and Roghmann, K. J. (1992) Immunization opportunities missed among urban poor children. *Pediatrics* **89,** 1019–1026.

42. Lannon, C., Brack, V., Stuart, J., Caplow, M., McNeill, A., Bordley, C., and Margolis, P. (1995) What mothers say about why poor children fall behind on immunizations. *Arch Pediatr. Adolesc. Med.* **149,** 1070–1075.

43. Bloom, B. R. (1995) A perspective on issues relating to future vaccines. *Ann. NY Acad. Sci.* **754,** 388–395.

INDEX